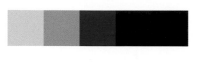

A PRACTICAL MANUAL OF

Diabetic Retinopathy Management

A PRACTICAL MANUAL OF
Diabetic Retinopathy Management

Peter H. Scanlon
MD, MRCOphth, DCH, FRCP

Consultant Ophthalmologist, Gloucestershire and Oxford Eye Units
Lecturer, Harris Manchester College
University of Oxford
Oxford, UK

Charles P. Wilkinson
MD

Chairman, Department of Ophthalmology, Greater Baltimore Medical Center
Professor of Ophthalmology, Johns Hopkins University
Baltimore, USA

Stephen J. Aldington
DMS, FBIPP

Gloucestershire Education and Research Development Manager, Cheltenham, UK

David R. Matthews
MA (Oxon), DPhil, BM, BCh, FRCP

Professor of Diabetic Medicine, University of Oxford
Chairman, Oxford Centre for Diabetes, Endocrinology & Metabolism
Oxford, UK

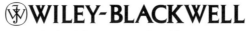

WILEY-BLACKWELL

A John Wiley & Sons, Ltd., Publication

Library of Congress Cataloging-in-Publication Data
A practical manual of diabetic retinopathy management / Peter H. Scanlon . . . [et al.].
        p. ; cm.
    Includes bibliographical references and index.
    ISBN 978-1-4051-7035-2
    1. Diabetic retinopathy—Diagnosis—Handbooks, manuals, etc.   2. Diabetic retinopathy—Treatment—Handbooks,
manuals, etc.   I. Scanlon, Peter H.
    [DNLM: 1. Diabetic Retinopathy—diagnosis.   2. Diabetic Retinopathy—therapy. WK 835 P895 2009]
    RE661.D5P73 2009
    617.7′35—dc22

                                                                                                        2008026360

ISBN: 978-1-4051-7035-2

A catalogue record for this book is available from the British Library.

Set in 9.25/11.5pt Minion by Graphicraft Limited, Hong Kong
Printed and bound in Singapore by Fabulous Printers Pte Ltd.

1   2009

Contents

Acknowledgements

I am grateful to my colleagues in Gloucestershire who have provided very useful examples of conditions that have enhanced the quality of this book and also provided some text where their knowledge was superior to my own. I am particularly grateful for the contributions from the following people:

- Lisa Collins (Lead Optometrist) was of great assistance in the sections about ultrasound B scan and perimetry.
- Rob Johnston (Consultant Ophthalmologist) for providing examples from his patients and writing a paragraph on electronic patient records and ocular anaesthesia.
- Quresh Mohammed (Consultant Ophthalmologist) for providing expertise and ocular coherence tomography (OCT) images of patients with diabetic retinopathy.
- Susan Carter (Senior Optometrist) for writing a section on low vision rehabilitation.
- Mark Histed (Gloucestershire Screening Programme Manager) for taking numerous photographs for the book and assisting in obtaining some of the old photographs from our archive files.
- David Mordant (Research Fellow in Ophthalmology) and Professor Andrew McNaught (Consultant Ophthalmologist) for writing a section on oximetry.
- Nigel Kirkpatrick (Consultant Ophthalmologist) for allowing me to use examples of his patients.
- Dr Janet Ropner (Consultant Haematologist, Gloucestershire Royal Hospital) for providing some haematology images.
- Jenny Sykes (researcher), Liz Dawes and Alex Purcell (Clinical Audit) for tirelessly working on the provision of background research, patient histories, patient consent forms and information in support of the writing of this book.

I am grateful to Dr Bahram Jafar-Mohammadi from the Oxford Centre for Diabetes, Endocrinology and Metabolism for providing a case history of a patient with HNF-1α MODY and my brother Dr John Scanlon, a Consultant Paediatrician at Worcestershire Royal Hospital, for his advice on a paediatric case history. I am also grateful to Dr Brendan McDonald, Consultant Ocular Pathologist at the John Radcliffe Hospital in Oxford, for providing pathology images.

I would like to acknowledge my appreciation of Martin Joyce (Consultant Ophthalmologist) who taught me in the early stages of my ophthalmology career and has provided images for this book and Tim Hart (Consultant Ophthalmologist) who was a great support and encouraged me to use one of the early digital fundus fluorescein cameras. I would like to acknowledge the support of the Gloucestershire Eye Therapy Trust, who generously provided the first digital fundus fluorescein camera, the first screening cameras and the first OCT equipment for the Gloucestershire Eye Unit, which has enabled the department to be at the forefront of modern ophthalmic imaging.

We thank the editors for their support.

We are very grateful to all the patients who have allowed photographs of their eyes and some case histories to be included in this book.

We are grateful to our wives and partners for their patience and understanding and I am particularly grateful to my wife Sally for her support.

Peter H. Scanlon

Prologue

Peter H. Scanlon

THE SCOPE OF THE PROBLEM OF THE EPIDEMIC OF DIABETES

In 1997, Amos[1] estimated that 124 million people worldwide have diabetes, 97% non-insulin-dependent diabetes mellitus (NIDDM), and that by 2010 the total number with diabetes is projected to reach 221 million. The regions with the greatest potential increases are Asia and Africa, where diabetes rates could rise to 2 or 3 times those experienced in 1997.

In 2000, Sorensen[2] reported that the World Health Organization has recognized that there is a 'global epidemic of obesity' and the prevalence of type 2 diabetes is rising in parallel.

The International Diabetes Federation have estimated the prevalence of diabetes in 2003 in the 20–79 age groups and projected this to an estimate in 2025. This is shown in Fig. 1.

North America

Reports from the USA and Canada have shown the following rises.

1 In 2000, Burrows[3] reported that the number of native Americans and Alaska natives with diagnosed diabetes increased by 29% from 43,262 to 64,474 individuals between 1990 and 1997. By 1997, the prevalence was 5.4%, and the age-adjusted prevalence was 8.0%.

2 In 2000, Mokdad[4,5] reported the results of the Behavioral Risk Factor Surveillance System in the USA 1990–98. The prevalence of diabetes rose from 4.9% in 1990 to 6.5% in 1998 and to 6.9% in 1999. The prevalence of diabetes was highly correlated with the prevalence of obesity ($r = 0.64$, $p < 0.001$).

3 In 2001, Boyle[6] estimated that the number of Americans with diagnosed diabetes is projected to increase 165%, from 11 million in 2000 (prevalence of 4.0%) to 29 million in 2050 (prevalence of 7.2%).

4 In 2007, Lipscombe[7] reported the prevalence of diabetes in Ontario, Canada to have increased substantially during the past 10 years, and by 2005 to have already exceeded the global rate that was predicted for 2030. Using population-based data from the province of Ontario, Canada, age-adjusted and sex-adjusted diabetes prevalence increased from 5.2% of the population in 1995 to 6.9% in 2000 and to 8.8% of the population in 2005.

The UK

Reports from the UK have shown the following rises.

1 In 2000, Ehtisham[8] reported type 2 diabetes emerging in UK children.

2 In 2001, Farouhi[9] constructed an epidemiological model by applying age-, sex-, and ethnic-specific prevalence rates to resident populations of England at national, regional and PCT level. The estimated prevalence of total diabetes for all people in England was 4.41% in 2001 equating to 2.168 million people. Type 2 92.3% and type 1 7.7% (166,000 people).

3 In 2002, Feltbower[10] reported an increasing incidence of type 1 diabetes in south Asians in Bradford.

4 In 2006, the latest data[11] in England for people diagnosed with diabetes have shown a national prevalence of diabetes of 3.35%.

5 In 2007, Evans[12] reported that a diabetes clinical information system in Tayside, Scotland, showed a doubling in incidence and prevalence of type 2 diabetes between 1993 and 2004, with statistically significant increasing trends of 6.3 and 6.7% per year respectively.

Worldwide reports

1 In 2000, Sidibe[13] reported that the rise in complications of diabetes mellitus in Africa has gone hand in hand with the growing disease prevalence.

2 In 2001, Zimmet[14] reviewed the global and societal implications of the diabetes epidemic.

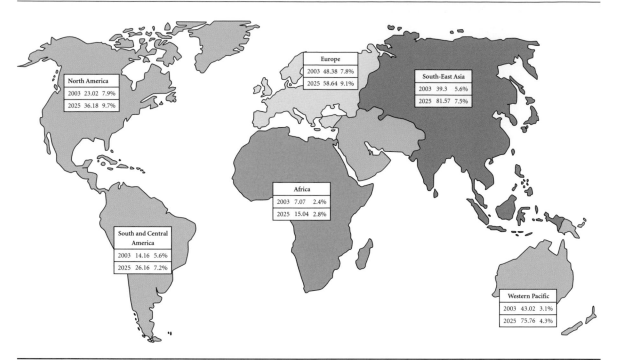

Fig. 1 World map and table showing the International Diabetes Federation prevalence estimates of diabetes in 2003 and 2025 in 20–79 age group.

Region	Year	Number with diabetes (millions)	% of population with diabetes
Africa	2003	7.07	2.4%
	2025	15.04	2.8%
Eastern Mediterranean and Middle East region	2003	19.24	7%
	2025	39.41	8%
Europe	2003	48.38	7.8%
	2025	58.64	9.1%
North America	2003	23.02	7.9%
	2025	36.18	9.7%
South and Central American region	2003	14.16	5.6%
	2025	26.16	7.2%
South-East Asian region	2003	39.3	5.6%
	2025	81.57	7.5%
Western Pacific region	2003	43.02	3.1%
	2025	75.76	4.3%

3 In 2001, Aspray[15] reported that the prevalence of diabetes in sub-Saharan Africa varied from 1% of the rural population to 5.3% of the urban population.

4 In 2004, Wild[16] reported the prevalence of diabetes for all age groups worldwide was estimated to be 2.8% in 2000 and 4.4% in 2030.

The total number of people with diabetes is projected to rise from 171 million in 2000 to 366 million in 2030.

The prevalence of diabetes is higher in men than in women, but there are more women with diabetes than men. The urban population in developing countries is projected to double between 2000 and 2030. The most important demographic change to diabetes prevalence across the world appears to be the increase in the proportion of people over 65 years of age.

These findings indicate that the 'diabetes epidemic' will

continue even if levels of obesity remain constant. Given the increasing prevalence of obesity, it is likely that these figures provide an underestimate of future diabetes prevalence.

In 2006 Cugati[17] reported data from the Blue Mountains Eye Study (BMES) in Australia that examined 3654 residents (82.4% response) aged over 49 years in BMES I (1992–1994). Survivors (n = 2335) and newly eligible residents (n = 1174) were examined in BMES II (1997–2000). Diabetes was defined by history or fasting plasma glucose $\geq$7.0 mmol/L. The overall diabetes prevalence increased from 7.8 to 9.9% (p = 0.002).

THE PREVALENCE OF SIGHT-THREATENING DIABETIC RETINOPATHY WORLDWIDE

See Fig. 2.

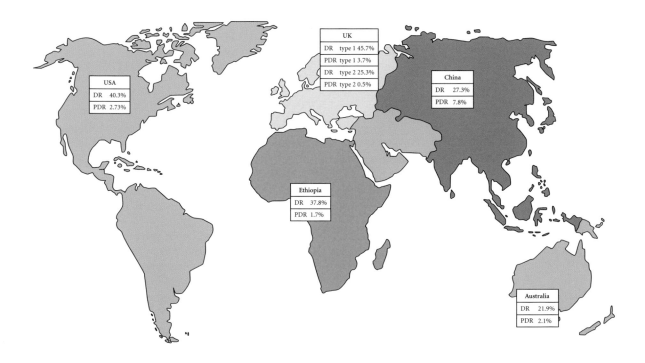

USA		Ethiopia	
Prevalence of DR	40.3%	Prevalence of DR	37.8%
Prevalence of proliferative DR	2.73%	Prevalence of proliferative DR	1.7%
UK		China	
Prevalence of DR in type 1	45.7%	Prevalence of DR	27.3%
Prevalence of proliferative DR in type 1	3.7%	Prevalence of proliferative DR	7.8%
Prevalence of DR in type 2	25.3%	Oman	
Prevalence of proliferative DR in type 2	0.5%	Prevalence of DR	14.4%
India		Prevalence of proliferative DR	2.7%
Prevalence of DR	13. 4%	Australia	
Prevalence of proliferative DR	1.9%	Prevalence of DR	21.9%
		Prevalence of proliferative DR	2.1%

Variations in screening methodology may explain some of these differences.

Fig. 2 World map and table showing the reported prevalence of diabetic retinopathy (DR) and proliferative DR.

The USA

Reports have shown that diabetic retinopathy (DR) continues to be prevalent in the USA.

1 In 1992, Klein[18] reported results from the Wisconsin Epidemiological Study of Diabetic Retinopathy (WESDR study). This was a population-based study in southern Wisconsin of 996 insulin-taking younger-onset diabetic persons (given diagnoses of diabetes under 30 years) and 1370 patients given diagnoses of diabetes at age 30 years or older who were examined using standard protocols to determine the prevalence and severity of DR and associated risk variables. Proliferative diabetic retinopathy (PDR) was found to be a prevalent complication: 23% in the younger-onset group, 10% in the older-onset group that were taking insulin, and 3% in the group not taking insulin.

2 In 1995 Klein[19] reported the incidence of macular oedema over a 10-year period. This was 20.1% in the younger-onset group, 25.4% in the older-onset group taking insulin, and 13.9% in the older-onset group not taking insulin.

3 In 2001, West[20] studied Hispanic patients with diabetes over 40 years in Arizona. The prevalences were any DR 48%, and moderate to severe non-proliferative DR (NPDR) and PDR 32%.

4 In 2003, Brown[21] reported that, despite improvement in levels of glycaemia and blood pressure, PDR remains prevalent.

5 In 2004, Kempen[22] reported that, among an estimated 10.2 million US adults 40 years and older known to have diabetes, the estimated crude prevalence rates for retinopathy and vision-threatening retinopathy were 40.3% and 8.2%, respectively.

6 In 2006 Wong[23] reported on a multiethnic population of 778 individuals from ages 45 to 85 years with diabetes; the prevalence of any retinopathy was 33.2% and of macular oedema 9.0%.

In WESDR,[24] one-third of the eyes that developed vision-threatening DR had proliferative DR and two-thirds had clinically significant macular oedema. Hence, taking the estimated crude prevalence rates for vision-threatening retinopathy of 8.2% from the paper by Kempen,[22] the estimated crude prevalence rates for PDR would be 2.73%.

The UK

Reports from the UK have shown that sight-threatening DR is prevalent in the UK.

1 In 1998, Kohner[25] reported baseline retinopathy levels in 2964 patients with diabetes enrolled in the United Kingdom Prospective Diabetes Study (UKPDS). Retinopathy, defined as microaneurysms or worse lesions in at least one eye, was present in 39% of men and 35% of women. Marked retinopathy with cotton wool spots or intraretinal microvascular abnormalities was present in 8% of men and 4% of women.

2 In 2002, Younis[26,27] reported baseline results from population screening in Liverpool of 831 people with type 1 diabetes and 7231 people with type 2 diabetes. The results showed a baseline for the type 1 diabetes group of any DR 45.7%, PDR 3.7% and STED 16.4%, and for the type 2 group of any DR 25.3%, PDR 0.5% and sight threatening eye disease (STED) 6.0%.

Worldwide reports

Worldwide reports have shown that sight-threatening DR is prevalent worldwide.

1 In 1997, Kernell[28] reported the youngest child in the literature (11.8 years) at that time with preproliferative DR to be from Sweden.

2 In 1999, Donaghue[29] described the youngest child reported in the literature to have background DR at that time (1999) to be 7.9 years (duration 5.6 years, HbA1c 8.9%) and from Australia.

3 In 2000, McKay[30] reported results of 4744 people over 40 years from nine randomly selected Melbourne clusters and four randomly selected rural Victorian clusters in Australia. The prevalence of any DR among people with self-reported diabetes was 29.1% and untreated vision-threatening retinopathy was 2.8%.

4 In 2000, Ramachandran[31] studied 617 patients with type 1 diabetes in India reporting a prevalence of any DR of 13. 4% and proliferative DR of 1.9%.

5 In 2001, Hesse[32] reported on 2801 people with diabetes employed by Volkswagen in Germany. Of 263 patients aged over 40 years, 18.8% had mild or moderate NPDR, 3.3% severe NPDR and 2.2% PDR. Of 2228 patients aged over 40 years, 11.9% mild or moderate NPDR, 2.6% severe NPDR and 0.9% PDR.

6 In 2001, Seyoum[33] studied 302 patients with diabetes in Ethiopia, reporting a prevalence of 37.8% any DR and 1.7% PDR.

7 In 2002, Liu[34] found a prevalence of any DR 27.3%, and PDR 7.8% among 773 newly diagnosed patients in Beijing, China.

8 In 2003, in the Australian Diabetes, Obesity and Lifestyle study (AusDiab) of 11,247 adults over 25 years in 42 randomly selected areas of Australia, Tapp[35] showed a prevalence of any DR of 21.9% in those with known type 2 diabetes and 6.2% in those newly diagnosed. The prevalence of PDR was 2.1% in those with known diabetes.

9 In 2003, Khandekar[36] found that amongst 2249 patients with diabetes in Oman, 14.39% were found to have any DR and the prevalence of, PDR was 2.66%.

10 In 2006, Knudsen[37] reported the point prevalence of proliferative retinopathy in the county of North Jutland, Denmark to be 0.8% and 0.3% for type 1 and type 2 diabetes. Equivalent prevalence rates of clinically significant macular oedema were 7.9% and 12.8%, respectively.

11 A published systematic review by Williams[38] in 2004 on the epidemiology of DR and macular oedema concluded that studies of sufficient size to stratify for age and duration of eye disease show an increase in DR in older age groups with long-standing disease.

ADVANCES IN THE MANAGEMENT OF DIABETES

Advances in management of diabetes have had a substantial impact on DR. These are discussed in detail in Chapter 2.

The demonstration by the Diabetes Control and Complications Trial[39] that retinopathy in type 1 diabetes could be reduced by intensive treatment of blood glucose has led to much better control and retinopathy progression has been reduced.

Studies[40,41] in the early 1990s showed the link between hypertension in type 1 diabetes and a higher occurrence of retinopathy and progression of pre-existing retinopathy.

A similar demonstration in the United Kingdom Prospective Diabetes Study[42] (UKPDS) that in type 2 diabetes the development of retinopathy (incidence) was strongly associated with baseline glycaemia and glycaemic exposure and that progression was associated with hyperglycaemia (as evidenced by a higher HbA1c) has led to better control in type 2 diabetes and in reduction in retinopathy progression. The UKPDS[43] also demonstrated that high blood pressure is detrimental to every aspect of DR in type 2 diabetes and that a tight blood pressure control policy reduces the risk of clinical complications from diabetic eye disease (see Fig. 3).

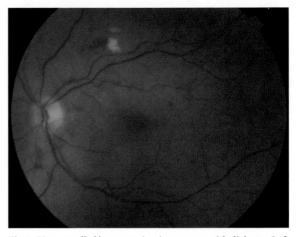

Fig. 3 Uncontrolled hypertension in a person with diabetes. Left macular colour photograph showing flame haemorrhages and cotton wool spots.

ADVANCES IN THE MANAGEMENT OF DIABETIC RETINOPATHY

Since Spalter[44] described the photocoagulation of circinate maculopathy in DR, clear evidence for the efficacy of laser treatment for diabetic eye disease has been shown from the Diabetic Retinopathy Study[45–49] and the Early Treatment Diabetic Retinopathy Study[50–58]. In 1981 they reported[47] that photocoagulation, as used in the study, reduced the 2-year risk of severe visual loss by 50% or more (see Fig. 4).

In 1985, a report[50] from the Early Treatment Diabetic Retinopathy Study showed that focal photocoagulation of 'clinically significant' diabetic macular oedema (CSMO) substantially reduced the risk of visual loss.

Smiddy[59] wrote an excellent review in 1999 when he noted that, according to the Early Treatment Diabetic Retinopathy Study, at least 5% of eyes receiving optimal medical treatment will still have progressive retinopathy that requires laser treatment and pars plana vitrectomy. He also noted that, although vitrectomy improves the prognosis for a favourable visual outcome, preventive measures, such as improved control of glucose levels and timely application of panretinal photocoagulation, are equally important in the management. Vitrectomy clearly does have a place in the management of diabetic eye disease (Fig. 5). Evidence of improving visual results during the last 20 years following vitrectomy has been shown in studies reported by Blankenship,[60] Thompson,[61–64] Sigurdsson,[65] Flynn,[66] Nakazawa,[67] Karel,[68] Harbour,[69]

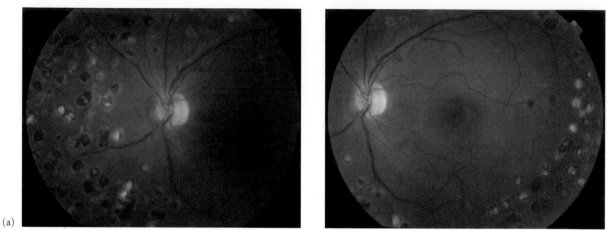

Fig. 4 Stable treated eye after panretinal photocoagulation for NVD: (a) left nasal view; (b) left macular view.

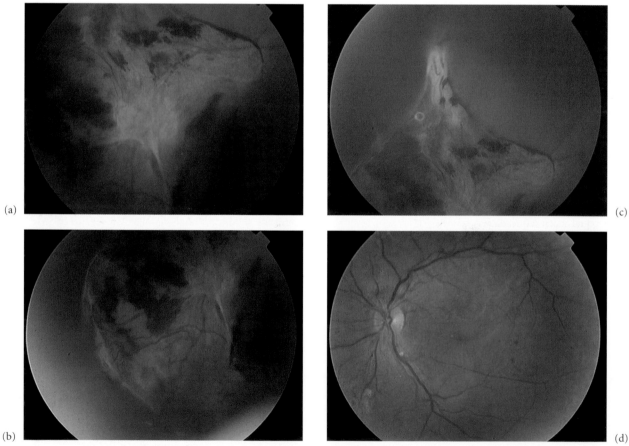

Fig. 5 Extensive tractional detachment with haemorrhage: (a) left macular view; (b) left nasal view; (c) left superior view; (d) same eye after vitrectomy.

Pendergast,[70] La Heij,[71] Yamamoto,[72] Amino,[73] Lewis,[74] Lahey,[75] Treumer,[76] Schrey,[77] and Diolaiuti.[78] However, a restriction in driving field has recently been reported in over two-thirds of patients in a small series of patients by Barsam[79].

Developments in techniques of laser treatment are discussed in later chapters of this book as are the novel treatments for diabetic macular oedema (e.g. corticosteroids and anti-vascular endothelial growth factor drugs). Laser photocoagulation, however, remains the standard of care and the only treatment with proven efficacy in a large-scale clinical trial.

Despite the available treatments, many patients present late in the course of the disease when treatment is more difficult. There have been considerable advances in early detection in the last 10 years with the advent of systematic screening programmes for DR.

The St Vincent Declaration, a joint initiative on diabetes care and research of the World Health Organization (Europe) and the International Diabetes Federation (Europe), included 5-year targets for improvement in diabetes outcomes. One of these targets was to reduce diabetes-related blindness by one-third or more over the next 5 years.

A conference took place in Liverpool, UK on 17–18 November 2005 to review progress in the prevention of visual impairment due to DR in Europe. The conference recommended the following steps in the development of systematic screening programmes for sight-threatening DR.

Step 1

Access to effective treatment:
- minimum number of lasers per 100,000 population
- equal access for all patient groups
- maximum time to treatment from diagnosis 3 months.

Step 2

Establish opportunistic screening:
- dilated fundoscopy at time of attendance for routine care
- annual review
- national guidelines on referral to an ophthalmologist.

Step 3

Establish systematic screening:
- establish and maintain disease registers
- systematic call and recall for all people with diabetes
- annual screening
- test used has sensitivity of ≥80% and specificity of ≥90%
- coverage ≥80%.

Step 4

Establish systematic screening with full quality assurance and full coverage:
- digital photographic screening
- all personnel involved in screening will be certified as competent
- 100% coverage
- quality assurance at all stages
- central/regional data collection for monitoring and measurement of effectiveness.

PRACTICE POINTS

- There is an epidemic of diabetes worldwide.
- The prevalence of diabetic retinopathy is rising as a consequence of the epidemic of diabetes.
- Effective treatments are available but are dependent on the stage of diagnosis.
- Systematic screening programmes can be set up to detect diabetic retinopathy at an appropriate stage to reduce the incidence and prevalence of blindness.

REFERENCES

1 Amos AF, McCarty DJ, Zimmet P. The rising global burden of diabetes and its complications: estimates and projections to the year 2010. *Diabet Med* 1997; **14**(Suppl 5): S1–S5.

2 Sorensen TI. The changing lifestyle in the world. Body weight and what else? *Diabetes Care* 2000; **23**(Suppl 2): B1–4.

3 Burrows NR, Geiss LS, Engelgau MM, Acton KJ. Prevalence of diabetes among Native Americans and Alaska Natives, 1990–1997: an increasing burden. *Diabetes Care* 2000; **23**(12): 1786–90.

4 Mokdad AH, Ford ES, Bowman BA, Nelson DE, Engelgau MM, Vinicor F *et al.* Diabetes trends in the US: 1990–1998. *Diabetes Care* 2000; **23**(9): 1278–83.

5 Mokdad AH, Ford ES, Bowman BA, Nelson DE, Engelgau MM, Vinicor F *et al.* The continuing increase of diabetes in the US. *Diabetes Care* 2001; **24**(2): 412.

6 Boyle JP, Honeycutt AA, Narayan KM, Hoerger TJ, Geiss LS, Chen H *et al.* Projection of diabetes burden through 2050: impact of changing demography and disease prevalence in the U.S. *Diabetes Care* 2001; **24**(11): 1936–40.

7 Lipscombe LL, Hux JE. Trends in diabetes prevalence, incidence, and mortality in Ontario, Canada 1995–2005: a population-based study. *Lancet* 2007; **369**(9563): 750–6.

8 Ehtisham S, Barrett TG, Shaw NJ. Type 2 diabetes mellitus in UK children – an emerging problem. *Diabet Med* 2000; **17**(12): 867–71.

9 Farouhi NG, Merrick D, Goyder E, Ferguson BA, Abbas J, Lachowycz K *et al.* Diabetes prevalence in England, 2001 – estimates from an epidemiological model. *Diabet Med* 2006; **23**(2): 189–97.

10 Feltbower RG, Bodansky HJ, McKinney PA, Houghton J, Stephenson CR, Haigh D. Trends in the incidence of childhood diabetes in south Asians and other children in Bradford, UK. *Diabet Med* 2002; **19**(2): 162–6.

11 QoF. Quality and Outcomes Framework data from all four countries for the year 2004/5. http://www.gpcontract.co.uk Accessed January 2008

12 Evans JM, Barnett KN, Ogston SA, Morris AD. Increasing prevalence of type 2 diabetes in a Scottish population: effect of increasing incidence or decreasing mortality? *Diabetologia* 2007; **50**(4): 729–32.

13 Sidibe EH. Main complications of diabetes mellitus in Africa. *Ann Med Interne (Paris)* 2000; **151**(8): 624–8.

14 Zimmet P, Alberti KG, Shaw J. Global and societal implications of the diabetes epidemic. *Nature* 2001; **414**(6865): 782–7.

15 Aspray TJ, Unwin N. Diabetes in sub-Saharan Africa. *Adv Exp Med Biol* 2001; **498**: 21–6.

16 Wild S, Roglic G, Green A, Sicree R, King H. Global prevalence of diabetes: estimates for the year 2000 and projections for 2030. *Diabetes Care* 2004; **27**(5): 1047–53.

17 Cugati S, Kifley A, Mitchell P, Wang JJ. Temporal trends in the age-specific prevalence of diabetes and diabetic retinopathy in older persons: population-based survey findings. *Diabetes Res Clin Pract* 2006; **74**(3): 301–8.

18 Klein R, Klein BE, Moss SE. Epidemiology of proliferative diabetic retinopathy. *Diabetes Care* 1992; **15**(12): 1875–91.

19 Klein R, Klein BE, Moss SE, Cruickshanks KJ. The Wisconsin Epidemiologic Study of Diabetic Retinopathy. XV. The long-term incidence of macular edema. *Ophthalmology* 1995; **102**(1): 7–16.

20 West SK, Klein R, Rodriguez J, Munoz B, Broman AT, Sanchez R *et al*. Diabetes and diabetic retinopathy in a Mexican-American population: Proyecto VER. *Diabetes Care* 2001; **24**(7): 1204–9.

21 Brown JB, Pedula KL, Summers KH. Diabetic retinopathy: contemporary prevalence in a well-controlled population. *Diabetes Care* 2003; **26**(9): 2637–42.

22 Kempen JH, O'Colmain BJ, Leske MC, Haffner SM, Klein R, Moss SE *et al*. The prevalence of diabetic retinopathy among adults in the United States. *Arch Ophthalmol* 2004; **122**(4): 552–63.

23 Wong TY, Klein R, Islam FM, Cotch MF, Folsom AR, Klein BE *et al*. Diabetic retinopathy in a multi-ethnic cohort in the United States. *Am J Ophthalmol* 2006; **141**(3): 446–55.

24 Klein R, Meuer SM, Moss SE, Klein BE. Retinal microaneurysm counts and 10-year progression of diabetic retinopathy. *Arch Ophthalmol* 1995; **113**(11): 1386–91.

25 Kohner EM, Aldington SJ, Stratton IM, Manley SE, Holman RR, Matthews DR *et al*. United Kingdom Prospective Diabetes Study, 30: diabetic retinopathy at diagnosis of non-insulin-dependent diabetes mellitus and associated risk factors. *Arch Ophthalmol* 1998; **116**(3): 297–303.

26 Younis N, Broadbent DM, Harding SP, Vora JP. Incidence of sight-threatening retinopathy in type 1 diabetes in a systematic screening programme. *Diabet Med* 2003; **20**(9): 758–65.

27 Younis N, Broadbent DM, Vora JP, Harding SP. Incidence of sight-threatening retinopathy in patients with type 2 diabetes in the Liverpool Diabetic Eye Study: a cohort study. *Lancet* 2003; **361**(9353): 195–200.

28 Kernell A, Dedorsson I, Johansson B, Wickstrom CP, Ludvigsson J, Tuvemo T *et al*. Prevalence of diabetic retinopathy in children and adolescents with IDDM. A population-based multicentre study. *Diabetologia* 1997; **40**(3): 307–10.

29 Donaghue KC, Fairchild JM, Chan A, Hing SJ, Howard NJ, Silink M. Diabetes complication screening in 937 children and adolescents. *J Pediatr Endocrinol Metab* 1999; **12**(2): 185–92.

30 McKay R, McCarty CA, Taylor HR. Diabetic retinopathy in Victoria, Australia: the Visual Impairment Project. *Br J Ophthalmol* 2000; **84**(8): 865–70.

31 Ramachandran A, Snehalatha C, Sasikala R, Satyavani K, Vijay V. Vascular complications in young Asian Indian patients with type 1 diabetes mellitus. *Diabetes Res Clin Pract* 2000; **48**(1): 51–6.

32 Hesse L, Grusser M, Hoffstadt K, Jorgens V, Hartmann P, Kroll P. Population-based study of diabetic retinopathy in Wolfsburg. *Ophthalmologe* 2001; **98**(11): 1065–8.

33 Seyoum B, Mengistu Z, Berhanu P, Abdulkadir J, Feleke Y, Worku Y *et al*. Retinopathy in patients of Tikur Anbessa Hospital diabetic clinic. *Ethiop Med J* 2001; **39**(2): 123–31.

34 Liu DP, Molyneaux L, Chua E, Wang YZ, Wu CR, Jing H *et al*. Retinopathy in a Chinese population with type 2 diabetes: factors affecting the presence of this complication at diagnosis of diabetes. *Diabetes Res Clin Pract* 2002; **56**(2): 125–31.

35 Tapp RJ, Shaw JE, Harper CA, de Courten MP, Balkau B, McCarty DJ *et al*. The prevalence of and factors associated with diabetic retinopathy in the Australian population. *Diabetes Care* 2003; **26**(6): 1731–7.

36 Khandekar R, Al Lawatii J, Mohammed AJ, Al Raisi A. Diabetic retinopathy in Oman: a hospital based study. *Br J Ophthalmol* 2003; **87**(9): 1061–4.

37 Knudsen LL, Lervang HH, Lundbye-Christensen S, Gorst-Rasmussen A. The North Jutland County Diabetic Retinopathy Study: population characteristics. *Br J Ophthalmol* 2006; **90**(11): 1404–9.

38 Williams R, Airey M, Baxter H, Forrester J, Kennedy-Martin T, Girach A. Epidemiology of diabetic retinopathy and macular oedema: a systematic review. *Eye* 2004; **18**(10): 963–83.

39 The effect of intensive treatment of diabetes on the development and progression of long-term complications in insulin-dependent diabetes mellitus. The Diabetes Control and Complications Trial Research Group. *N Engl J Med* 1993; **329**(14):977–86.

40 Chase HP, Garg SK, Jackson WE, Thomas MA, Harris S, Marshall G *et al*. Blood pressure and retinopathy in type I diabetes. *Ophthalmology* 1990; **97**(2): 155–9.

41 Joner G, Brinchmann-Hansen O, Torres CG, Hanssen KF. A nationwide cross-sectional study of retinopathy and microalbuminuria in young Norwegian type 1 (insulin-dependent) diabetic patients. *Diabetologia* 1992; **35**(11): 1049–54.

42 Stratton IM, Kohner EM, Aldington SJ, Turner RC, Holman RR, Manley SE *et al.* UKPDS 50: risk factors for incidence and progression of retinopathy in type II diabetes over 6 years from diagnosis. *Diabetologia* 2001; **44**(2): 156–63.

43 Matthews DR, Stratton IM, Aldington SJ, Holman RR, Kohner EM. Risks of progression of retinopathy and vision loss related to tight blood pressure control in type 2 diabetes mellitus: UKPDS 69. *Arch Ophthalmol* 2004; **122**(11): 1631–40.

44 Spalter HF. Photocoagulation of circinate maculopathy in diabetic retinopathy. *Am J Ophthalmol* 1971; **1**(1 Part 2): 242–50.

45 The Diabetic Retinopathy Study Research Group. Preliminary report on effects of photocoagulation therapy. *Am J Ophthalmol* 1976; **81**(4): 383–96.

46 The Diabetic Retinopathy Study Research Group Photocoagulation treatment of proliferative diabetic retinopathy: the second report of diabetic retinopathy study findings. *Ophthalmology* 1978; **85**(1): 82–106.

47 The Diabetic Retinopathy Study Research Group. Photocoagulation treatment of proliferative diabetic retinopathy. Clinical application of Diabetic Retinopathy Study (DRS) findings, DRS Report Number 8. *Ophthalmology* 1981; **88**(7): 583–600.

48 The Diabetic Retinopathy Study Research Group. Four risk factors for severe visual loss in diabetic retinopathy. The third report from the Diabetic Retinopathy Study. *Arch Ophthalmol* 1979; **97**(4): 654–5.

49 The Diabetic Retinopathy Study Research Group. Indications for photocoagulation treatment of diabetic retinopathy: Diabetic Retinopathy Study Report no. 14. *Int Ophthalmol Clin* 1987; **27**(4): 239–53.

50 Early Treatment Diabetic Retinopathy Study Research Group. Photocoagulation for diabetic macular edema. Early Treatment Diabetic Retinopathy Study report number 1. *Arch Ophthalmol* 1985; **103**(12): 1796–806.

51 Early Treatment Diabetic Retinopathy Study Research Group. Treatment techniques and clinical guidelines for photocoagulation of diabetic macular edema. Early Treatment Diabetic Retinopathy Study Report Number 2. *Ophthalmology* 1987; **94**(7): 761–74.

52 Early Treatment Diabetic Retinopathy Study Research Group. Fundus photographic risk factors for progression of diabetic retinopathy. ETDRS report number 12. *Ophthalmology* 1991; **98**(5 Suppl): 823–33.

53 Early Treatment Diabetic Retinopathy Study Research Group. Classification of diabetic retinopathy from fluorescein angiograms. ETDRS report number 11. *Ophthalmology* 1991; **98**(5 Suppl): 807–22.

54 Early Treatment Diabetic Retinopathy Study Research Group. Grading diabetic retinopathy from stereoscopic color fundus photographs – an extension of the modified Airlie House classification. ETDRS report number 10. *Ophthalmology* 1991; **98**(5 Suppl): 786–806.

55 Early Treatment Diabetic Retinopathy Study Research Group. Early photocoagulation for diabetic retinopathy. ETDRS report number 9. *Ophthalmology* 1991; **98**(5 Suppl): 766–85.

56 Early Treatment Diabetic Retinopathy Study Research Group. Effects of aspirin treatment on diabetic retinopathy. ETDRS report number 8. *Ophthalmology* 1991; **98**(5 Suppl): 757–65.

57 Early Treatment Diabetic Retinopathy Study design and baseline patient characteristics. ETDRS report number 7. *Ophthalmology* 1991; **98**(5 Suppl): 741–56.

58 Early Treatment Diabetic Retinopathy Study Research Group. Fluorescein angiographic risk factors for progression of diabetic retinopathy. ETDRS report number 13. *Ophthalmology* 1991; **98**(5 Suppl): 834–40.

59 Smiddy WE, Flynn HW Jr. Vitrectomy in the management of diabetic retinopathy. *Surv Ophthalmol* 1999; **43**(6): 491–507.

60 Blankenship GW, Machemer R. Long-term diabetic vitrectomy results. Report of 10 year follow-up. *Ophthalmology* 1985; **92**(4): 503–6.

61 Thompson JT, de Bustros S, Michels RG, Rice TA, Glaser BM. Results of vitrectomy for proliferative diabetic retinopathy. *Ophthalmology* 1986; **93**(12): 1571–4.

62 Thompson JT, de Bustros S, Michels RG, Rice TA. Results and prognostic factors in vitrectomy for diabetic vitreous hemorrhage. *Arch Ophthalmol* 1987; **105**(2): 191–5.

63 Thompson JT, de Bustros S, Michels RG, Rice TA. Results and prognostic factors in vitrectomy for diabetic traction retinal detachment of the macula. *Arch Ophthalmol* 1987; **105**(4): 497–502.

64 Thompson JT, de Bustros S, Michels RG, Rice TA. Results and prognostic factors in vitrectomy for diabetic traction-rhegmatogenous retinal detachment. *Arch Ophthalmol* 1987; **105**(4): 503–7.

65 Sigurdsson H, Baines PS, Roxburgh ST. Vitrectomy for diabetic eye disease. *Eye* 1988; **2**(Pt 4): 418–23.

66 Flynn HW Jr, Chew EY, Simons BD, Barton FB, Remaley NA, Ferris FL 3rd. Pars plana vitrectomy in the Early Treatment Diabetic Retinopathy Study. ETDRS report number 17. The Early Treatment Diabetic Retinopathy Study Research Group. *Ophthalmology* 1992; **99**(9): 1351–7.

67 Nakazawa M, Kimizuka Y, Watabe T, Kato K, Watanabe H, Yamanobe S *et al.* Visual outcome after vitrectomy for diabetic retinopathy. A 5-year follow-up. *Acta Ophthalmol (Copenh)* 1993; **71**(2): 219–23.

68 Karel I, Kalvodova B. Long-term results of pars plana vitrectomy and silicone oil for complications of diabetic retinopathy. *Eur J Ophthalmol* 1994; **4**(1): 52–8.

69 Harbour JW, Smiddy WE, Flynn HW, Jr., Rubsamen PE. Vitrectomy for diabetic macular edema associated with a thickened and taut posterior hyaloid membrane. *Am J Ophthalmol* 1996; **121**(4): 405–13.

70 Pendergast SD, Hassan TS, Williams GA, Cox MS, Margherio RR, Ferrone PJ *et al.* Vitrectomy for diffuse diabetic macular edema associated with a taut premacular posterior hyaloid. *Am J Ophthalmol* 2000; **130**(2): 178–86.

71 La Heij EC, Hendrikse F, Kessels AG, Derhaag PJ. Vitrectomy results in diabetic macular oedema without evident

vitreomacular traction. *Graefes Arch Clin Exp Ophthalmol* 2001; **239**(4): 264–70.

72 Yamamoto T, Akabane N, Takeuchi S. Vitrectomy for diabetic macular edema: the role of posterior vitreous detachment and epimacular membrane. *Am J Ophthalmol* 2001; **132**(3): 369–77.

73 Amino K, Tanihara H. Vitrectomy combined with phacoemulsification and intraocular lens implantation for diabetic macular edema. *Jpn J Ophthalmol* 2002; **46**(4): 455–9.

74 Lewis H. The role of vitrectomy in the treatment of diabetic macular edema (editorial). *Am J Ophthalmol* 2001; **131**(1): 123–5.

75 Lahey JM, Francis RR, Kearney JJ. Combining phacoemulsification with pars plana vitrectomy in patients with proliferative diabetic retinopathy: a series of 223 cases. *Ophthalmology* 2003; **110**(7): 1335–9.

76 Treumer F, Bunse A, Rudolf M, Roider J. Pars plana vitrectomy, phacoemulsification and intraocular lens implantation. Comparison of clinical complications in a combined versus two-step surgical approach. *Graefes Arch Clin Exp Ophthalmol* 2006; **244**(7): 808–15.

77 Schrey S, Krepler K, Wedrich A. Incidence of rhegmatogenous retinal detachment after vitrectomy in eyes of diabetic patients. *Retina* 2006; **26**(2): 149–52.

78 Diolaiuti S, Senn P, Schmid MK, Job O, Maloca P, Schipper I. Combined pars plana vitrectomy and phacoemulsification with intraocular lens implantation in severe proliferative diabetic retinopathy. *Ophthalmic Surg Lasers Imaging* 2006; **37**(6): 468–74.

79 Barsam A, Laidlaw A. Visual fields in patients who have undergone vitrectomy for complications of diabetic retinopathy. A prospective study. *BMC Ophthalmol* 2006; **6**: 5.

1 Introduction

Peter H. Scanlon

In this book the fundamental approach is to describe the classification of diabetes, risk factors for diabetic retinopathy and lesions of diabetic retinopathy, and explain the significance of these lesions in terms of progression of the disease, recommended treatment and consequences for vision. Methods of screening for diabetic retinopathy and other retinal conditions that are more frequent in diabetes or have similar appearances to diabetic retinopathy are also discussed.

The four main themes in this introductory chapter are:
1 practical assessment consisting of history, examination and non-ocular investigations
2 multidisciplinary management
3 investigative techniques to assess diabetic retinopathy
4 the application of lasers in diabetic retinopathy.

PRACTICAL ASSESSMENT

History

The history can be divided into the following sections:
- presenting complaint
- past ocular history
- diabetic history
- complications of diabetes
- past medical history
- drug history
- family history
- psychosocial history.

Presenting complaint
Many patients with diabetic retinopathy are asymptomatic until the more advanced stages of the disease. When symptoms do occur they are usually a gradual blurring of vision in diabetic maculopathy or a sudden onset of visual symptoms with a vitreous haemorrhage in proliferative diabetic retinopathy. Patients notice a streak or a sudden onset of floaters in one eye, which increases with progressive visual loss over the next hour as the vitreous haemorrhage progresses. The amount of visual loss depends on the amount or position of the vitreous haemorrhage. If the vitreous or preretinal haemorrhage is in the visual axis of the eye then visual loss is usually quite marked.

Past ocular history
- Visual symptoms
- Cataract or strabismus surgery
- Laser treatment
- Vitrectomy.

Diabetic history
- Type of diabetes
- Duration of diabetes
- Treatment of diabetes – diet, oral hypoglycaemics, insulin or a combination.

Complications of diabetes
- Nephropathy – renal impairment, peritoneal dialysis, haemodialysis
- Cardiovascular – angina, myocardial infarction, coronary artery bypass
- Cerebrovascular – transient ischaemic attack, stroke.

Past medical history
- Serious illnesses
- Operations.

Drug history
- Present medication
- Allergies.

Family history
- Diabetes
- Other illnesses.

A Practical Manual of Diabetic Retinopathy Management.
Peter H Scanlon, Charles P Wilkinson, Stephen J Aldington and David R Matthews. Published 2009 by Blackwell Publishing, ISBN 978-1-4051-7035-2.

Psychosocial
- Occupation
- Number of cigarettes smoked per day

- Units of alcohol consumed per day
- Any history of psychiatric illness
- Home circumstances – type of accommodation, whether lives alone, etc.

Eye examination

1 Assessment of visual acuity

The first part of the eye exam is an assessment of visual acuity (VA). A Snellen or LogMar chart is used and should be back-surface illuminated in order to provide accurate measurements (Figs 1.1 & 1.2).
- The unaided VA is recorded first.
- The VA with current distance spectacle correction is recorded.
- The VA with current distance spectacle correction and a pinhole is recorded.

The best VA of the above three measurements is the best recorded VA.

A refraction may be performed if required.

2 Assessment of colour vision

People with diabetes can develop an acquired colour vision defect (typically a blue loss initially) before showing any significant features of diabetic retinopathy. One patient who appeared to have mild non-proliferative diabetic retinopathy had developed pronounced loss of colour vision and this meant that he was unable to continue in his current employment as a train driver.

The most appropriate test for identifying and quantifying acquired colour vision loss is the Farnsworth–Munsell

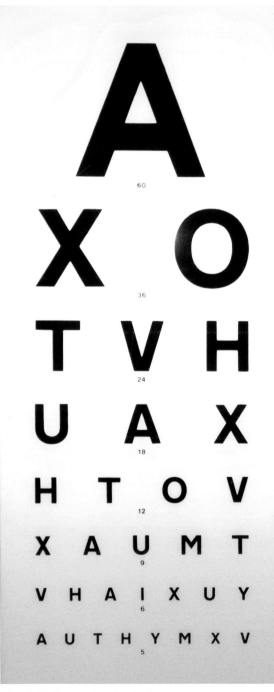

Fig. 1.1 Snellen visual acuity chart.

Fig. 1.2 LogMar visual acuity chart.

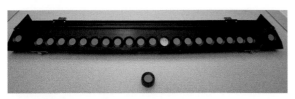

Fig. 1.3 Farnsworth–Munsell 100 hue discrimination test.

100 hue discrimination test (Fig. 1.3). In clinical practice, however, this test is often not available and the Ishihara test, which is designed for detecting congenital (red/green) colour vision defects, is applied. If the Ishihara test is used for the assessment of acquired colour vision defects, clinicians need to be cautious in interpreting test results since it produces a high false-negative rate, so passing the test is not necessarily consistent with normal colour vision.

3 Inspection of external structures

4 Visual fields to confrontation
The patient is asked to cover one eye and stare at the examiner's eye. The examiner's finger/hand or an object like a hat pin with a white or coloured head is moved out of the patient's visual field and brought back in, and the patient asked to indicate when the finger/hand or object comes back into view. This can be used as a simple preliminary test and can be useful particularly if a hemianopia is suspected. More minor degrees of field loss usually require formal testing using automated perimetry or a tangent screen examination.

5 Ocular movement
Patients with diabetes do develop nerve palsies that affect ocular movement but this is usually apparent from the history of sudden onset of diplopia.

6 Pupillary reactions to light and accommodation

7 Red reflex with an ophthalmoscope
This helps to determine whether a media opacity is present such as cataract or vitreous haemorrhage.

8 Preparing for slit-lamp biomicroscopy of the eye

Check that a clear binocular image of the slit beam can be obtained
Check that clear monocular images can be obtained from each eyepiece. A frequent reason for blurred vision is

that the previous operator has left these eye pieces at an unusual focus. The eyepiece construction allows for the distance between both eyepieces to be modified to reflect the interpupillary distance of the user. A sharply defined single image of the slit should be seen.

Patient instructions and positioning
Clear instructions need to be given to the patient and the patient needs to be comfortable. This may require:
- adjusting the patient height
- adjusting the height of the chin rest so that the outer canthus of the patient's eye is aligned to the marker
- ensuring that the patient's head is central
- using a fixation target for the eye not being examined.

Illumination
Controlling the light levels falling on the eye is also an important part of any slit-lamp routine. This can be achieved by altering the power, adding a filter or altering the slit width and height.

Magnification level
The magnification can be adjusted depending on the type of slit-lamp used.

9 Examination of the following structures is routinely undertaken:
- lids and lashes
- conjunctiva, cornea and sclera
- tear film assessment
- anterior chamber
- iris – it is important in diabetic retinopathy to check the iris for rubeosis
- lens – cataract is more common in people with diabetes.

10 Measurement of intraocular pressure is often undertaken using the Goldmann tonometer

11 Both pupils are dilated with G. tropicamide 1% and in most patients G. phenylephrine 2.5% as well

12 Direct ophthalmoscopy
Direct ophthalmoscopy is an examination method commonly used by physicians and general practitioners. It provides magnified views of retinal details, such as the optic disc, individual retinal vessels and the fovea. It is fast and easy to perform, and images appear upright and in normal orientation. It has a limited two-dimensional field of view and has been shown to have a limited sensitivity and specificity for the detection of sight-threatening

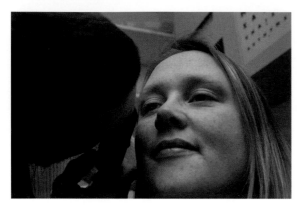

Fig. 1.4 Direct ophthalmoscopy.

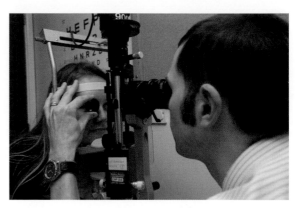

Fig. 1.5 Slit-lamp biomicroscopy with 78D lens.

diabetic retinopathy. It is, however, useful for ad hoc detection of diabetic retinopathy (Fig. 1.4).

13 Slit-lamp biomicroscopy of the retina

Slit-lamp biomicroscopy is the commonest method employed by ophthalmologists to diagnose and monitor retinal disease. A well-dilated pupil is very important for obtaining an adequate view of the posterior segment with the slit-lamp biomicroscope. Several condensing lenses enable the desired magnification to be achieved. These lenses fall into two categories: non-contact lenses and fundus contact lenses.

Non-contact lenses, such as the 60D, 78D, and 90D, provide a magnified stereoscopic view and an inverted, reversed image of the retina. The 60D lens provides the highest magnification, while the 90D lens provides the lowest magnification but the largest visual field view, and the 78D lens is between the two. Newer lenses have been produced, which the manufacturers claim have a higher magnification without sacrificing much of the visual field view (e.g. the Superfield NC, the Digital Wide Field and the Digital 1.0× imaging lenses provided by Volk). See Fig. 1.5.

Fundus contact lenses (contact lens biomicroscopy) are used if thickening or oedema is suspected but is not obvious using the non-contact lenses (Fig. 1.6). The Goldmann three- or four-mirror lenses and the contact ruby lens are commonly used fundus contact lenses that provide images at the same orientation as the retina. Lenses commonly used for laser such as the Volk Area Centralis and the Ocular Mainster (Standard) focal/grid lens provide an inverted image.

For scanning the retina, moderate illumination and a wider slit-lamp beam are used. For evaluating retinal thickness in the macular area and elsewhere, a thin, elong-

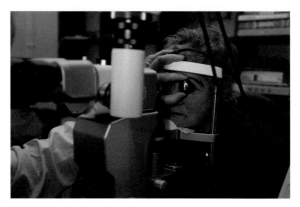

Fig. 1.6 Contact lens biomicroscopy.

ated slit-lamp beam with bright illumination is used. Patients who are sensitive to light can be examined using a red-free filter. When a red-free filter is used, choroidal naevi are more difficult to visualize but haemorrhages, intraretinal microvascular abnormality (IRMA) and neovascularization are usually easily visible.

14 Binocular indirect ophthalmoscopy

Binocular indirect ophthalmoscopy (BIO) is useful for evaluating the posterior segment and retinal periphery (Figs 1.7 & 1.8). A larger area can be viewed than with slit-lamp biomicroscopy but this view is less magnified.

The binocular indirect ophthalmoscope (BIO) is adjusted for the operator's interpupillary distance and the illumination system is usually placed in the upper third of the field for the superior retina examination and the lower third for the inferior retina. Lens powers used for binocular indirect ophthalmoscopy vary from +14D to +40D lenses. The 20D lens is often used as it provides adequate magnification and field of view in most situations.

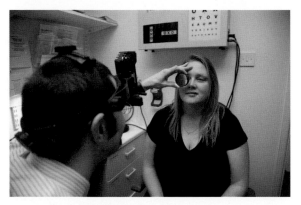

Fig. 1.7 Binocular indirect ophthalmoscopy.

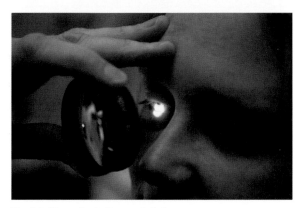

Fig. 1.8 Binocular indirect ophthalmoscopy.

As the lens dioptre increases the width of the field of view increases. The lower the power of the condensing lens the further from the eye it must be held; the stronger the power of the condensing lens the closer to the eye it must be held. To achieve high magnification with any lens, the lens is kept stationary, and the operator should move closer to it.

When BIO is performed, the best position for the patient is reclined. The addition of scleral depression enables one to further evaluate the retinal periphery when required.

MULTIDISCIPLINARY MANAGEMENT

There are a number of risk factors for progression of diabetic retinopathy that do not usually come within the remit of the ophthalmologist's management of the patient such as control of blood glucose, blood pressure and lipids. It is very important for the ophthalmologist to be aware of the control of these risk factors in the individual patient and to have good communication with the diabetic physician or general practitioner who is looking after this aspect of the patient's management.

A rapid improvement in diabetic retinopathy can sometimes be seen when a previously uncontrolled hypertensive receives adequate treatment for their blood pressure. Similarly, a patient who has had poor renal function who commences renal dialysis may show an improvement in their diabetic retinopathy independent of their blood pressure control.

It is important for the ophthalmologist to be involved when a patient who has had poor glucose control and high HbA1c values for a number of years suddenly decides to dramatically improve their control with the assistance of their diabetic physician. Monitoring for a deterioration of their diabetic retinopathy in the first 6–12 months following the rapid improvement of diabetic control caused by the 'early worsening phenomenon' (described in the later chapters of this book) is required, particularly if any diabetic retinopathy is present at baseline.

INVESTIGATIVE TECHNIQUES TO ASSESS DIABETIC RETINOPATHY

Retinal photography

Digital colour retinal photography is increasingly being used as a record of retinal lesions when a patient is being monitored in a retinal clinic by an ophthalmologist. Locations of hard exudates and haemorrhages in the macular area can easily be compared to previous appearances from the photographs taken at the last visit (Fig. 1.9a,b). Similarly, the location and appearances of different levels of non-proliferative and proliferative diabetic retinopathy can also be compared.

Fundus fluorescein angiography

This is a diagnostic procedure in which sodium fluorescein 10% or 20% injection is given rapidly into the antecubital vein or a vein in the forearm or back of the hand, taking precautions to avoid extravasation. (If the needle has extravasated the injection is stopped as the dye is very painful when injected subcutaneously.) Fluorescein dye produces a yellow fluorescence in blue light; blue light is therefore shone into the eye and the resultant yellow fluorescence is photographed through a yellow filter. The dye usually appears in the choroidal and retinal vasculature within 10–20 seconds. If a vein on the back of the hand is used, it may take longer than 20 seconds to appear.

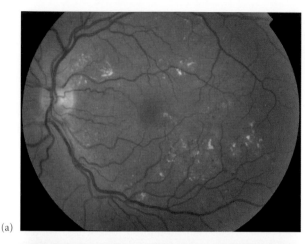

(a)

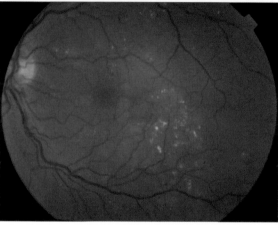

(b)

Fig. 1.9 (a) Exudates in macular area before treatment.
(b) Exudates in macular area after treatment with laser.

The fluorescein dye causes few side-effects, the most common being nausea and vomiting. Syncope is not uncommon and resolves quickly provided the patient is laid horizontally. Skin rashes and itching are seen at times. More serious side-effects are bronchospasm, anaphylactic shock and cardiac arrest. However, these more serious events are extremely rare.

After injection, the skin shows a temporary yellow discolouration, which lasts for 24–48 hours until the dye is excreted in the urine. It has a photosensitizing effect on the skin and the patient should avoid exposure to direct sunlight during this period of time. If the patient is not warned that their urine will be an orange-green colour this might also be a cause of concern.

The fluorescein dye also gives a false high glucose reading on self-testing of the urine and blood. Patients should be warned not to adjust their insulin dose on the basis of

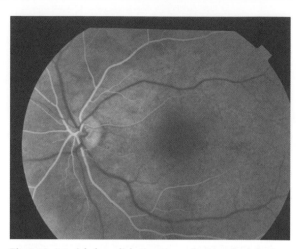

Fig. 1.10 Arterial phase diabetic retinopathy 24 s after injection.

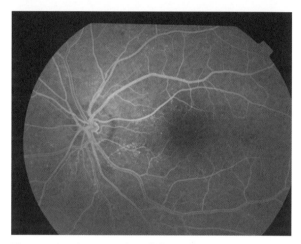

Fig. 1.11 Arteriovenous phase diabetic retinopathy 32 s after injection.

their self-testing results for 48 hours after the fluorescein angiogram.

An example of a normal fluorescein angiogram demonstrating the different phases of the angiogram (choroidal, arterial, arteriovenous and venous) is shown in Chapter 5 on the normal eye.

Figures 1.10–1.12 show the pattern in diabetic retinopathy.

Ocular coherence tomography

Optical coherence tomography (OCT) is an imaging technique that interprets the 'time of flight' and intensity of reflected optical waves using interferometry. OCT uses wavelengths between 600 nm and 2000 nm, and the

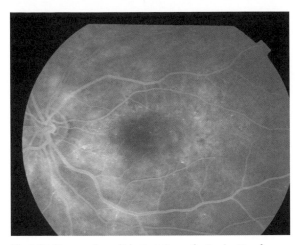

Fig. 1.12 Venous phase diabetic retinopathy 2 min 48 s after injection.

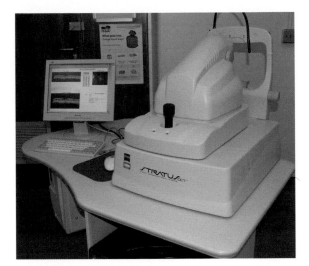

Fig. 1.13 An optical coherence tomography (OCT) machine.

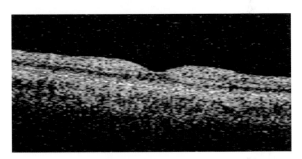

Fig. 1.14 Normal OCT B-mode image.

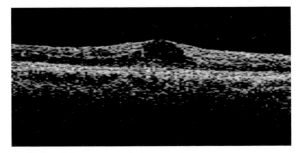

Fig. 1.15 Clinically significant macular oedema (CSMO) B-mode image.

modern light sources vary between superluminescent diodes, mode-locked lasers and photonic crystal fibres.[1]

OCT has an increasing role to play in the assessment and monitoring of patients with diabetic macular oedema. As a result of the high level of resolution, OCT is particularly suitable for retinal thickness measurements offering penetration to approximately 2–3 mm with micrometer-scale axial and lateral resolution. Neubauer[2] and Goebel[3] both compared the OCT and the retinal thickness analyser (RTA) and concluded that the OCT seemed to be more suitable in the clinical screening for macular oedema. OCT has been principally applied to create longitudinal images (similar to ultrasound B-scan) that are in-depth measurements through the retina. See Figs 1.13–1.15.

OCT images can be presented either as cross-sectional images or as tomographic maps (Figs 1.16 & 1.17). A cross-sectional or B-mode image is constructed from many A-scans, which are a combination of reflectivity profiles and depth. To facilitate interpretation a false colour scheme is added in which bright colours such as red and green correspond to highly reflective areas and darker colours such as blue and black correspond to areas of lower reflectivity. With the early OCT machines that use the above principles of A- and B-mode imaging, tomographic maps are produced by obtaining six consecutive cross-sectional scans at 30° angular orientations in a radial spoke pattern centred on the fovea. A similar false colour scheme to aid interpretation, as described above for the B-mode images, is used for the tomographic maps.

In a clinical setting, Yang[4] found that OCT may be more sensitive than a clinical examination in assessing diabetic macular oedema and that it could be used as a quantita-tive tool for documenting changes in macular thickening. Frank[5] found that although changes in macular thickness over the course of the day did not occur in all subjects, the 8 am value, obtained just after waking, was significantly higher (p = 0.0005) than any of the three later values.

The ability to capture images similar to OCT depth information in slices of the tissue at orientations

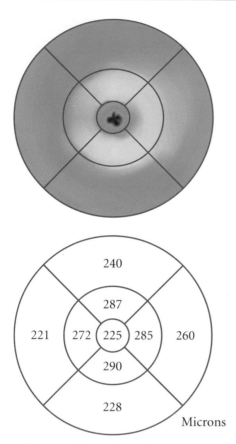

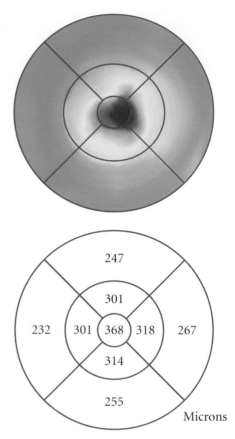

Fig. 1.16 Tomographic map of normal eye.

Fig. 1.17 Tomographic map of above patient with CSMO.

perpendicular to the optic axis (*en face* images, or C-scans) was described by Podoleanu,[6] and later T scanning (transverse priority) images were described by Cucu.[7] This and other methods have provided three-dimensional (3D) OCT images, which have provided the ability to construct 3D volumes at different depths. The application of these techniques is further discussed in Chapter 15 on 'Future advances in the management of diabetic retinopathy'.

Ultrasound B-scan examination

Ocular ultrasound is a means of visualizing the eye and retrobulbar region involving the placement of a high-frequency 10-MHz probe onto the eye or eyelid. Multiple two-dimensional images, obtained by taking a series of scan sections of the eye, enable the clinician to assess the anatomical features of the posterior segment of the eye (Figs 1.18–1.20).

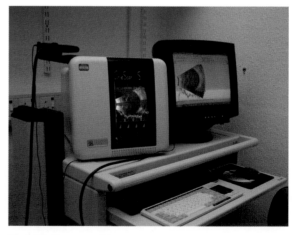

Fig. 1.18 B-scan machine.

Ultrasound echoes are produced at the interface between adjacent ocular tissues of different densities. The greater the difference in tissue density, the higher the

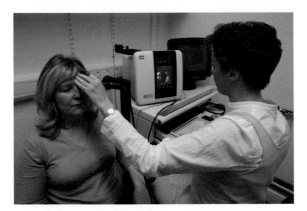

Fig. 1.19 B-scan being performed.

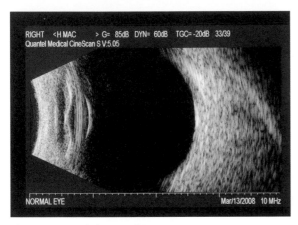

Fig. 1.20 Normal ultrasound B-scan.

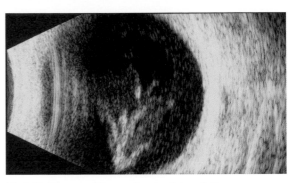

Fig. 1.21 Ultrasound B-scan showing intragel vitreous haemorrhage with normal retina.

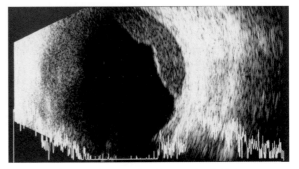

Fig. 1.22 Ultrasound B-scan showing retrohyaloid vitreous haemorrhage with normal retina.

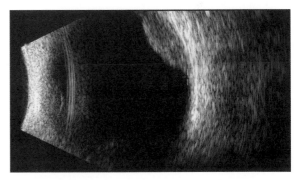

Fig. 1.23 Ultrasound B-scan showing peripheral primary melanoma.

intensity (amplitude) of the returning echo. This can allow differentiation between membranes; for example posterior vitreous detachment (low-amplitude echo) and retinal detachment (high-amplitude echo).

Ultrasound examination is particularly helpful in determining the density and extent of a vitreous haemorrhage, the presence of vitreoretinal attachments, fibrovascular membranes, tractional retinal detachment and large proliferative vessel fronds. Serial ultrasound examinations of a vitreous haemorrhage, over a period of weeks, normally demonstrate a reduction in the extent and density of blood, as the haemorrhage is absorbed. Any vulnerable areas of retinal traction can be identified and monitored carefully during the period when an ophthalmoscopic retinal examination is not possible (Figs 1.21–1.23).

In diabetic eyes with advanced proliferative changes, the ultrasound image may be complex and difficult to interpret, particularly when fibrovascular membranes and tractional or rhegmatogenous retinal detachments

coexist. The membrane's shape, echo amplitude, reflectivity characteristics and dynamic assessment, during and immediately after eye movement, contribute to an accurate diagnosis.

An ocular ultrasound examination is an appropriate investigation for any patient with an obscured fundal view. It is also particularly helpful to the vitreoretinal surgeon when planning for and performing a vitrectomy procedure.

Ultrasound A-scan examination provides a one-dimensional section of the eye that produces an accurate measurement of the size, length and thickness of the ocular features. A-scan is used most commonly for the measurement of axial length, required for the calculation of intraocular lens implant power in cataract surgery, but with appropriate standardized calibration, it can also be used in conjunction with B-scan to quantify retinal features and solid lesions.

Perimetry

Perimetry is the systematic measurement of differential light sensitivity in the visual field by the detection of the presence of test targets on a defined background in order to map and quantify the visual field.

There are two main methods for undertaking perimetry: (i) kinetic perimetry and (ii) static perimetry.

Goldmann kinetic perimetry

The most common visual field equipment used for kinetic assessment is the Goldmann perimeter. It is a large hemispherical bowl of radius 30 cm with a standardized white interior brightness onto which stimuli of various sizes and brightness are projected. Patients are required to maintain fixation on a central target while a stimulus of specified size (from 1 mm to 5 mm diameter) and brightness is moved slowly from the patient's peripheral area of 'non-seeing' into the area of 'seeing'. When the patient first detects the light stimulus they respond by pressing a buzzer to alert the operator (Fig. 1.24).

The stimulus is moved systematically by the perimetrist to examine areas of the visual field. Points of equal retinal sensitivity are mapped onto a chart, which when joined

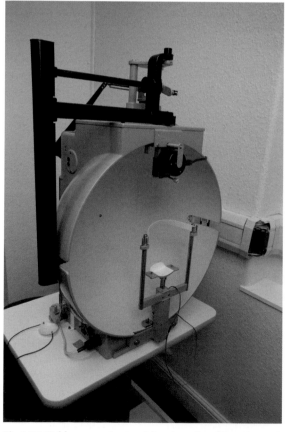

(a)

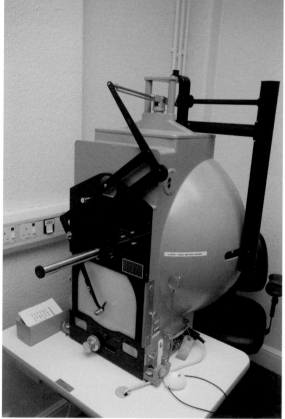

(b)

Fig. 1.24 Goldmann perimeter: (a) patient view; (b) operator view.

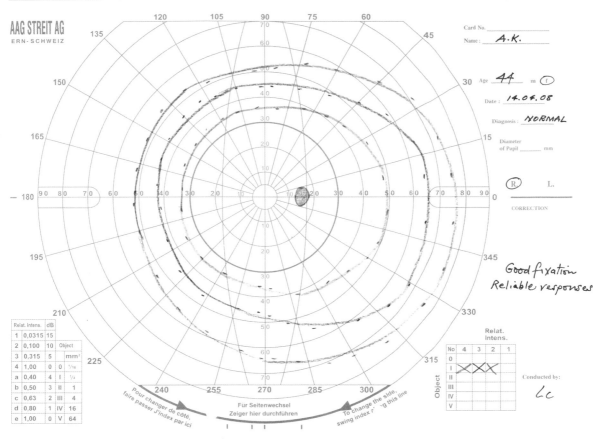

AAG STREIT AG
ERN-SCHWEIZ

Card No. _____
Name : *A.K.*
Age *44* m ⓕ
Date : *14.04.08*
Diagnosis : *NORMAL*
Diameter of Pupil _____ mm

Ⓡ   L.

CORRECTION

Good fixation
Reliable responses

Relat. Intens.	dB			
1	0,0315	15		
2	0,100	10	Object	
3	0,315	5	mm²	
4	1,00	0	0	1/16
a	0,40	4	I	1/4
b	0,50	3	II	1
c	0,63	2	III	4
d	0,80	1	IV	16
e	1,00	0	V	64

Relat. intens.

No	4	3	2	1
0				
I				
II	✕	✕	✕	
III				
IV				
V				

Conducted by: *Lc*

Pour changer de côté, faire passer J'index par ici

Für Seitenwechsel
Zeiger hier durchführen

To change the side, swing index ... g this line

Fig. 1.25 Example of a normal Goldmann visual field.

together produce a 'contour' line, called an isopter. Any contraction of the visual field, area of reduced sensitivity or blind spot becomes evident as they are mapped out (Fig. 1.25).

Goldmann perimetry is particularly helpful in the detection and diagnosis of neurological visual field defects such as quadrantinopia and hemianopia. Due to the subjectivity and versatility of the examination procedure, the assessment requires an experienced and skilled perimetrist.

Automated static perimetry

Automated perimeters use static light stimuli, of various intensities at fixed locations within a hemispherical bowl, to provide an accurate measurement of retinal sensitivity. Automated perimeters are particularly effective in identifying and quantifying defects within the central visual field and are used routinely for screening for abnormality and for quantifying progression of defects. The equip-

ment employs various testing strategies, which are selected by the clinician based on the underlying pathology, suspected pathology and the level of detail required (i.e. screening or detailed quantification of defects).

The testing procedure involves presenting single or multiple patterned, static light stimuli in a preselected, random order, to minimize patient prediction. Once the stimulus is observed, the patient responds, either verbally or via means of a buzzer. The pattern of stimuli presented and the time taken for completing the test is dependent on the strategy selected. Visual field examination can be time-consuming for the patient, who may be required to concentrate for long periods of time. Optimizing the length of testing time to reduce patient fatigue and to maximize performance is an important factor in test selection and in obtaining reliable results.

The Humphrey visual field analyser is generally considered to be the most common visual field equipment in use in UK ophthalmology departments (Fig. 1.26).

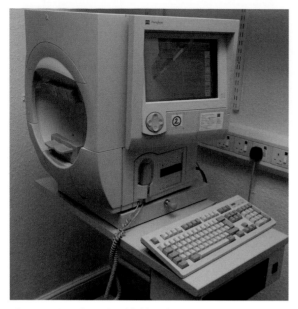 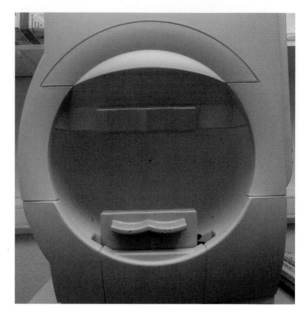

Fig. 1.26 Humphrey visual field analyser.

Normal visual field examination requires each eye to be tested independently (Fig. 1.27). One eye is covered while the other maintains accurate, central fixation for the duration of the test. Occasionally, binocular visual field testing is required for patients who have undergone panretinal photocoagulation, resulting in peripheral visual field constriction or defects within the central 20°. This may impact on a person's ability to meet the UK Driver and Vehicle Licensing Agency (DVLA) visual field standard. This requires a binocular assessment to be undertaken, using the Esterman grid testing pattern. A series of 120 points, at a specified light intensity, are presented individually across a rectangular area extending over 150° of the horizontal binocular visual field. Holders of a UK driver's licence are required to meet the standard of a horizontal visual field of at least 120°, with no significant central defect (Fig. 1.28). (For detailed information on the visual standards required for driving, please refer to the DVLA website: www.dvla.gov.uk.)

THE APPLICATION OF LASERS IN DIABETIC RETINOPATHY

Laser is defined as *l*ight *a*mplification by *s*imulated *e*mission of *r*adiation.

Coherence is one of the unique properties of laser light. It arises from the stimulated emission process, which provides the amplification, and the emitted photons are 'in step' and have a definite phase relation to each other.

Spatial coherence tells us how uniform the phase of the wave front is, which gives us the ability to precisely focus the laser beam to apply very small burns to pathological tissue with minimal disturbance to surrounding tissue.

Temporal coherence tells us how monochromatic a source is and this gives us the ability to select a very narrow bandwidth of light that is preferentially absorbed by the pathological tissue site.

With improvements of laser technology, different types of laser are now used in the diagnosis and treatment of many eye disorders. Laser–tissue interactions can occur in several ways but are broadly grouped under photothermal, photochemical and photoionizing effects.

When lasers are used for treatment of diabetic retinopathy, they rely principally on the effect of photocoagulation.

Photocoagulation (photothermal effect)

Photocoagulation causes denaturation of proteins when temperatures rise sufficiently. The temperature rise in tissues is proportional to the amount of light absorbed by that tissue. The retinal pigment epithelium absorbs light because of its melanin content, and blood vessels absorb light because of their haemoglobin content.

Lasers commonly used for photocoagulation are argon, krypton and diode Nd : YAG lasers.

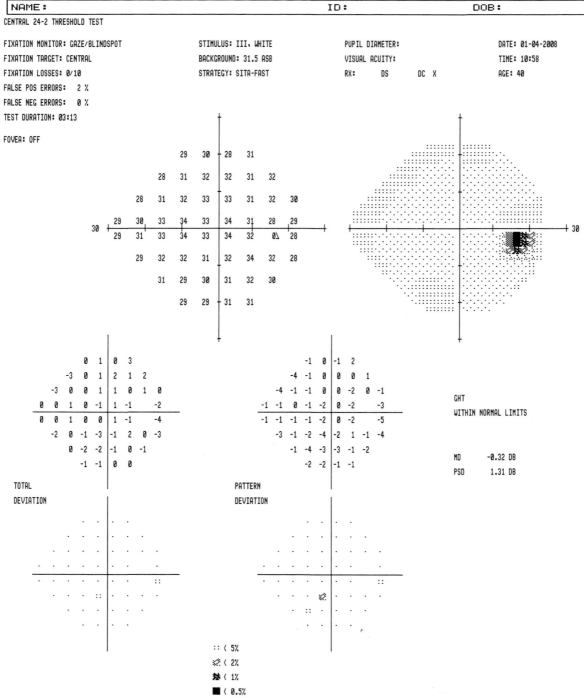

SINGLE FIELD ANALYSIS   EYE: RIGHT

NAME :   ID :   DOB :

CENTRAL 24-2 THRESHOLD TEST

FIXATION MONITOR: GAZE/BLINDSPOT   STIMULUS: III, WHITE   PUPIL DIAMETER: DATE: 01-04-2008
FIXATION TARGET: CENTRAL   BACKGROUND: 31.5 ASB   VISUAL ACUITY: TIME: 10:58
FIXATION LOSSES: 0/10   STRATEGY: SITA-FAST   RX: DS   DC X   AGE: 40
FALSE POS ERRORS: 2 %
FALSE NEG ERRORS: 0 %
TEST DURATION: 03:13

FOVEA: OFF

GHT
WITHIN NORMAL LIMITS

MD   -0.32 DB
PSD   1.31 DB

TOTAL
DEVIATION

PATTERN
DEVIATION

:: (5%
⚼ (2%
⬚ (1%
■ (0.5%

Fig. 1.27 Example of a normal Humphrey visual field. (*Continued on p. 14*)

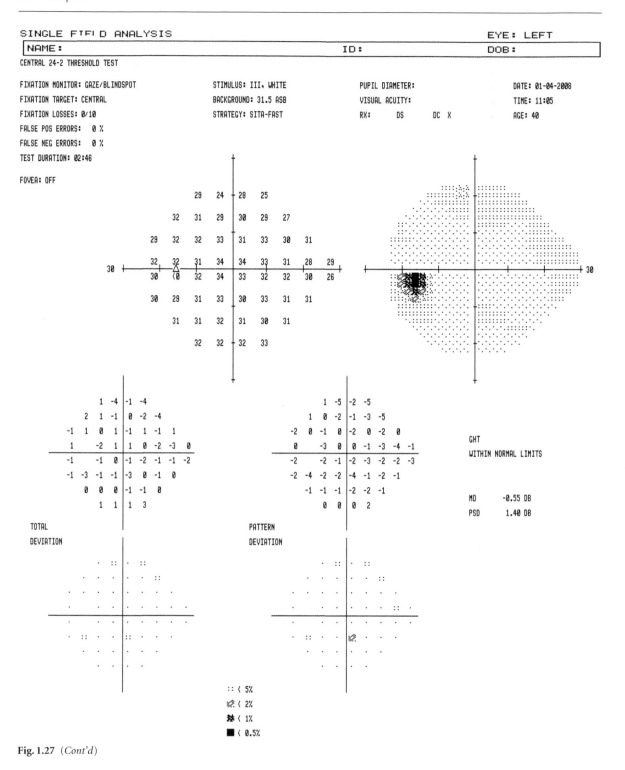

SINGLE FIELD ANALYSIS   EYE: LEFT

| NAME: | ID: | DOB: |

CENTRAL 24-2 THRESHOLD TEST

FIXATION MONITOR: GAZE/BLINDSPOT   STIMULUS: III, WHITE   PUPIL DIAMETER: DATE: 01-04-2008

FIXATION TARGET: CENTRAL   BACKGROUND: 31.5 ASB   VISUAL ACUITY: TIME: 11:05

FIXATION LOSSES: 0/10   STRATEGY: SITA-FAST   RX: DS   DC X   AGE: 40

FALSE POS ERRORS: 0 %

FALSE NEG ERRORS: 0 %

TEST DURATION: 02:46

FOVEA: OFF

```
                    29   24    28   25
               32   31   29    30   29   27
          29   32   32   33    31   33   30   31
     30   32   32   31   34    34   33   31   28   29
          30  <0    32   34    33   32   32   30   26
          30   29   31   33    30   33   31   31
               31   31   32    31   30   31
                    32   32    32   33
```

```
        1   -4  -1  -4                      1   -5  -2  -5
    2   1   -1   0  -2  -4              1   0  -2  -1  -3  -5
-1  1   0   1  -1   1  -1   1      -2   0  -1   0  -2   0  -2   0
1      -2   1   1   0  -2  -3   0      0      -3   0   0  -1  -3  -4  -1        GHT
-1     -1   0  -1  -2  -1  -1  -2      -2     -2  -1  -2  -3  -2  -2  -3        WITHIN NORMAL LIMITS
-1 -3  -1  -1  -3   0  -1   0      -2 -4  -2  -2  -4  -1  -2  -1
    0   0   0  -1  -1   0              -1  -1  -1  -2  -2  -1                    MD      -0.55 DB
        1   1   1   3                      0   0   0   2                        PSD      1.40 DB
```

TOTAL   PATTERN

DEVIATION   DEVIATION

```
            .  ::  .  ::                      .  ::  .  ::
        .   .   .  .  .   ::               .   .   .  .  .   ::
    .   .   .  .  .   .                 .   .   .  .  .   .
    .   .   .  .  .   .  .              .   .   .  .  .   .  .  ::  .
    .   .   .  .  .   .                 .   .   .  .  .   .
    .  ::  .   .  ::  .   .  .          .  ::  .   .  ⊠  .   .  .
        .   .  .  .   .  .                 .   .  .  .   .  .
            .   .  .  .                        .   .  .  .
```

```
                    ::  < 5%
                    ⊠  < 2%
                    ▨  < 1%
                    ■  < 0.5%
```

Fig. 1.27 *(Cont'd)*

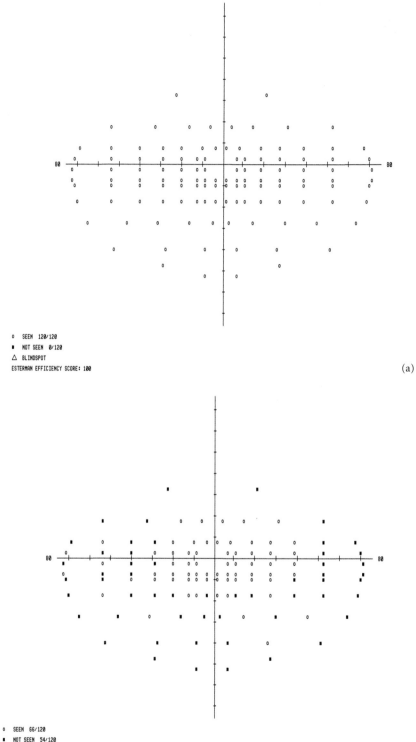

Fig. 1.28 (a) Example of a normal Esterman visual field. (b) Example of a restricted Esterman field in a diabetic patient. The case history of this patient is described in Case History 1, Chapter 9 on proliferative and advanced diabetic retinopathy.

Two other clinical effects of lasers commonly used in ophthalmology are photodisruption and photoablation.

Photodisruption (photoionizing effect)

Short-pulsed, high-power lasers disrupt tissues by delivering irradiance to tissue targets such as the peripheral iris producing a laser iridotomy for the prevention of angle closure glaucoma using an Nd : YAG Q-switched laser.

Photoablation (photochemical effect)

Tissue is removed in some way by light, such as when inter-molecular bands of biological tissues are broken, disintegrating target tissues, and the disintegrated molecules are volatilized. The excimer laser uses photoablation in photo-refractive procedures such as photorefractive keratectomy (PRK) and laser subepithelial keratectomy (LASEK).

Active laser media are available in the following states:
• solid – crystalline or amorphous (e.g. Nd : YAG laser)
• liquid (e.g. dye laser)
• gaseous (e.g. argon ion laser, CO_2 laser, excimer laser)
• other (e.g. diode laser).

A laser gain medium is the active medium of the laser which can amplify the power of light. The term gain refers to the amount of amplification. Energy is pumped into the active medium in a very disorganized form and is partially transformed into radiation energy, which is highly ordered.

Light wavelengths produced by different lasers

Argon blue-green lasers produce light over a narrow bandwidth, the main peaks being at 488 and 514 nm. This laser is the commonest laser used for both panretinal laser and macular laser treatment of diabetic retinopathy.

The Pascal pattern scan laser is a frequency-doubled Nd : YAG diode-pumped solid state laser producing light of wavelength 532 nm. This laser was introduced in June 2006 and it is unique in that it allows the operator to apply multiple spots almost simultaneously in prechosen patterns of up to 25 spots.

Diode lasers were introduced in 1993. These were laser-emitting diodes of gallium-aluminium-arsenide, which were portable and had a wavelength of emission of 810 nm. Most of the laser energy from the diode laser is absorbed by the pigment in the melanocytes in the choroid, which makes it more difficult for the operator to define the correct treatment power to use and, because of the depth of penetration, the diode laser appears to be more painful for patients than the argon blue-green or the Pascal laser.

PRACTICE POINT

• Over the last 30 years, modern technology has produced major advances in the investigations and treatment that can be undertaken in our diabetic patients. However, a carefully taken history and high-quality clinical examination are still vital components of the care of any patient with diabetic retinopathy.

REFERENCES

1 Podoleanu AG. Optical coherence tomography. *Br J Radiol* 2005; **78**(935): 976–88.
2 Neubauer AS, Priglinger S, Ullrich S, Bechmann M, Thiel MJ, Ulbig MW *et al.* Comparison of foveal thickness measured with the retinal thickness analyzer and optical coherence tomography. *Retina* 2001; **21**(6): 596–601.
3 Goebel W, Franke R. Retinal thickness in diabetic retinopathy: comparison of optical coherence tomography, the retinal thickness analyser, and fundus photography. *Retina* 2006; **26**(1): 49–57.
4 Yang CS, Cheng CY, Lee FL, Hsu WM, Liu JH. Quantitative assessment of retinal thickness in diabetic patients with and without clinically significant macular edema using optical coherence tomography. *Acta Ophthalmol Scand* 2001; **79**(3): 266–70.
5 Frank R, Schulz L, Abe K, Iezzi R. Variation in diabetic macular edema. *Ophthalmology* 2004; **111**(10): 1945–56.
6 Podoleanu AG, Dobre GM, Cucu RG, Rosen R, Garcia P, Nieto J *et al.* Combined multiplanar optical coherence tomography and confocal scanning ophthalmoscopy. *J Biomed Opt* 2004; **9**(1): 86–93.
7 Cucu R, Podoleanu A, Rogers J, Pedro J, Rosen R. Combined confocal/en face T-scan-based ultra high-resolution optical coherence tomography in vivo retinal imaging. *Optics Letters* 2006; **31**(11): 1684–6.

2 Diabetes

David R. Matthews & Peter H. Scanlon

Diabetes mellitus can be characterized as the chronic condition in which there is an excess of glucose circulating in the bloodstream. Glucose homeostasis is complex and is the result of the interplay of insulin secretion and insulin sensitivity. Typically the differences between type 1 diabetes mellitus (T1DM) and type 2 diabetes mellitus (T2DM) are characterized by the absolute deficiency of insulin in the former and the relative deficiency of insulin associated with insulin resistance in the latter. This insulin deficiency – either complete or partial – is the basic mechanism behind diabetes, though other factors have an influence and can sometimes be more important when considering treatment. Insulin resistance, defined as the reduced capacity of peripheral tissues and the liver to respond to insulin, is almost always found in diabetes, and is especially important in type 2 diabetes where insulin resistance compounds the secretory defects. Because insulin resistance can be such a feature of T2DM, hyper-insulinaemia may be found, though the high concentrations are still insufficient to control the glycaemia.

The body normally regulates glucose very precisely in the fasting state between about 4 and 5.5 mmol/L in the plasma. Blood glucose concentrations above the normal limits lead to excessive glycosylation of proteins and this is probably one of the main aetiologies of the long-term complications of diabetes. In particular, the risks of hyperglycaemia and hypertension are multiplicative for microvascular disease, of which the commonest is diabetic retinopathy.

CLASSIFICATION OF DIABETES

Diabetes mellitus is generally divided into the categories 'type 1 diabetes' and 'type 2 diabetes', with much rarer

A Practical Manual of Diabetic Retinopathy Management.
Peter H Scanlon, Charles P Wilkinson, Stephen J Aldington and David R Matthews. Published 2009 by Blackwell Publishing, ISBN 978-1-4051-7035-2.

additional categories of maturity-onset diabetes of the young (MODY) and secondary diabetes. The two major forms differ in their cause and in the urgency of treatment necessary (Table 2.1). It has even been suggested that the dichotomy is false as there is a grey area between the two types[1]. As a broad generalization, type 1 diabetes occurs in those who are generally younger (so teenagers are more likely to have type 1, and those in middle age type 2) and thinner (so being overweight is a risk for type 2 diabetes and not for type 1). Type 1 diabetes has a rapid onset, and symptoms can be severe. Prompt medical intervention is almost always necessary. Type 2 diabetes is quite strongly genetic (being found in families from one generation to the next, and in brothers and sisters as they get to middle age or older) and is also related to becoming overweight or not taking enough exercise or both. Type 2 diabetes can have a very slow and insidious onset, and the diagnosis may be missed for many months or be found by chance on routine medical screening or during health-check medical investigations. In the UKPDS study it was observed that up to 50% of patients had some detectable form of tissue damage at diagnosis, the majority of this being background diabetic retinopathy[2].

CASE HISTORY 1
Type 1 diabetes with retinopathy

A 5-year-old girl presented with thirst, polyuria and weight loss. Her father had type 1 diabetes mellitus. She had an elevated blood glucose of 23 mmol/L and a slightly elevated urea, but no signs of diabetic ketoacidosis. She was started on a standard mixture of 30% soluble insulin and 70% isophane insulin with a estimated dose of 0.6 units/kg of body weight per day (total). This was split into two-thirds in the morning and one-third at night (i.e. 0.4 units/kg in the morning and 0.2 units/kg in the evening). Stabilization occurred over the next few weeks. Two years later she was requiring 1 unit/kg of body weight per day, and a small increase was required during puberty.

Table 2.1 Differences between type 1 and type 2 diabetes.

	Type 1 diabetes	Type 2 diabetes
Older and alternative names	Juvenile-onset diabetes Insulin-dependent diabetes mellitus (IDDM)	Maturity-onset diabetes Non-insulin-dependent diabetes mellitus (NIDDM)
Onset	Any time in life, but teenagers and children are most likely to have this type	Generally diagnosed over the age of 40, but can occur in the overweight or in some genetic conditions in younger people
Symptoms at onset	Thirst, tiredness, weight loss, polyuria, ketoacidosis in extremis	Tiredness, nocturia, thrush and skin infections
Body type	Generally normal-weight or thin	Generally overweight
Speed of onset	Usually becomes critical and needs urgent attention within a few weeks (or even days) of the first symptoms	May not be noticed as a problem. Onset can be insidious. Diagnosis made often incidental to other pathology
Genetics	Some genetic propensity to run in families, but not caused by a single gene	Quite a strong genetic propensity to run in families, but not caused by a single gene
Triggered by	Autoimmunity. GAD antibody and ICA positive	Relative insulin deficiency where the beta-cells have insufficient function in an internal environment characterized by insulin resistance
Treated by	Optimizing lifestyle. Will need insulin very early in the treatment plan	Optimizing lifestyle, which may initially be enough. Generally will need oral agents initially. Progress onto insulin is usual at a median duration of diabetes of about 6 years
How common	About 0.2% of the population (2 cases per 1000 people)	Up to 4% of UK population, up to 8% in USA, up to 20% in parts of Asia and up to 50% in Pima and Nauru Indians
Retinopathy	Rare in the first 5 years if the diabetes is treated adequately. Some background retinopathy usual by 15 years duration	33% of patients have background retinopathy at diagnosis

The diabetes was reasonably well controlled with regular attendance at the paediatric diabetic clinic until she reached the age of 14, when her parents divorced, the control deteriorated and her clinic visits became irregular. At the age of 16 she was admitted with diabetic ketoacidosis but she discharged herself 2 days later when she felt that she could manage again at home. During her teenage years she found that whenever she controlled her diabetes well she had a tendency to put on weight and hence tended to run her blood sugars on the high side in order to stay slim. She had been discharged from the paediatric clinic at the age of 16 years and, following her episode of diabetic ketoacidosis, she was supposed to attend the adult clinic but never attended. Her family doctor prescribed her insulin and checked her blood pressure, and looked in her fundi once a year with a direct ophthalmoscope.

At the age of 21 years she had a sudden onset of a floater in her left eye and presented as an emergency to the eye department. Photographs were taken 2 days after the initial presentation (Fig. 2.1a,b). These showed proliferative diabetic retinopathy in both eyes. Laser treatment was commenced for both eyes. She had one laser treatment on each eye but failed to attend follow-up appointments that were sent.

The following year (aged 22 years) she presented with a sudden loss of vision in her left eye (Fig. 2.1c,d). Her left eye required a vitrectomy and her right eye laser treatment under general anaesthesia. She has subsequently had a vitrectomy in her right eye. She has attended most of her follow-up visits after the vitrectomy but has now developed renal problems and is under the care of the renal physician.

AETIOPATHOLOGY OF DIABETES

Type 1 diabetes

Type 1 diabetes is autoimmune in its aetiology, usually involving the generation of detectable islet cell antibodies (ICAs) or glutamic acid decarboxylase antibodies (GADAs). Detection of such antibodies helps to confirm the autoimmune nature of the process, but the presence of the antibodies is neither necessary nor sufficient in the

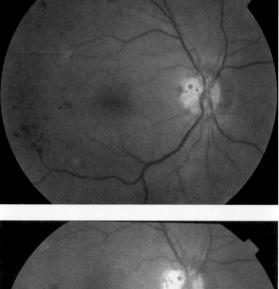

(a)

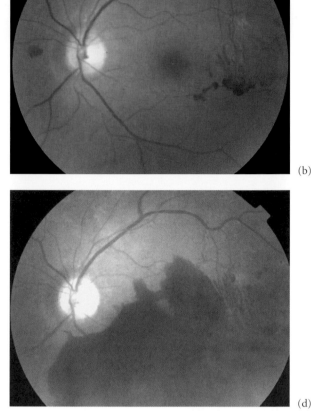

(b)

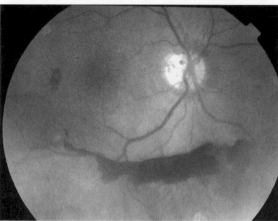

(c)

(d)

Fig. 2.1 Case history 1. (a) Right macular colour photograph at presentation. (b) Left macular colour photograph at presentation. (c) Right macular red-free photograph 1 year after presentation. (d) Left macular red-free photograph 1 year after presentation.

process. Some classic type 1 diabetes occurs without such antibodies being detectable, and some subjects will have antibodies for many years without developing the clinical condition. There is continuing debate about the triggering effects of other proteins or of infections in sensitizing the autoimmune system. Some associations – such as those with milk proteins and cytomegalovirus – are recurrent in the literature, but again the exposure seems neither necessary nor sufficient. There are genetic propensities, but even identical twins have a discordance rate of 70%.

Type 2 diabetes

Type 2 diabetes is common – 20 times as common as type 1 diabetes – and has an obscure pathophysiology. The risks of the disease are related to obesity; those with a BMI greater than 35 have a 37 times greater risk than those with a BMI less than 22. The condition seems to be genetically coded and concordance between identical twins over time converges towards about 90%. Many theories have been propounded: lipotoxicity, glucose toxicity, amyloidosis secondary to islet-associated polypeptide beta-pleating and insulin resistance are all currently under close scrutiny. What has become clear, however, is that there is always some element of beta-cell failure whenever type 2 diabetes is diagnosed. Because the pathophysiology tends to be indolent, symptoms can sometimes be slight or so slow in onset that they are not recognized as being pathological – nocturia is the classic example of this. The consequence is that the body may have been exposed to several years of hyperglycaemia and the result is the finding of tissue damage at diagnosis. Retinopathy is the commonest finding, with about 30% of all subjects newly diagnosed having detectable retinal lesions.

CASE HISTORY 2
Type 2 diabetes presenting with neuropathy and retinopathy

A 53-year-old man presented to his GP with a year's history of tingling and soreness in his feet. On examination he was hypertensive with a blood pressure of 180/94 mmHg, his random blood glucose was 15.4 mmol/L and his HbA1c result 11.4%. He was not obese, with a BMI of 24.8. His cholesterol was raised at 8.6 mmol/L with an HDL of 1.6 mmol/L and LDL of 5.2 mmol/L. His renal function was normal with an albumin creatinine ratio of 0.8 mg/mmol. He was referred to diabetic eye screening at which point photographs showed extensive diabetic maculopathy in both eyes (Fig. 2.2).

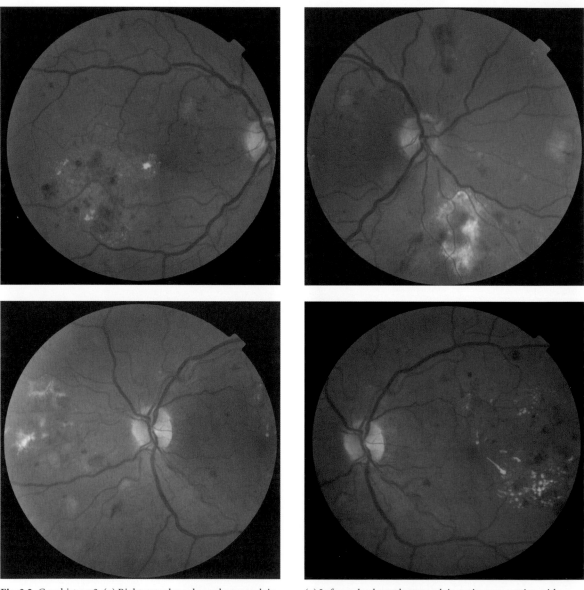

(a)

(b)

(c)

(d)

Fig. 2.2 Case history 2. (a) Right macular colour photograph in patient presenting with type 2 diabetes. (b) Right nasal colour photograph in patient presenting with type 2 diabetes. (c) Left nasal colour photograph in patient presenting with type 2 diabetes. (d) Left macular colour photograph in patient presenting with type 2 diabetes.

His family doctor treated him with metformin 2 g daily, aspirin 75 mg daily, simvastatin 40 mg daily, gliclazide 80 mg daily and ramipril 2.5 mg daily, and his HbA1c gradually improved over a 3-month period to 8.6.

He received focal laser treatment to each eye.

Maturity-onset diabetes of the young

There are some important monogenic forms of diabetes that have been recognized. About 2% of all diabetes appears similar to type 2 diabetes but is diagnosed in the teenage years and early 20s – this has been given the oxymoron 'maturity-onset diabetes of the young' or 'MODY'. MODY types 1–6 are recognized as having specific monogenic aetiologies (Table 2.2) and they have markedly different outcomes in terms of progression and complications. The commonest type (MODY-3) is caused by hepatic nuclear factor (HNF-1α) abnormalities, and responds well to low-dose sulphonylureas. MODY-2 (about 20% of all MODY) is important to diagnose because it is a well-regulated hyperglycaemic state with a norm set at about 6 mmol/L rather than 4 mmol/L fasting. Because sustained hyperglycaemia is not a feature, those with MODY-2 rarely have macrovascular complications or significant retinopathy.

Recent discoveries[3,4] of ABCC8 (SUR1) and INS (insulin) gene mutations presenting in patients clinically defined as having MODY will have implications for clinical management.

CASE HISTORY 3
HNF-1α MODY diabetes

A 46-year-old man, who attended the eye clinic for monitoring of moderate non-proliferative diabetic retinopathy (preproliferative) was diagnosed with type 1 diabetes at the age of 18, having presented with a 4-month

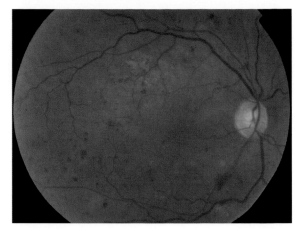

Fig. 2.3 Case history 3. Right macular image from a patient with MODY.

history of tiredness, polydipsia and polyuria (Fig. 2.3). A random blood glucose at diagnosis was 16.0 mmol/L and he had a BMI of 24 kg/m^2. He has a positive family history of diabetes, with his sister, father and paternal grandfather having been diagnosed with type 1 diabetes in their late teens (Fig. 2.4). His father had relatively good glycaemic control despite not being fully compliant with his insulin therapy.

He was initially treated with basal bolus insulin regimen and responded well with good glycaemic control and an HbA1c of 6.7% one month after diagnosis.

At one follow-up appointment 14 years later, he mentioned forgetting to take his insulin for 4 days whilst on a camping trip. He remained well, and monitored his blood glucose which never rose above 12.0 mmol/L. He was also noted to be requiring small doses of insulin and have persistent glycosuria despite blood glucose levels in the normal range. A C-peptide level was checked and was found to be positive. Following this, a GAD (glutamic acid

Table 2.2 Classification of MODY (maturity onset diabetes of the young).

MODY type	Monogenic cause	Complications and features
MODY-1	HNF-4α	Diabetes deteriorates. Complications as common as with T2DM
MODY-2	Glucokinase defect (heterozygotic)	About 20% of all MODY. Mild hyperglycaemia. Non-progressive form of diabetes. Complications mild or none
MODY-3	HNF-1α	About 60% of all MODY. Commonest of the MODY gene defects. Responds well to low-dose sulphonylurea
MODY-4	IPF-1	Very rare
MODY-5	HNF-1β	May present with renal disease
MODY-x	Monogenic, but target unidentified	Not known

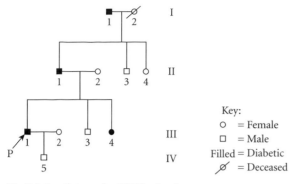

Key:
○ = Female
□ = Male
Filled = Diabetic
⌀ = Deceased

Fig. 2.4 Family tree of an HNF1α family.

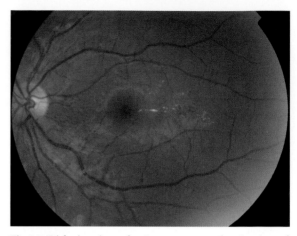

Fig. 2.5 Diabetic retinopathy. A young woman showing signs of maculopathy developing and reflections.

decarboxylase) antibody level was checked and found to be negative. At this point he was investigated for a genetic aetiology and found to have the P291fsinsC mutation of HNF1α. He was commenced on a low dose of gliclazide 40 mg once daily and his insulin therapy was stopped. He responded very well to this dosage with excellent glycaemic control. He has continued on this medication since, although requiring increased dosage, and his HbA1c remains at 6.5%. His family members with diabetes have undergone a genetic test for the specific HNF1α mutation and are all mutation positive. All except his grandfather have been switched to gliclazide therapy and their insulin stopped.

Secondary diabetes

Secondary diabetes occurs as a result of trauma to the pancreas (surgery, pancreatitis, obstruction) or from the exposure of the body to agents that may affect beta-cell function (major tranquillizers, beta-blockers, thiazide diuretics) or induce insulin resistance (steroids). There are hormone diseases associated with secondary diabetes – Cushing's disease, acromegaly, phaeochromocytoma – where the secretory product induces insulin resistance. Beta-cell failure can be caused by haemochromatosis and by tropical calcific disease. Secondary diabetes may often need insulin treatment, and the incidence of complications is essentially the same as for type 1 and type 2 diabetes.

TISSUE COMPLICATIONS OF DIABETES

The tissue complications of diabetes are divided into macrovascular (cardiac, cerebrovascular and peripheral vascular) and microvascular (retinopathy, neuropathy and nephropathy). The complications tend to occur together for the obvious reason that processes affecting small vessels in the eye are likely to be affecting small vessels in the nerves and kidney as well. Retinopathy is often the easiest complication to detect because the smallest of lesions (microaneurysms) can be visualized long before any change to the subjective function of the eye would be apparent. Retinopathy tracks closely with nephropathy, and so careful screening of renal function needs to be carried out in those who have retinopathy and vice versa.

Pregnancy can sometimes accelerate retinopathy for reasons that are unclear. Because there is no clear way of distinguishing those who may have fast-developing changes it is recommended that careful initial and subsequent screening is carried out during pregnancy (Fig. 2.5).

RISK FACTORS FOR DIABETIC RETINOPATHY

Modifiable risk factors

Blood glucose
In 1976, Cahill[5] wrote that the weight of evidence strongly supports the concept that the microvascular complications of diabetes are decreased by reduction of glucose concentrations. In 1981, Hyman[6] recommended a nationally coordinated clinical study of sufficient duration to resolve the issue. Evidence for the link between poor glucose control and greater progression of diabetic retinopathy (DR) was provided by Frank,[7] Dahl-Jorgensen,[8] Brinchmann-Hansen,[9] Joner,[10] Klein,[11–13] Goldstein,[14] Danne,[15] Davis[16] and Fong.[17]

The study that changed opinion and confirmed that intensive blood glucose control reduces the risk of new-onset DR and slows the progression of existing DR for patients with IDDM was the Diabetes Control and Complications Trial (DCCT).[18–22] The trial included 1441 people with type 1 diabetes, 726 with no DR at baseline (the primary prevention cohort) and 715 with mild retinopathy (the secondary intervention cohort), with mean follow-up of 6.5 years. For the primary prevention cohort, intensive therapy reduced the mean risk for the development of DR by 76% (95% CI), compared with conventional therapy. For the secondary intervention cohort, intensive therapy slowed the progression of DR by 54% (95% CI) and reduced the development of proliferative diabetic retinopathy (PDR) or severe non-proliferative diabetic retinopathy (NPDR) by 47% (95% CI).

The equivalent study for patients with type 2 diabetes was the United Kingdom Prospective Diabetes Study (UKPDS).[23–25] This study recruited 5012 people with type 2 diabetes, and the effect of intensive blood glucose control with sulphonylureas or insulin was compared with conventional treatment. Compared with the conventional group, there was a 25% risk reduction in the intensive group (95% CI 7–40%, p = 0.0099) in microvascular endpoints, including the need for retinal photocoagulation. Patients allocated metformin had risk reductions of 32% compared with the conventional group (95% CI 13–47%, p = 0.002) for any diabetes-related endpoint. Despite an early loss of glycaemic differences, a continued reduction in microvascular risk and emergent risk reductions for myocardial infarction and death from any cause were observed during 10 years of post-trial follow up.[26] A continued benefit after metformin therapy was evident among overweight patients.

CASE HISTORY 4
Improving glycaemic control

A 43-year-old woman who had had type 1 diabetes since the age of 26 years (when she was started on insulin during her third pregnancy), began insulin pump therapy. Before the pump therapy her HbA1c results had been 9.3% and 8.6%, her BMI 76.8 kg/m^2 and her blood pressure 164/98 mmHg. Figure 2.6(a) shows a photograph taken 6 months after she started insulin pump therapy.

Over the next 3 years her HBA1c improved gradually to readings of 6.9% and 7.1% and her blood pressure improved to 145/75 mmHg with increased antihypertensive medication.

She was then on approximately 50 units humalog per

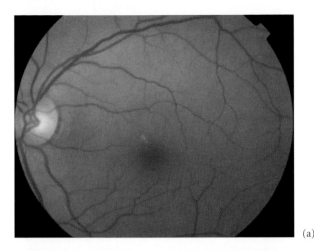
(a)

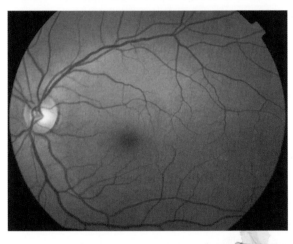
(b)

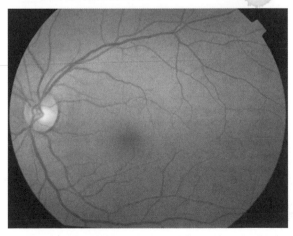
(c)

Fig. 2.6 Case history 4. (a) Exudates in left macular area. (b) Clearing of exudates in macular area. (c) Red free photograph showing clearing of exudates in left macular area.

day. The pump delivered 30 units over 24 hours, and the rest was given as a bolus dependent on carbohydrate intake or exercise. She determined the bolus amount herself, calculating 1 unit for every 8 g of carbohydrate.

Subsequent photographs showed a clearing of the exudates in her macular area (Fig. 2.6b,c).

Blood pressure

Control of systemic hypertension has been shown to reduce the risk of new-onset DR and slow the progression of existing DR in studies reported by Chase,[27] Joner,[10] Klein,[11] UKPDS,[25] Stratton,[28] Estacio[29] and Matthews[30]. In the early 1990s, Chase[27] and Joner[10] demonstrated in young subjects with type 1 diabetes that elevation in diastolic blood pressure, both alone and in combination with elevated systolic blood pressure, and higher mean arterial blood pressure correlated with the presence of retinopathy and progression of pre-existing retinopathy.

The UKPDS[25,30] described the effect of tight blood pressure control on the risk of microvascular complications in type 2 diabetes. After 7.5 years of follow-up the group assigned to tight blood pressure control had a 34% relative risk reduction (99% CI 11%–50% p = 0.0004) compared with the less tight blood pressure control group, using two step ETDRS graded retinopathy deterioration as the event marker. There was also a reduced risk of 37% (99% CI 8%–58%) over 9 years of visual deterioration in the tight vs less tight control groups as assessed by deterioration in visual acuity by three lines of the early treatment of diabetic retinopathy study (ETDRS) chart (Fig. 2.7).

Lipid levels

Evidence that elevated serum lipids are associated with macular exudates and that moderate visual loss and partial regression of hard exudates may be possible by reducing elevated lipid levels comes from studies reported by Chew,[31] Fong,[17] Klein,[32] Sen,[33] Cusick[34] and Lyons[35].

In 1996 Chew[31] reported an association of elevated serum lipid levels with retinal hard exudates in diabetic patients from the ETDRS and Fong[17] later reported that patients with persistent severe visual loss in the ETDRS had higher levels of cholesterol (244.1 vs. 228.5 mg/dL, p = 0.0081) at baseline. Sen[33] and Cusick[34] described the regression of retinal hard exudates in patients with diabetic maculopathy after correction of dyslipidaemia. In 2004, Lyons[35] demonstrated in the Diabetes Control and Complications Trial/Epidemiology of Diabetes Interventions and Complications Study cohort new associations between serum lipoproteins and severity of retinopathy in type 1 diabetes (Fig. 2.8).

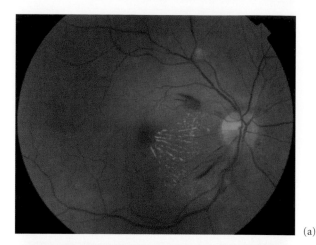

(a)

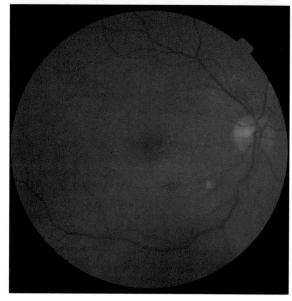

(b)

Fig. 2.7 (a) Uncontrolled hypertension in a person with diabetes. Right macular colour photograph showing flame haemorrhages, cotton wool spots and exudate encroaching in the right macular area. (b) Improvement in right macular appearance following control of blood pressure.

Smoking

There is some evidence that smoking may be a risk factor in progression of diabetic retinopathy in type 1 diabetes as described by Muhlhauser[36,37] and Karamanos.[38] However, in type 2 disease the evidence is controversial and smoking may protect[22] against the progression of retinopathy in some patients despite the fact that it is an independent risk factor for cardiovascular disease in all patients with diabetes.

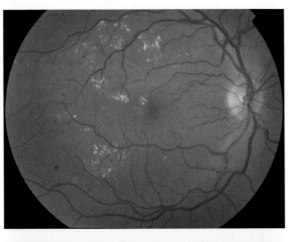

(a)

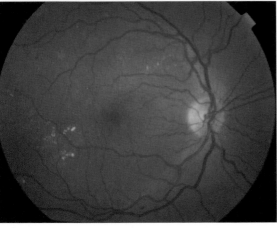

(b)

Fig. 2.8 (a) Macular exudates in diabetic retinopathy before treatment. (b) Macular exudates in diabetic retinopathy after treatment with laser treatment and a statin.

Non-modifiable risk factors

Duration

Among the non-modifiable risk factors, the major determinant of progression of diabetic retinopathy is duration of diabetes. This has been demonstrated in studies by Palmberg,[39] Frank,[7] Klein,[13,40–46] Burger,[47] Kohner,[48] Orchard,[49] ETDRS,[50,51] Goldstein,[14] McNally,[52] UKPDS,[28,53] Vitale,[54] d'Annunzio,[55] Donaghue,[56,57] Kernell,[58] Vitale,[59] Danne,[60] Davis,[16] Henricsson,[61] Ling,[62] Liu,[63] and Younis.[64,65]

In 1981, Palmberg[39] investigated a group of 461 people with juvenile-onset type 1 diabetes: at diagnosis no DR was identified, at 7 years 50% were found to have DR, and at 17–50 years 90% were found to have DR. PDR was first seen at 13 years, and 26% were found to have PDR at 26–50 years. In the Wisconsin Epidemiological Study of Diabetic Retinopathy (WESDR), Klein[40,41] demonstrated in 1984 that in 996 subjects with younger-onset type 1 diabetes any DR was found in 17% when their diabetes was of less than 5 years' duration, while those with diabetes of at least 15 years' duration had a prevalence of 97.5%. Proliferative DR was found in 1.2% of those with less than 10 years' duration and 67% of those with at least 35 years' duration.

In 1986, Burger[47] studied 231 people with juvenile-onset IDDM in the Berlin retinopathy study who had 1–6 examinations with fluorescein angiography over 5 years: 47% developed retinal changes, half of which were classified as minimal (<5 microaneurysms). The median individual risk for development of early DR was 9.1 years of diabetes duration.

In 1989 Klein[44,45] reported that in 271 people with type 1 diabetes diagnosed aged ≤30 years with no DR observed at the first visit, 59% developed DR after 4 years. Of 713 people with no proliferative DR at first visit, 11% developed proliferative DR after 4 years. Worsening of DR occurred in 41% and improvement in only 7%. The incidence of proliferative DR rose to 14% after 13 years of diabetes.

Of 154 people with type 1 diabetes diagnosed at ≥30 years with no DR at first visit, 47% developed DR after 4 years. Of 418 with no proliferative DR at first visit, 7% developed proliferative DR after 4 years and worsening of DR in 34%.

Of 320 people with type 2 diabetes diagnosed at ≥30 years with no DR at first visit, 34% developed DR after 4 years. Of 486 with no proliferative DR at first visit, 2% developed proliferative DR after 4 years and worsening of DR occurred in 25%.

Age

The Wisconsin Epidemiological Study[40,41,66] demonstrated that in those whose age of diagnosis was less than 30 years and who had diabetes of 10 years duration or less, the severity of retinopathy was related to older age at examination. When the age at diagnosis was 30 or more years, the severity of retinopathy was related to younger age at diagnosis. In those taking insulin divided by age group into those diagnosed before the age of 30 years, and those diagnoses at or beyond 30 years, the 10-year incidence of retinopathy was 89% and 79%, progression of retinopathy 76% and 69%, and progression to proliferative retinopathy 30% and 24%, respectively. In the UKPDS,[28] in those who already had retinopathy, progression was associated with older age.

Genetic predisposition

Diabetic retinopathy progresses from mild non-proliferative DR to proliferative DR and is considered to develop as a consequence of long duration of diabetes, poor glycaemic control, high blood pressure and several genetic factors. Early studies of identical twins with diabetes mellitus suggest familial clustering of diabetic retinopathy. An association between severity of diabetic retinopathy and HLA antigens has been suggested in a number of studies,[67–69] although this has not been uniformly accepted.[70] The Diabetes Control and Complications Trial (DCCT) suggested that, as well as environmental factors, the severity of diabetic retinopathy is influenced by familial factors, probably of genetic origin. Researchers have been searching for many years for the genes responsible for retinopathy. Generally, genes which encode factors involved in the pathogenesis of diabetic retinopathy are considered as candidates. For example, angiotensin I-converting enzyme,[71] nitric oxide synthase (NOS2A and NOS3),[72] vascular endothelial growth factor (VEGF),[73–76] pigmented epithelium-derived factor (PEDF), protein kinase C-beta (PKC-beta) and receptor for advanced glycation end products (RAGE)[77–80] have all been implicated in the pathogenesis of DR. The majority of candidate genes studied exhibit weak or no association with retinopathy status, and where associations have been detected these results have not been replicated in multiple populations.

Ethnicity

Emanuele[81] reported ethnicity, race and baseline retinopathy correlates in the veterans affairs diabetes trial, which has a cohort enriched with approximately 20% Hispanics and 20% African Americans. The prevalence of diabetic retinopathy scores greater than 40 was higher for Hispanics (36%) and African Americans (29%) than for non-Hispanic whites (22%). The differences between Hispanics and non-Hispanic whites and between African Americans and non-Hispanic whites were both significant (p < 0.05 in each case). These differences could not be accounted for by an imbalance in traditional risk factors such as age, duration of diagnosed diabetes, HbA1c, and blood pressure. Simmons[82] compared ethnic differences in the prevalence of diabetic retinopathy in European, Maori and Pacific peoples with diabetes in Auckland, New Zealand. They demonstrated that moderate or more severe retinopathy is more common in Polynesians than in Europeans and this difference could not be explained by differences in diabetes duration, insulin therapy, the extent of renal disease, blood pressure or glycaemic control.

PRACTICE POINTS

- Diabetic retinopathy is integrally linked to glycaemic control, blood pressure control, lipid levels and other non-modifiable risk factors such as duration of diabetes.
- It is very important to have good communication between the ophthalmologist, diabetologist and any other health professional looking after someone with diabetic microvascular complications.
- Some patients are diagnosed with type 2 diabetes when they present with sight-threatening diabetic retinopathy and have clearly had diabetes for many years without their knowledge.

REFERENCES

1 Gale EA. Declassifying diabetes. *Diabetologia* 2006; **49**(9): 1989–95.
2 Kohner EM, Aldington SJ, Stratton IM, Manley SE, Holman RR, Matthews DR et al. United Kingdom Prospective Diabetes Study, 30: diabetic retinopathy at diagnosis of non-insulin-dependent diabetes mellitus and associated risk factors. *Arch Ophthalmol* 1998; **116**(3): 297–303.
3 Molven A, Ringdal M, Nordbo AM, Raeder H, Stoy J, Lipkind GM et al. Mutations in the insulin gene can cause MODY and autoantibody-negative type 1 diabetes. *Diabetes* 2008; **57**(4): 1131–5.
4 Babenko AP, Polak M, Cave H, Busiah K, Czernichow P, Scharfmann R et al. Activating mutations in the ABCC8 gene in neonatal diabetes mellitus. *N Engl J Med* 2006; **355**(5): 456–66.
5 Cahill GF Jr, Etzwiler LD, Freinkel N. Editorial: 'Control' and diabetes. *N Engl J Med* 1976; **294**(18): 1004–5.
6 Hyman BN. The prevention of diabetic retinopathy. *Ophthalmology* 1981; **88**: 35A–37A.
7 Frank RN, Hoffman WH, Podgor MJ, Joondeph HC, Lewis RA, Margherio RR et al. Retinopathy in juvenile-onset type I diabetes of short duration. *Diabetes* 1982; **31**(10): 874–82.
8 Dahl-Jorgensen K, Brinchmann-Hansen O, Hanssen KF, Ganes T, Kierulf P, Smeland E et al. Effect of near normoglycaemia for two years on progression of early diabetic retinopathy, nephropathy, and neuropathy: the Oslo study. *BMJ* 1986; **293**(8 November 1986): 1195–9.
9 Brinchmann-Hansen O, Dahl-Jorgensen K, Sandvik L, Hanssen KF. Blood glucose concentrations and progression of diabetic retinopathy: the seven year results of the Oslo study. *BMJ* 1992; **304**(6818): 19–22.
10 Joner G, Brinchmann-Hansen O, Torres CG, Hanssen KF. A nationwide cross-sectional study of retinopathy and micro-albuminuria in young Norwegian type 1 (insulin-dependent) diabetic patients. *Diabetologia* 1992; **35**(11): 1049–54.
11 Klein R, Klein BE, Moss SE. Epidemiology of proliferative diabetic retinopathy. *Diabetes Care* 1992; **15**(12): 1875–91.

12 Klein R, Klein BE, Moss SE, Cruickshanks KJ. The Wisconsin Epidemiologic Study of Diabetic Retinopathy. XV. The long-term incidence of macular edema. *Ophthalmology* 1995; **102**(1): 7–16.

13 Klein R, Klein BE, Moss SE, Cruickshanks KJ. The Wisconsin Epidemiologic Study of Diabetic Retinopathy: XVII. The 14-year incidence and progression of diabetic retinopathy and associated risk factors in type 1 diabetes. *Ophthalmology* 1998; **105**(10): 1801–15.

14 Goldstein DE, Blinder KJ, Ide CH, Wilson RJ, Wiedmeyer HM, Little RR *et al.* Glycemic control and development of retinopathy in youth-onset insulin-dependent diabetes mellitus. Results of a 12-year longitudinal study. *Ophthalmology* 1993; **100**(8): 1125–31; discussion 1131–2.

15 Danne T, Weber B, Hartmann R, Enders I, Burger W, Hovener G. Long-term glycemic control has a nonlinear association to the frequency of background retinopathy in adolescents with diabetes. Follow-up of the Berlin Retinopathy Study. *Diabetes Care* 1994; **17**(12): 1390–6.

16 Davis MD, Fisher MR, Gangnon RE, Barton F, Aiello LM, Chew EY *et al.* Risk factors for high-risk proliferative diabetic retinopathy and severe visual loss: Early Treatment Diabetic Retinopathy Study Report #18. *Invest Ophthalmol Vis Sci* 1998; **39**(2): 233–52.

17 Fong DS, Ferris FL 3rd, Davis MD, Chew EY. Causes of severe visual loss in the early treatment diabetic retinopathy study: ETDRS report no. 24. Early Treatment Diabetic Retinopathy Study Research Group. *Am J Ophthalmol* 1999; **127**(2): 137–41.

18 The Diabetes Control and Complications Trial Research Group. The effect of intensive treatment of diabetes on the development and progression of long-term complications in insulin-dependent diabetes mellitus. *N Engl J Med* 1993; **329**(14): 977–86.

19 Diabetes Control and Complications Trial Research Group. Effect of intensive diabetes treatment on the development and progression of long-term complications in adolescents with insulin-dependent diabetes mellitus: Diabetes Control and Complications Trial. *J Pediatr* 1994; **125**(2): 177–88.

20 The Diabetes Control and Complications Trial. The effect of intensive diabetes treatment on the progression of diabetic retinopathy in insulin-dependent diabetes mellitus. *Arch Ophthalmol* 1995; **113**(1): 36–51.

21 Early worsening of diabetic retinopathy in the Diabetes Control and Complications Trial. *Arch Ophthalmol* 1998; **116**(7): 874–86.

22 The Diabetes Control and Complications Trial/ Epidemiology of Diabetes Interventions and Complications Research Group. Retinopathy and nephropathy in patients with type 1 diabetes four years after a trial of intensive therapy. *N Engl J Med* 2000; **342**(6): 381–9.

23 UK Prospective Diabetes Study (UKPDS) Group. Intensive blood-glucose control with sulphonylureas or insulin compared with conventional treatment and risk of complications in patients with type 2 diabetes (UKPDS 33). *Lancet* 1998; **352**(9131): 837–53.

24 UK Prospective Diabetes Study (UKPDS) Group. Effect of intensive blood-glucose control with metformin on complications in overweight patients with type 2 diabetes (UKPDS 34). *Lancet* 1998; **352**(9131): 854–65.

25 UK Prospective Diabetes Study (UKPDS) Group. Tight blood pressure control and risk of macrovascular and microvascular complications in type 2 diabetes: UKPDS 38. *BMJ* 1998; **317**(7160): 703–13.

26 Holman RR, Paul SK, Bethel MA, Matthews DR, Neil HA. 10-Year follow-up of intensive glucose control in Type 2 diabetes. *N Engl J Med*. 2008; Sep 10. [Epub ahead of print]

27 Chase HP, Garg SK, Jackson WE, Thomas MA, Harris S, Marshall G *et al.* Blood pressure and retinopathy in type I diabetes. *Ophthalmology* 1990; **97**(2): 155–9.

28 Stratton IM, Kohner EM, Aldington SJ, Turner RC, Holman RR, Manley SE *et al.* UKPDS 50: risk factors for incidence and progression of retinopathy in type II diabetes over 6 years from diagnosis. *Diabetologia* 2001; **44**(2): 156–63.

29 Estacio RO, Jeffers BW, Gifford N, Schrier RW. Effect of blood pressure control on diabetic microvascular complications in patients with hypertension and type 2 diabetes. *Diabetes Care* 2000; **23 Suppl 2**: B54–64.

30 Matthews DR, Stratton IM, Aldington SJ, Holman RR, Kohner EM. Risks of progression of retinopathy and vision loss related to tight blood pressure control in type 2 diabetes mellitus: UKPDS 69. *Arch Ophthalmol* 2004; **122**(11): 1631–40.

31 Chew EY, Klein ML, Ferris FL 3rd, Remaley NA, Murphy RP, Chantry K *et al.* Association of elevated serum lipid levels with retinal hard exudate in diabetic retinopathy. Early Treatment Diabetic Retinopathy Study (ETDRS) Report 22. *Arch Ophthalmol* 1996; **114**(9): 1079–84.

32 Klein R, Sharrett AR, Klein BE, Moss SE, Folsom AR, Wong TY *et al.* The association of atherosclerosis, vascular risk factors, and retinopathy in adults with diabetes : the atherosclerosis risk in communities study. *Ophthalmology* 2002; **109**(7): 1225–34.

33 Sen K, Misra A, Kumar A, Pandey RM. Simvastatin retards progression of retinopathy in diabetic patients with hypercholesterolemia. *Diabetes Res Clin Pract* 2002; **56**(1): 1–11.

34 Cusick M, Chew EY, Chan CC, Kruth HS, Murphy RP, Ferris FL 3rd. Histopathology and regression of retinal hard exudates in diabetic retinopathy after reduction of elevated serum lipid levels. *Ophthalmology* 2003; **110**(11): 2126–33.

35 Lyons TJ, Jenkins AJ, Zheng D, Lackland DT, McGee D, Garvey WT *et al.* Diabetic retinopathy and serum lipoprotein subclasses in the DCCT/EDIC cohort. *Invest Ophthalmol Vis Sci* 2004; **45**(3): 910–18.

36 Muhlhauser I. Cigarette smoking and diabetes: an update. *Diabet Med* 1994; **11**(4): 336–43.

37 Muhlhauser I, Bender R, Bott U, Jorgens V, Grusser M, Wagener W *et al.* Cigarette smoking and progression of

retinopathy and nephropathy in type 1 diabetes. *Diabet Med* 1996; **13**(6): 536–43.

38 Karamanos B, Porta M, Songini M, Metelko Z, Kerenyi Z, Tamas G *et al.* Different risk factors of microangiopathy in patients with type I diabetes mellitus of short versus long duration. The EURODIAB IDDM Complications Study. *Diabetologia* 2000; **43**(3): 348–55.

39 Palmberg P, Smith M, Waltman S, Krupin T, Singer P, Burgess D *et al.* The natural history of retinopathy in insulin-dependent juvenile-onset diabetes. *Ophthalmology* 1981; **88**(7): 613–18.

40 Klein R, Klein BE, Moss SE, Davis MD, DeMets DL. The Wisconsin epidemiologic study of diabetic retinopathy. II. Prevalence and risk of diabetic retinopathy when age at diagnosis is less than 30 years. *Arch Ophthalmol* 1984; **102**(4): 520–6.

41 Klein R, Klein BE, Moss SE, Davis MD, DeMets DL. The Wisconsin epidemiologic study of diabetic retinopathy. III. Prevalence and risk of diabetic retinopathy when age at diagnosis is 30 or more years. *Arch Ophthalmol* 1984; **102**(4): 527–32.

42 Klein R, Klein BE, Moss SE, Davis MD, DeMets DL. Retinopathy in young-onset diabetic patients. *Diabetes Care* 1985; **8**(4): 311–15.

43 Klein R, Klein BE, Moss SE, Davis MD, DeMets DL. The Wisconsin Epidemiologic Study of Diabetic Retinopathy. VII. Diabetic nonproliferative retinal lesions. *Ophthalmology* 1987; **94**(11): 1389–400.

44 Klein R, Klein BE, Moss SE, Davis MD, DeMets DL. The Wisconsin Epidemiologic Study of Diabetic Retinopathy. IX. Four-year incidence and progression of diabetic retinopathy when age at diagnosis is less than 30 years. *Arch Ophthalmol* 1989; **107**(2): 237–43.

45 Klein R, Klein BE, Moss SE, Davis MD, DeMets DL. The Wisconsin Epidemiologic Study of Diabetic Retinopathy. X. Four-year incidence and progression of diabetic retinopathy when age at diagnosis is 30 years or more. *Arch Ophthalmol* 1989; **107**(2): 244–9.

46 Klein R, Meuer SM, Moss SE, Klein BE. Retinal microaneurysm counts and 10-year progression of diabetic retinopathy. *Arch Ophthalmol* 1995; **113**(11): 1386–91.

47 Burger W, Hovener G, Dusterhus R, Hartmann R, Weber B. Prevalence and development of retinopathy in children and adolescents with type 1 (insulin-dependent) diabetes mellitus. A longitudinal study. *Diabetologia* 1986; **29**(1): 17–22.

48 Kohner EM, Sleightholm M. Does microaneurysm count reflect severity of early diabetic retinopathy? *Ophthalmology* 1986; **93**(5): 586–9.

49 Orchard TJ, Dorman JS, Maser RE, Becker DJ, Drash AL, Ellis D *et al.* Prevalence of complications in IDDM by sex and duration. Pittsburgh Epidemiology of Diabetes Complications Study II. *Diabetes* 1990; **39**(9): 1116–24.

50 Early Treatment Diabetic Retinopathy Study Research Group. Fundus photographic risk factors for progression of diabetic retinopathy. ETDRS report number 12. *Ophthalmology* 1991; **98**(5 Suppl): 823–33.

51 Early Treatment Diabetic Retinopathy Study design and baseline patient characteristics. ETDRS report number 7. *Ophthalmology* 1991; **98**(5 Suppl): 741–56.

52 McNally PG, Raymond NT, Swift PG, Hearnshaw JR, Burden AC. Does the prepubertal duration of diabetes influence the onset of microvascular complications? *Diabet Med* 1993; **10**(10): 906–8.

53 Aldington SJ, Stratton IM, Matthews DR, Kohner EM. Relationship of retinal microaneurysm count to progression of retinopathy over 3 and 6 years in non-insulin dependent diabetes. *Diabetic Med* 1995; **12**(Suppl 1): 3.

54 Vitale S, Maguire MG, Murphy RP, Hiner CJ, Rourke L, Sackett C *et al.* Clinically significant macular edema in type I diabetes. Incidence and risk factors. *Ophthalmology* 1995; **102**(8): 1170–6.

55 d'Annunzio G, Malvezzi F, Vitali L, Barone C, Giacchero R, Klersy C *et al.* A 3–19-year follow-up study on diabetic retinopathy in patients diagnosed in childhood and treated with conventional therapy. *Diabet Med* 1997; **14**(11): 951–8.

56 Donaghue KC, Fung AT, Hing S, Fairchild J, King J, Chan A *et al.* The effect of prepubertal diabetes duration on diabetes. Microvascular complications in early and late adolescence. *Diabetes Care* 1997; **20**(1): 77–80.

57 Donaghue KC, Fairchild JM, Chan A, Hing SJ, King J, Howard NJ *et al.* Diabetes microvascular complications in prepubertal children. *J Pediatr Endocrinol Metab* 1997; **10**(6): 579–85.

58 Kernell A, Dedorsson I, Johansson B, Wickstrom CP, Ludvigsson J, Tuvemo T *et al.* Prevalence of diabetic retinopathy in children and adolescents with IDDM. A population-based multicentre study. *Diabetologia* 1997; **40**(3): 307–10.

59 Vitale S, Maguire MG, Murphy RP, Hiner C, Rourke L, Sackett C *et al.* Interval between onset of mild nonproliferative and proliferative retinopathy in type I diabetes. *Arch Ophthalmol* 1997; **115**(2): 194–8.

60 Danne T, Kordonouri O, Enders I, Hovener G. Monitoring for retinopathy in children and adolescents with type 1 diabetes. *Acta Paediatr Suppl* 1998; **425**: 35–41.

61 Henricsson M, Berntorp K, Fernlund P, Sundkvist G. Progression of retinopathy in insulin-treated type 2 diabetic patients. *Diabetes Care* 2002; **25**(2): 381–5.

62 Ling R, Ramsewak V, Taylor D, Jacob J. Longitudinal study of a cohort of people with diabetes screened by the Exeter Diabetic Retinopathy Screening Programme. *Eye* 2002; **16**(2): 140–5.

63 Liu WJ, Lee LT, Yen MF, Tung TH, Williams R, Duffy SW *et al.* Assessing progression and efficacy of treatment for diabetic retinopathy following the proliferative pathway to blindness: implication for diabetic retinopathy screening in Taiwan. *Diabet Med* 2003; **20**(9): 727–33.

64 Younis N, Broadbent DM, Harding SP, Vora JP. Incidence of sight-threatening retinopathy in type 1 diabetes in a systematic screening programme. *Diabet Med* 2003; **20**(9): 758–65.

65 Younis N, Broadbent DM, Vora JP, Harding SP. Incidence of sight-threatening retinopathy in patients with type 2 diabetes in the Liverpool Diabetic Eye Study: a cohort study. *Lancet* 2003; **361**(9353): 195–200.

66 Klein R, Klein BE, Moss SE, Cruickshanks KJ. The Wisconsin Epidemiologic Study of diabetic retinopathy. XIV. Ten-year incidence and progression of diabetic retinopathy. *Arch Ophthalmol* 1994; **112**(9): 1217–28.

67 Birinci A, Birinci H, Abidinoglu R, Durupinar B, Oge I. Diabetic retinopathy and HLA antigens in type 2 diabetes mellitus. *Eur J Ophthalmol* 2002; **12**(2): 89–93.

68 Mimura T, Funatsu H, Uchigata Y, Kitano S, Shimizu E, Amano S *et al.* Glutamic acid decarboxylase autoantibody prevalence and association with HLA genotype in patients with younger-onset type 1 diabetes and proliferative diabetic retinopathy. *Ophthalmology* 2005; **112**(11): 1904–9.

69 Dornan TL, Ting A, McPherson CK, Peckar CO, Mann JI, Turner RC *et al.* Genetic susceptibility to the development of retinopathy in insulin-dependent diabetics. *Diabetes* 1982; **31**(3): 226–31.

70 Wong TY, Cruickshank KJ, Klein R, Klein BE, Moss SE, Palta M *et al.* HLA-DR3 and DR4 and their relation to the incidence and progression of diabetic retinopathy. *Ophthalmology* 2002; **109**(2): 275–81.

71 Matsumoto A, Iwashima Y, Abiko A, Morikawa A, Sekiguchi M, Eto M *et al.* Detection of the association between a deletion polymorphism in the gene encoding angiotensin I-converting enzyme and advanced diabetic retinopathy. *Diabetes Res Clin Pract* 2000; **50**(3): 195–202.

72 Kumaramanickavel G, Sripriya S, Vellanki RN, Upadyay NK, Badrinath SS, Rajendran V *et al.* Inducible nitric oxide synthase gene and diabetic retinopathy in Asian Indian patients. *Clin Genet* 2002; **61**(5): 344–8.

73 Awata T, Inoue K, Kurihara S, Ohkubo T, Watanabe M, Inukai K *et al.* A common polymorphism in the 5′-untranslated region of the VEGF gene is associated with diabetic retinopathy in type 2 diabetes. *Diabetes* 2002; **51**(5): 1635–9.

74 Ideno J, Mizukami H, Kakehashi A, Saito Y, Okada T, Kume A *et al.* 187. Adeno-associated virus vector-mediated soluble flt-1 gene transfer prevents diabetic retinopathy in spontaneously diabetic rat model. *Molecular Therapy* 2004; **9**(Suppl 1): 72.

75 Ray D, Mishra M, Ralph S, Read I, Davies R, Brenchley P. Association of the VEGF gene with proliferative diabetic retinopathy but not proteinuria in diabetes. *Diabetes* 2004; **53**(3): 861–4.

76 Zhang SX, Ma JX, Sima J, Chen Y, Hu MS, Ottlecz A *et al.* Genetic difference in susceptibility to the blood–retina barrier breakdown in diabetes and oxygen-induced retinopathy. *Am J Pathol* 2005; **166**(1): 313–21.

77 Hudson BI, Stickland MH, Futers TS, Grant PJ. Effects of novel polymorphisms in the RAGE gene on transcriptional regulation and their association with diabetic retinopathy. *Diabetes* 2001; **50**(6): 1505–11.

78 Petrovic GM, Steblovnik K, Peterlin B, Petrovic D. The - 429 T/C and - 374 T/A gene polymorphisms of the receptor of advanced glycation end products gene are not risk factors for diabetic retinopathy in Caucasians with type 2 diabetes. *Klin Monatsbl Augenheilkd* 2003; **220**(12): 873–6.

79 Kashiwagi A, Araki S. Relation between polymorphisms G1704T and G82S of RAGE gene and diabetic retinopathy in Japanese type 2 diabetic patients. *Intern Med* 2005; **44**(5): 397–8.

80 Yoshioka K, Yoshida T, Takakura Y, Umekawa T, Kogure A, Toda H *et al.* Relation between polymorphisms G1704T and G82S of rage gene and diabetic retinopathy in Japanese type 2 diabetic patients. *Intern Med* 2005; **44**(5): 417–21.

81 Emanuele N, Sacks J, Klein R, Reda D, Anderson R, Duckworth W *et al.* Ethnicity, race, and baseline retinopathy correlates in the veterans affairs diabetes trial. *Diabetes Care* 2005; **28**(8): 1954–8.

82 Simmons D, Clover G, Hope C. Ethnic differences in diabetic retinopathy. *Diabet Med* 2007; **24**(10): 1093–8.

3 Lesions and classifications of diabetic retinopathy

Peter H. Scanlon

Diabetic retinopathy refers to pathology of the capillaries, arterioles and venules in the retina and the subsequent effects of leakage from or occlusion of the small vessels.

Diabetes can affect larger blood vessels of the head and neck and of the retina, but pathology of the larger blood vessels does not come under the classification of diabetic retinopathy. Changes that occur within the retinal capillary wall include:

1 thickening of the basement membrane
2 pericyte loss
3 epithelial cell dysfunction (loss of epithelial tight junctions)
4 loss of endothelial cells.

ETDRS CLASSIFICATION

The Early Treatment Diabetic Retinopathy Study[1,2] (ETDRS) classified a number of lesions of diabetic retinopathy and described the progression of diabetic retinopathy in relation to the development of these lesions (Tables 3.1 & 3.2).

The lesions that the ETDRS described as critical to the stages of progression of diabetic retinopathy were as follows.

1 Microaneurysms.
2 Small retinal haemorrhages.
3 HMa (haemorrhage/microaneurysm).
4 Other larger retinal haemorrhages:
 • flame haemorrhages
 • blot haemorrhages
5 Hard exudates (sometimes now just referred to as exudates).
6 Cotton wool spots (referred to as soft exudates or SE in the ETDRS but this term is now rarely used).

A Practical Manual of Diabetic Retinopathy Management.
Peter H Scanlon, Charles P Wilkinson, Stephen J Aldington and David R Matthews. Published 2009 by Blackwell Publishing, ISBN 978-1-4051-7035-2.

7 Intraretinal microvascular abnormality.
8 Venous abnormalities:
 • venous loops
 • venous reduplication
 • venous beading (VB)
 • venous dilation
 • venous narrowing
 • opacification of the venous wall
 • perivenous exudate.
9 Arteriolar abnormalities:
 • arteriolar narrowing
 • opacification of arteriolar walls ('sheathing and white threads')
 • arteriovenous nipping – this is often a feature of hypertension that is associated with diabetes.
10 Fibrous proliferation at the disc (FPD).
11 Fibrous proliferation elsewhere (FPE).
12 New vessels on disc (NVD).
13 New vessels elsewhere (NVE).
14 Vitreous haemorrhage (VH).
15 Preretinal haemorrhage (PRH).
16 Post-laser treatment – laser scars.

Microaneurysms, small retinal haemorrhages and HMa

The ETDRS defined microaneurysm and haemorrhage as follows.

1 A microaneurysm is defined as a red spot <125 microns (approx width of vein at disc margin) with sharp margins.
2 Haemorrhage is defined as a red spot, which has irregular margins and/or uneven density, particularly when surrounding a smaller central lesion considered to be a microaneurysm. If a red lesion is >125 microns in its longest dimension it is usually a haemorrhage unless features such as round shape, smooth margins and a central light reflex suggest it is possibly a microaneurysm.

Table 3.1 ETDRS diabetic retinopathy classification of progression to proliferative diabetic retinopathy (PDR) based on $7 \times 30°$ field stereo photographs of each eye.

ETDRS final retinopathy severity scale[3]	ETDRS (final) grade	Lesions	Risk of progression to PDR in 1 year (ETDRS interim)	Practical clinic follow-up intervals (not ETDRS)
No apparent retinopathy	10 14, 15	DR absent DR questionable		1 year
Mild NPDR	20	Microaneurysms only		1 year
	35 a b c d e	One or more of the following: venous loops ≥definite in 1 field SE, IRMA, or VB questionable retinal haemorrhages present HE ≥definite in 1 field SE ≥definite in 1 field	Level 30 = 6.2%	6–12 months
Moderate NPDR	43a b	HMa moderate in 4–5 fields or severe in 1 field or IRMA definite in 1–3 fields	Level 41 = 11.3%	6 months
Moderately severe NPDR	47 a b c d	Both level 43 characteristics: HMa moderate in 4–5 fields or severe in 1 field and IRMA definite in 1–3 fields **or** any one of the following: IRMA in 4–5 fields HMa severe in 2–3 fields VB definite in 1 field	Level 45 = 20.7%	4 months
Severe NPDR	53 a b c d	One or more of the following: ≥2 of the three level 47 characteristics HMa severe in 4–5 fields IRMA ≥moderate in 1 field VB ≥definite in 2–3 fields	Level 51 = 44.2% Level 55 = 54.8%	3 months
Mild PDR	61a b	FPD or FPE present with NVD absent or NVE = definite	1976. Diabetic Retinopathy Study[4] Protocol changed to treat untreated eyes with high risk characteristics	
Moderate PDR	65a b	**1** NVE ≥moderate in 1 field or definite NVD with VH and PRH absent or questionable or **2** VH or PRH definite and NVE <moderate in 1 field and NVD absent	1981. Diabetic Retinopathy Study[5] recommendation to treat eyes with new vessels on or within 1 DD of the optic disc (NVD) ≥0.25–0.33 disc area, even	
High risk PDR	71 a b c d	Any of the following: **3** VH or PRH ≥moderate in 1 field **4** NVE ≥moderate in 1 field and VH or PRH definite in 1 field **5** NVD = 2 and VH or PRH definite in 1 field **6** NVD ≥moderate	in the absence of preretinal or vitreous haemorrhage. Photocoagulation, as used in the study, reduced the risk of severe visual loss by 50% or more.	
High risk PDR	75	NVD ≥moderate and definite VH or PRH		
Advanced PDR	81	Retina obscured due to VH or PRH		

Table 3.2 ETDRS maculopathy classification.

Early Treatment Diabetic Retinopathy Study	Outcome
Clinically significant macular oedema[6] as defined by:	
A zone or zones of retinal thickening one disc area or larger, any part of which is within one disc diameter of the centre of the macula	Consider laser
Retinal thickening at or within 500 microns of the centre of the macula	Consider laser
Hard exudates at or within 500 microns of the centre of the macula, if associated with thickening of the adjacent retina (not residual hard exudates remaining after disappearance of retinal thickening)	Consider laser

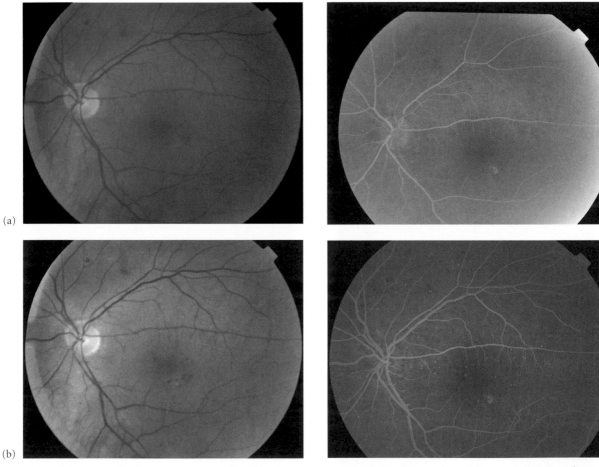

(a)

(b)

(c)

(d)

Fig. 3.1 (a) An example of microaneurysms and small haems. (b) The same example: red-free image. (c) The same example: fluorescein at 24 s and (d) at 32 s showing early fluorescence but no leakage at this stage and one old laser scar. (*Continued on facing page*)

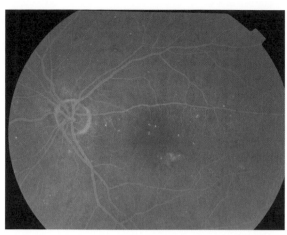

(e)

Fig. 3.1 (*Cont'd*) (e) The same example: fluorescein at 3 min 59 s showing leakage from some of the microaneurysms as shown by a fluffy fluorescence appearing around the microaneurysm.

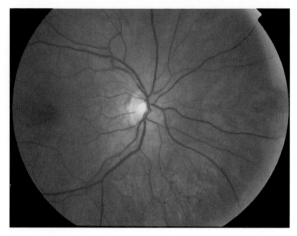

Fig. 3.3 HMas. Differentiation from microaneurysms is more difficult when fluorescein is not available.

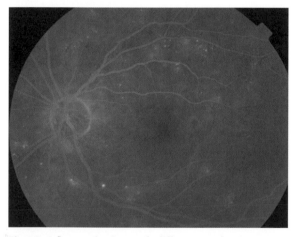

Fig. 3.2 A fluorescein picture of a different macular view showing the microaneurysms fluorescing and small haemorrhages not fluorescing.

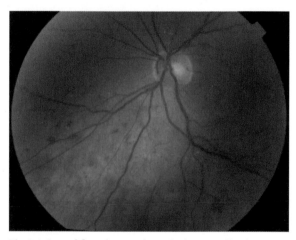

Fig. 3.4 Several flame haemorrhages in the nerve fibre layer.

3 Because the ETDRS recognized that it was very difficult to differentiate between microaneurysms and small haemorrhages, the concept of HMa was introduced, which is a small haemorrhage or microaneurysm (Figs 3.1–3.3).

Other larger retinal haemorrhages (Fig. 3.4)

Flame haemorrhages

Flame haemorrhages are superficial haemorrhages just under the nerve fibre layer that can be seen in relatively mild forms of diabetic retinopathy and are also seen in systemic hypertension.

Blot haemorrhages (Fig. 3.5)

Blot haemorrhages are deeper haemorrhages, which are a sign of retinal ischaemia in the area of the retina in which they occur and hence large numbers of blot haemorrhages are associated with significant retinal ischaemia.

Hard exudates (sometimes now just referred to as exudates) (Fig. 3.6)

The ETDRS defined hard exudates (HEs) as small white or yellowish-white deposits with sharp margins, located typically in the outer layers of the retina, but they may

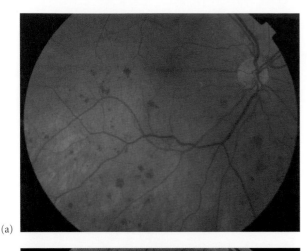

(a)

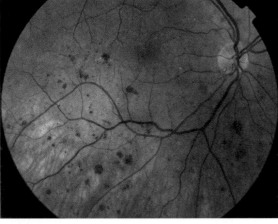

(b)

Fig. 3.5 (a) Blot haemorrhages in the right inferotemporal retina and a small patch of NVE. (b) Red-free photograph of the same patient with blot haemorrhages and small NVE.

be more superficial, particularly when retinal oedema is present.

Hard exudate rings were defined in the ETDRS according to whether 10%, 50% or 90% or more HEs present were part of a ring.

Cotton wool spots (referred to as soft exudates in the ETDRS but this term is now rarely used) (Fig. 3.7)

These are fluffy white opaque areas caused by an accumulation of axoplasm in the nerve fibre layer of the retina. This is caused by an arteriolar occlusion in that area of retina, which is apparent on a fluorescein angiogram.

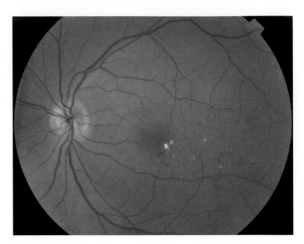

Fig. 3.6 (Hard) exudates encroaching on the central fovea.

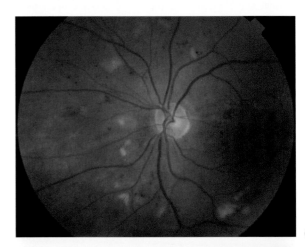

(a)

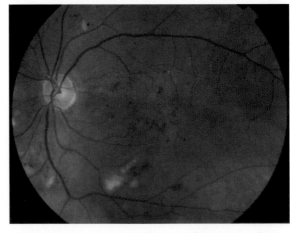

(b)

Fig. 3.7 Cotton wool spots (CWS): (a) in the nasal view; (b) in the macular view of the same patient. (*Continued on facing page*)

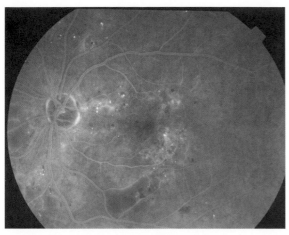

(c)

Fig. 3.7 (*Cont'd*) (c) Fluorescein of the same patient's macular view showing ischaemia in the areas of CWS.

Haemorrhages and intraretinal microvascular abnormalities are often seen in the retina adjacent to a cotton wool spot.

Intraretinal microvascular abnormality (IRMA) (Fig. 3.8)

Intraretinal microvascular abnormalities are defined as tortuous intraretinal vascular segments varying in calibre. By definition, intraretinal microvascular abnormalities are not on the surface of the retina and do not break through the internal limiting membrane.

Intraretinal microvascular abnormalities are derived from remodelling of the retinal capillaries and small collateral vessels in areas of microvascular occlusion. They are usually found on the borders of areas of non-perfused retina. They are, therefore, a sign of retinal ischaemia.

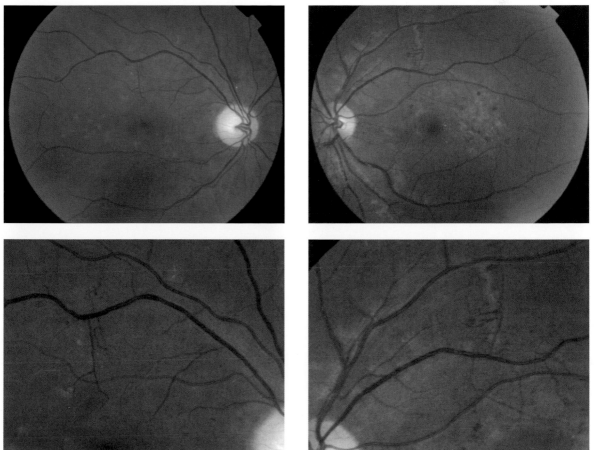

(a)

(b)

(c)

(d)

Fig. 3.8 IRMA: (a) colour photograph; (b) enlarged red-free photograph of area of IRMA in part (a); (c) colour photograph; (d) enlarged red-free photograph of area of IRMA in part (c).

Venous abnormalities

Venous loops and/or reduplication (Fig. 3.9)

In the ETDRS the definitions were as follows.

- Venous loop is an abrupt curving deviation of a vein from its normal path.
- Reduplication is dilation of a prexisting channel or proliferation of a new channel adjacent to and approxi-

mately the same calibre as the original vein (Figs 3.10 & 3.11).

Venous beading

In the ETDRS venous beading was described as a localized increase in calibre of the vein and the severity was dependent on the increase in calibre and the length of vein involved (Fig. 3.12).

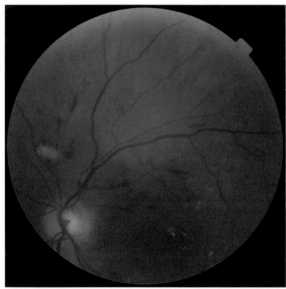

(a)

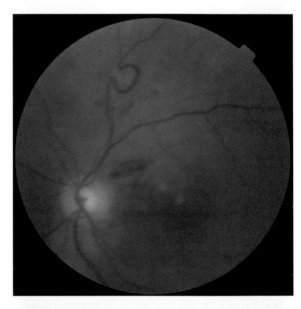

(c)

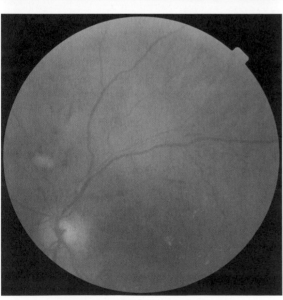

(b)

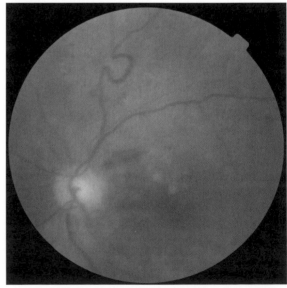

(d)

Fig. 3.9 An example of a venous loop developing: (a) year 1 colour photograph superior retina; (b) year 1 red-free photograph superior retina; (c) year 3 colour photograph superior retina; (d) year 3 red-free photograph superior retina; (*Continued on facing page*)

(e)

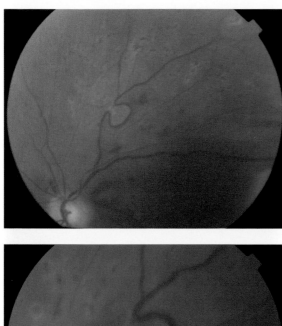

(f)

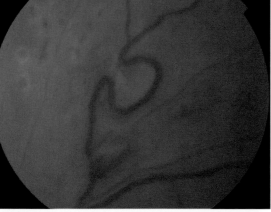

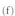(g)

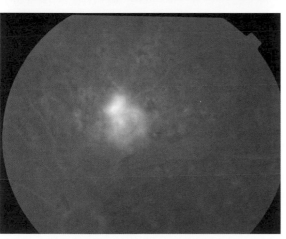

Fig. 3.9 (*Cont'd*) (e) year 4 colour photograph superior retina; (f) year 4 enlarged colour photograph superior retina; (g) fluorescein leak from the venous loop.

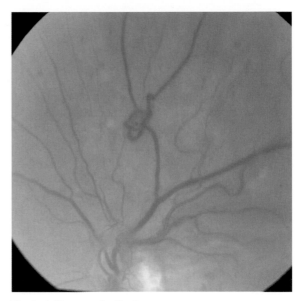

Fig. 3.10 Venous reduplication.

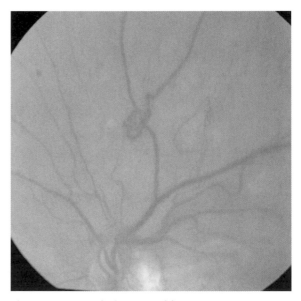

Fig. 3.11 Venous reduplication: red free.

Venous beading was found to be associated with retinal ischaemia. It is used for assessment of severity of diabetic retinopathy and response to laser treatment as venous dilation and beading do respond to scatter laser treatment.

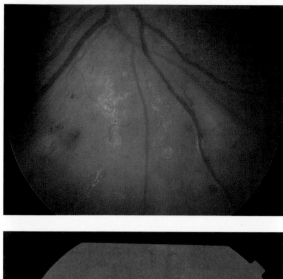

(a)

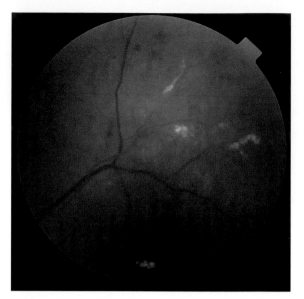

Fig. 3.13 Venous narrowing and perivenous exudate.

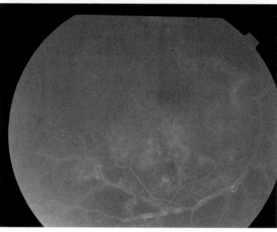

(b)

Fig. 3.12 (a) Venous dilation, venous beading and IRMA in an area of ischaemic retina. (b) Venous beading adjacent to an area of ischaemic retina in this fluorescein angiogram.

Other venous changes that occur in diabetic retinopathy are:

1 venous dilation – this is common in diabetic retinopathy and an obvious return to normal calibre is often apparent following panretinal photocoagulation for retinal neovascularization (see Fig. 3.12)
2 venous narrowing (Fig. 3.13)
3 opacification of the venous wall (venous sheathing/ 'white threads') (Fig. 3.14)
4 perivenous exudate (Fig. 3.15).

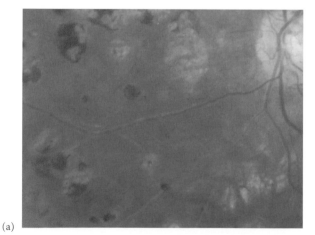

(a)

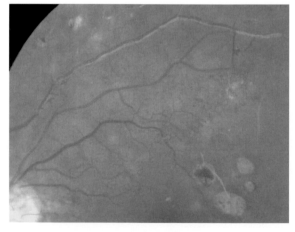

(b)

Fig. 3.14 Venous sheathing and pigmented laser scars: (a) inferonasal view left eye; (b) supertemporal view left eye.

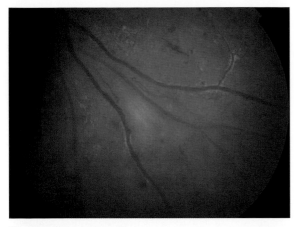

Fig. 3.15 Perivenous exudate.

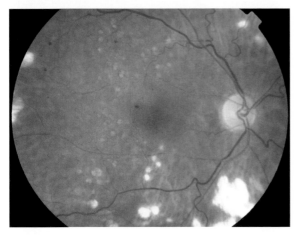

Fig. 3.16 Arteriolar narrowing.

Arteriolar abnormalities

Other arteriolar changes that occur in diabetic retinopathy are:

1 arteriolar narrowing (Fig. 3.16)
2 opacification of arteriolar walls ('sheathing and white threads') (Fig. 3.17)
3 arteriovenous nipping – narrowing of the venous diameter where it is crossed by a branch artery. It is often a feature of hypertension (Fig. 3.18).

Fibrous proliferation on or within 1 disc diameter of the disc margin

Fibrous proliferation at the disc (FPD) is fibrous tissue opaque enough to be seen at the disc or less than 1 disc diameter (DD) from the disc margin with or without accompanying new vessels (Fig. 3.19).

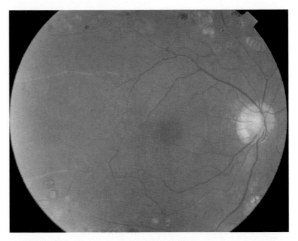

Fig. 3.17 Opacification of arteriolar walls.

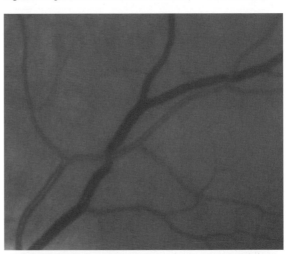

Fig. 3.18 Arteriovenous nipping.

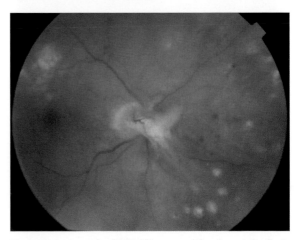

Fig. 3.19 An example of FPD (fibrous proliferation on the disc).

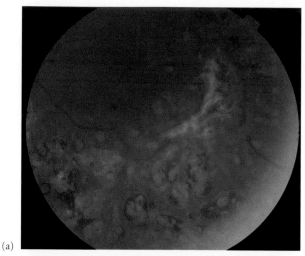

(a)

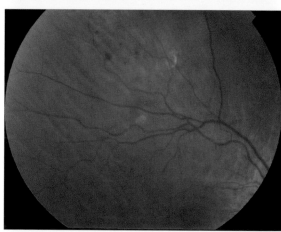

(b)

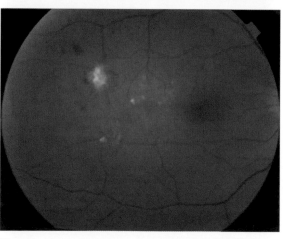

(c)

Fig. 3.20 Fibrous proliferation elsewhere (FPE): (a) FPE temporally following extensive laser treatment; (b) a localized area of FPE superiorly; (c) an area of FPE in the temporal retina.

Fibrous proliferation 'elsewhere'

Fibrous proliferation elsewhere (FPE) is fibrous tissue opaque enough to be seen more than 1 DD from the disc margin with or without accompanying new vessels (Fig. 3.20).

New vessels on and/or within 1 DD of the disc (NVD) (Fig. 3.21)

New vessels on the disc (NVD) are new immature vessels developing at the optic disc or within 1 disc diameter of the edge of the optic disc, which usually occur as a result of generalized retinal ischaemia. They have circular frond like tips and the activity of the new vessels after treatment can be determined by the relative size of the new vessels compared to before treatment and whether they have red blood corpuscles flowing through the circular frond

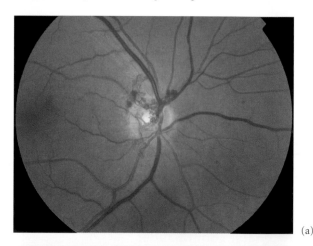

(a)

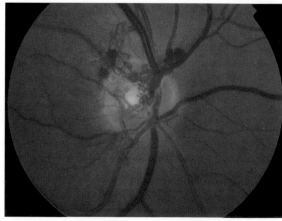

(b)

Fig. 3.21 (a) New vessels on disc (NVD); (b) NVD: magnified view.

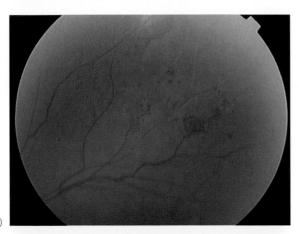

(a)

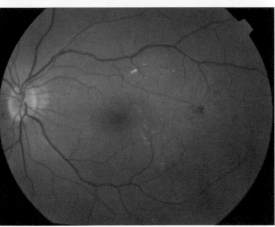

(b)

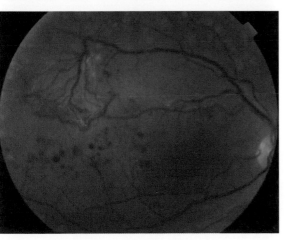

(c)

Fig. 3.22 (a) New vessels elsewhere (NVE) forming on the edge of an ischaemic area due to an occluded arteriole. (b) NVE forming in the left temporal retina. (c) Large NVE forming in the right temporal retina.

like tips of the new vessels. These abnormal vessels do not have an obvious purpose to their structure, unlike collateral vessels, which can be seen to be joining a vein above a blockage and then rejoining the vein below a blockage. Regression of new vessels after treatment is often accompanied by fibrosis.

New vessels 'elsewhere' (NVE) (Fig. 3.22)

New vessels elsewhere (NVE) are new immature vessels developing more than 1 disc diameter away from the edge of the optic disc and usually occurring on the edge of an area of retinal ischaemia peripheral to the NVE. They also have circular frond like tips and the activity of the new vessels after treatment can be determined by the relative size of the new vessels compared to before treatment and whether they have red blood corpuscles flowing through the circular frond like tips of the new vessels. Regression of new vessels after treatment is often accompanied by fibrosis.

Preretinal haemorrhage(PRH) (Fig. 3.23)

In the ETDRS, boat-shaped haemorrhages and roughly round, confluent or linear patches of haemorrhage just anterior to the retina or under the internal limiting membrane were included.

Vitreous haemorrhage (VH) (Figs 3.24 & 3.25)

A vitreous haemorrhage is a haemorrhage that is in the vitreous gel, having penetrated through the internal limiting membrane.

Post-maculopathy laser treatment – laser scars (Fig. 3.26)

Photocoagulation scars may be present after macular laser treatment. The best result would be clearing of clinically significant macular oedema and all hard exudates. Assessment of residual retinal oedema to decide whether further laser treatment is required will depend on an assessment of the amount of residual oedema, its location and the likely source and location of the leakage.

Post-scatter laser treatment for proliferative diabetic retinopathy – laser scars

Photocoagulation scars are usually visible following scatter laser treatment. The best result would be complete

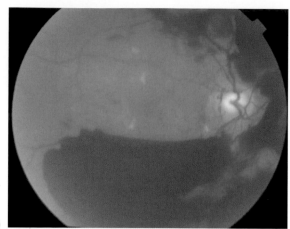

(a)

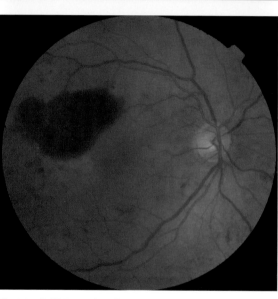

(b)

Fig. 3.23 (a,b) Examples of preretinal haemorrhage.

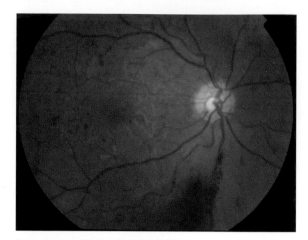

Fig. 3.24 A small vitreous haemorrhage.

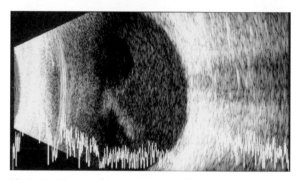

Fig. 3.25 A B-scan of a more pronounced vitreous haemorrhage.

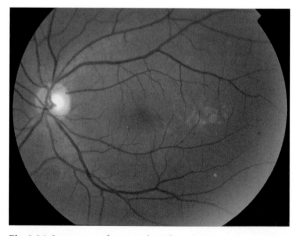

Fig. 3.26 Laser scars after maculopathy treatment.

regression of the new vessels. However, one is often left with partial regression of new vessels and a decision needs to be made as to the merits of further laser treatment. This decision will be based on the areas of retina that show laser photocoagulation scars, the appearance of the new vessels themselves (whether the frond-like tips still show circulation of red blood cells suggesting activity, whether the new vessels continue to grow or have shrunk, and what is the appearance of areas of retina). In an area of retina that has been adequately treated the venous calibre returns to normal, having very often shown signs of venous dilation and sometimes beading. There may also be areas of retina that show obvious signs of inadequate treatment as well as areas that show good treatment results as shown by the presence of photocoagulation scars and changes in venous calibre (Fig. 3.27).

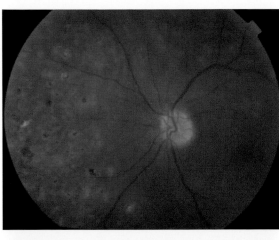

(a)

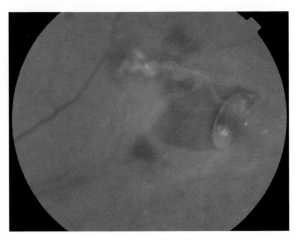

Fig. 3.28 Avulsion of NVE leaving horseshoe tear.

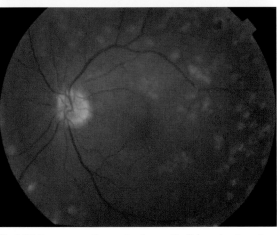

(b)

Fig. 3.27 Laser scars after scatter (panretinal) laser treatment: (a) left nasal view; (b) left macular view.

Posterior vitreous detachment

A posterior vitreous detachment (PVD) is a common condition of the eye in which the vitreous humour separates from the retina. The vitreous is attached to the retina, more strongly in some places than others, particularly around the optic nerve head and around the peripheral retina. In people with proliferative diabetic retinopathy, where new vessels have penetrated the internal limiting membrane, VH is the usual result. Once a complete posterior vitreous detachment has occurred, this removes the structure that new vessels rely on to proliferate anteriorly and a PVD can therefore be helpful in preventing further anterior neovascularization. This is, of course, one of the rationales behind vitrectomy surgery.

Rarely, a PVD can result in a retinal tear when the new vessel complex is pulled away from the retina. An example is shown in Fig. 3.28.

OTHER CLASSIFICATIONS

Because of the difficulty in correlating seven-field stereophotography to the clinical setting, particularly in the screening environment where the level of referral to an ophthalmologist needs to be clearly defined, two further simplified classifications have been developed. The International Classification has been developed for healthcare settings in countries like the USA where there are an adequate number of ophthalmologists to undertake the slit-lamp biomicroscopy examinations on patients with microaneurysms only. In England, the referral level has been defined to refer patients with retinopathy to an ophthalmologist at a later stage in the disease process (see Tables 3.3 & 3.4).

PRACTICE POINTS

- There are a number of different classifications of diabetic retinopathy, which have been developed to give indications of the risks of progression to proliferative diabetic retinopathy or vision-threatening maculopathy and the appropriate referral criteria, the latter depending on individual healthcare systems.
- The key factor in these classifications is accurate identification of the lesions that occur in diabetic retinopathy, which have been described in this chapter.

Table 3.3 International and English diabetic retinopathy classifications.

'International' clinical classification of diabetic retinopathy severity[7]	Recommended 'international' outcome	English screening programme levels[8]
Microaneurysms only	Optimize medical therapy, screen at least annually	R0 Screen annually No DR
More than just microaneurysms but less severe than severe NPDR	Refer to ophthalmologist	R1 Screen annually **Background** Microaneurysm(s) Retinal haemorrhage(s) ± any exudate
Severe NPDR Any of the following: a) Extensive intraretinal haem (>20) in 4 quadrants b) Definite venous beading in 2+ quadrants c) Prominent IRMA in 1+ quadrant And no signs of PDR	Consider scatter photocoagulation for type 2 diabetes	R2 Refer to ophthalmologist **Preproliferative** Venous beading Venous loop or reduplication Intraretinal microvascular abnormality (IRMA) Multiple deep, round or blot haemorrhages
Neovascularization Vitreous/preretinal haemorrhage	Scatter photocoagulation without delay for patients with vitreous haemorrhage or neovascularization within 1 DD of the optic nerve head	R3 Urgent referral to ophthalmologist **Proliferative** New vessels on disc (NVD) New vessels elsewhere (NVE) Preretinal or vitreous haemorrhage Preretinal fibrosis ± tractional retinal detachment

Table 3.4 International and English maculopathy classifications.

International classification[7]	Outcome	English classification[8]	Outcome
Diabetic macular oedema present as defined by some retinal thickening or hard exudates in the posterior pole and subclassified into:		Circinate or group of exudates within the macula (The macula is defined as that part of the retina which lies within a circle centred on the centre of the fovea whose radius is the distance between the centre of the fovea and the temporal margin of the disc)	Referral
Mild diabetic macular oedema Some retinal thickening or hard exudates in the posterior pole but distant from the macula	Referral	Any microaneurysm or haemorrhage within 1DD of the centre of the fovea only if associated with a best VA of ≤6/12 (if no stereo)	Referral
Moderate diabetic macular oedema Retinal thickening or hard exudates approaching the centre of the macula but not involving the centre	Referral	Exudate within 1 DD of the centre of the fovea	Referral
Severe diabetic macular oedema Retinal thickening or hard exudates involving the centre of the macula	Referral	Retinal thickening within 1 DD of the centre of the fovea (if stereo available)	Referral

REFERENCES

1 The Diabetic Retinopathy Study Research Group. Diabetic retinopathy study. Report Number 6. Design, methods, and baseline results. Report Number 7. A modification of the Airlie House classification of diabetic retinopathy. *Invest Ophthalmol Vis Sci* 1981; **21**(1 Pt 2): 1–226.

2 Early Treatment Diabetic Retinopathy Study Research Group. Grading diabetic retinopathy from stereoscopic color fundus photographs – an extension of the modified Airlie House classification. ETDRS report number 10. *Ophthalmology* 1991; **98**(5 Suppl): 786–806.

3 Early Treatment Diabetic Retinopathy Study Research Group. Fundus photographic risk factors for progression of diabetic retinopathy. ETDRS report number 12. *Ophthalmology* 1991; **98**(5 Suppl): 823–33.

4 Spalter HF. Photocoagulation of circinate maculopathy in diabetic retinopathy. *Am J Ophthalmol* 1971; **1**(1 Part 2): 242–50.

5 The Diabetic Retinopathy Study Research Group. Photocoagulation treatment of proliferative diabetic retinopathy. Clinical application of Diabetic Retinopathy Study (DRS) findings, DRS Report Number 8. *Ophthalmology* 1981; **88**(7): 583–600.

6 Early Treatment Diabetic Retinopathy Study Research Group. Treatment techniques and clinical guidelines for photocoagulation of diabetic macular edema. Early Treatment Diabetic Retinopathy Study Report Number 2. *Ophthalmology* 1987; **94**(7): 761–74.

7 Wilkinson CP, Ferris FL 3rd, Klein RE, Lee PP, Agardh CD, Davis M *et al.* Proposed international clinical diabetic retinopathy and diabetic macular edema disease severity scales. *Ophthalmology* 2003; **110**(9): 1677–82.

8 Harding S, Greenwood R, Aldington S, Gibson J, Owens D, Taylor R *et al.* Grading and disease management in national screening for diabetic retinopathy in England and Wales. *Diabet Med* 2003; **20**(12): 965–71.

4 Screening for diabetic retinopathy

Peter H. Scanlon

PRINCIPLES OF SCREENING

The *definition of screening* that was adopted by the WHO[1] in 1968 was 'the presumptive identification of unrecognized disease or defect by the application of tests, examinations or other procedures which can be applied rapidly. Screening tests sort out apparently well persons who probably have a disease from those who probably do not. A screening test is not intended to be diagnostic. Persons with positive or suspicious findings must be referred to their physicians for diagnosis and necessary treatment.'

The following principles for screening for human disease were derived from the public health papers produced by the WHO[1] in 1968.

1 The condition sought should be an important problem.
2 There should be an accepted treatment for patients with recognized disease.
3 Facilities for diagnosis and treatment should be available.
4 There should be a recognizable latent or early symptomatic stage.
5 There should be a suitable test or examination.
6 The test should be acceptable to the population.
7 The natural history of the condition, including development from latent to declared disease, should be adequately understood.
8 There should be an agreed policy on whom to treat as patients.
9 The cost of the case-finding programme (including early diagnosis and treatment of patients diagnosed) should be economically balanced in relation to possible expenditure on medical care as a whole.
10 Case-finding should be a continuing process and not a 'one-time' project.

A Practical Manual of Diabetic Retinopathy Management.
Peter H Scanlon, Charles P Wilkinson, Stephen J Aldington and David R Matthews. Published 2009 by Blackwell Publishing, ISBN 978-1-4051-7035-2.

Applying these principles to sight-threatening diabetic retinopathy raises the following questions.[2]

1 Is there evidence that sight-threatening diabetic retinopathy is an important public health problem?
2 Is there evidence that the incidence of sight-threatening diabetic retinopathy is going to remain the same or become an even greater public health problem?
3 Is there evidence that sight-threatening diabetic retinopathy has a recognizable latent or early symptomatic stage?
4 Is there evidence that treatment for sight-threatening diabetic retinopathy is effective and agreed universally?
5 Is a suitable and reliable screening test available, acceptable to both healthcare professionals and (more importantly) to the public?
6 Are the costs of screening and effective treatment of sight-threatening diabetic retinopathy balanced economically in relation to total expenditure on healthcare – including the consequences of leaving the disease untreated?

The evidence that sight-threatening diabetic retinopathy is an important public health problem

The UK Prospective Diabetes Study (UKPDS) reported a baseline prevalence of retinopathy in 39% of diabetic men and 35% of diabetic women. In 2002, Younis[3] reported baseline prevalence in the type 1 group of any diabetic retinopathy (DR), proliferative diabetic retinopathy (PDR) and sight-threatening diabetic retinopathy (STDR) as 45.7%, 3.7% and 16.4%, respectively. Baseline prevalence in the type 2 group of any DR, PDR and STDR was 25.3%, 0.5% and 6.0%, respectively.

In 1995, Evans[4] reported that diabetes was the most important cause of blindness in the working population (13.8%) in England with 11.9% due to diabetic retinopathy. In 2002, Kocur[5] reported that in European people of working age, diabetic retinopathy was the most frequently reported cause of serious visual loss. In the middle-income countries of Europe, diabetic retinopathy is the third most common cause, advanced cataract and glaucoma being more frequently observed.

The evidence that the incidence of sight-threatening diabetic retinopathy is going to remain the same or become an even greater public health problem

In 1997, Amos[6] estimated that 124 million people worldwide had diabetes, 97% of these having non-insulin-dependent diabetes mellitus (NIDDM). By the year 2010 the total number of people with diabetes is projected to reach 221 million. In 2000, Sorensen[7] reported that body weight and the prevalence of obesity were rising so rapidly in many countries that the WHO has recognized that there is a 'global epidemic of obesity.' The prevalence of type 2 diabetes is rising in parallel.

The evidence that sight-threatening diabetic retinopathy has a recognizable latent or early symptomatic stage (Fig. 4.1)

The Wisconsin Epidemiologic Study[8], the Berlin Retinopathy Study[9], the Early Treatment Diabetic Retinopathy Study[10] and the UKPDS[11] have all observed the natural history of diabetic retinopathy. In 2003, Younis[12,13] reported yearly and cumulative incidence of any retinopathy, maculopathy or sight-threatening diabetic retinopathy in patients with type 1 diabetes and type 2 diabetes who underwent 2742 and 20,570 screening events respectively. There is clear evidence from these studies that sight-threatening diabetic retinopathy has a recognizable latent or early symptomatic stage.

The evidence that treatment for sight-threatening diabetic retinopathy is effective and agreed universally

The evidence that laser treatment is effective
There is clear evidence from the following studies that laser treatment is effective and universally agreed.

The Diabetic Retinopathy Study Research Group[14–16] study provided evidence that photocoagulation treatment was of benefit in preventing severe visual loss in eyes with proliferative retinopathy. The Early Treatment Diabetic Retinopathy Study[17–19] (ETDRS) showed that focal photocoagulation of 'clinically significant' diabetic macular oedema substantially reduced the risk of visual loss.

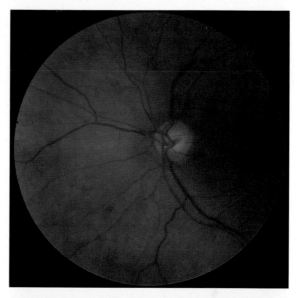

(a)

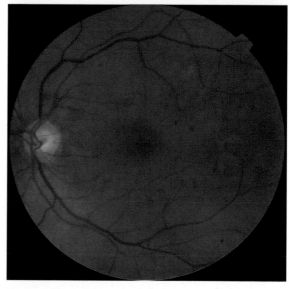

(b)

Fig. 4.1 Diabetic retinopathy detected during screening: (a) nasal view; (b) macular view.

Further reports[20–23] have shown favourable long-term visual results of photocoagulation (Figs 4.2–4.4).

The evidence that diabetic retinopathy can be prevented or the rate of deterioration reduced by improved control of blood glucose, blood pressure and lipid levels
The evidence that intensive blood glucose control reduces the risk of new-onset DR and slows the progression of

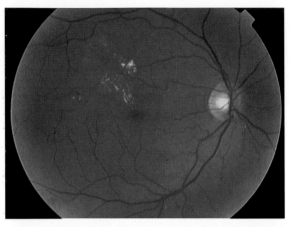

Fig. 4.2 Macular exudates before argon laser photocoagulation.

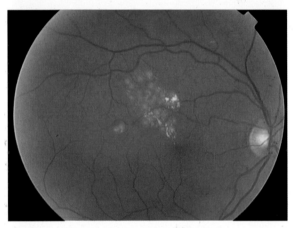

Fig. 4.3 Macular exudates immediately after laser photocoagulation.

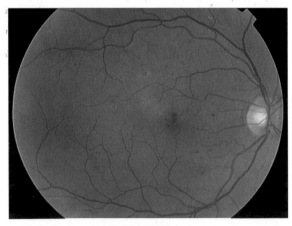

Fig. 4.4 Macular exudates 6 months after laser photocoagulation.

existing DR comes from the Diabetes Control and Complications Trial (DCCT)[24–26] and UKPDS.[11] The evidence that control of systemic hypertension reduces the risk of new-onset DR and slows the progression of existing DR comes from UKPDS[27–29] and other studies.[30,31] There is evidence that elevated serum lipids are associated with macular exudate[32] and prevention of moderate visual loss and partial regression of hard exudates may be possible by reducing elevated lipid levels.[33]

The evidence that a suitable and reliable screening test is available, acceptable to both healthcare professionals and (more importantly) to the public

There is widespread agreement that digital photography is the best method of screening for sight-threatening DR. The use of selective mydriasis and the number of fields captured have been more controversial. The reasons for digital photography being the preferred method are gained from the following studies.

Direct ophthalmoscopy

Studies of direct ophthalmoscopy against a recognized reference standard of seven-field stereo photography, an ophthalmologist using slit-lamp biomicroscopy or fluorescein angiography showed variable results in studies by Palmberg,[34] Sussman,[35] Foulds,[36] Moss,[37] Kleinstein,[38] Awh,[39] Nathan,[40] Pugh[41] and Harding.[42] The results are considered too variable across different professional groups, and even in the hands of a specialist registrar in ophthalmology[42] the sensitivity achieved for the detection of sight-threatening retinopathy was only 65% (95% CI 51–79%).

Optometrist's slit-lamp biomicroscopy

A number of studies have assessed the performance of optometrist's slit-lamp biomicroscopy including those by Hammond,[43] Burnett,[44] Prasad,[45] Hulme,[46] Olson,[47] Sharp,[48] Tu[49] and Warburton.[50] The best designed study is that of Olson[47] and Sharp[48] in which all those patients seen by an optometrist are also examined by a retinal specialist and a comparison is made with digital photography and 35-mm photography. In the Olson study, slit-lamp examination by optometrists for the detection of sight-threatening retinopathy (referable), achieved a sensitivity of 73% (95% CI 52–88%) and a specificity of 90% (95% CI 87–93%). No technical failure was reported. However, with two-field imaging, manual grading of red-free digital images achieved a sensitivity of 93% (95% CI 82–98%)

and a specificity of 87% (95% CI 84–90%). The technical failure rate for digital imaging reported was 4.4% of patients. Hence two-field digital photography as a method of screening achieved a higher sensitivity and specificity for screening than slit-lamp biomicroscopy by a number of trained optometrists.

Slit-lamp biomicroscopy schemes also have the disadvantage that, for quality assurance purposes, a percentage of patients require re-examination as opposed to re-examination of the images in a scheme using digital photography.

Mydriatic photography (<seven fields) using 35-mm film or Polaroid

Studies of mydriatic photography with 35-mm film or Polaroid against a recognized reference standard of seven-field stereo photography, an ophthalmologist using slit-lamp biomicroscopy or fluorescein angiography showed consistently good results by Kalm,[51] Lee,[52] Pugh,[41] Schachat,[53] Aldington,[54] Harding,[42] Kiri,[55] Taylor,[56] Broadbent,[57] Moller,[58] Stellingwerf,[59] Pandit,[60] Olson[47] and Sharp.[48] These studies have shown that consistently good results can be achieved, with sensitivities of >80% and high levels of specificity, using mydriatic photography with 35-mm film or Polaroid in screening for referable or sight-threatening diabetic retinopathy. In these studies, specificity does vary depending on whether ungradeable images are regarded as test positive but levels of >85% are consistently achieved.

Non-mydriatic photography

There have been strong proponents of non-mydriatic photography for many years. In 1993, ungradable image rates were reported as low as 4% by Leese.[61] However, it has been recognized in more recent years, following the publication of studies by Scanlon[62] and Murgatroyd,[63] that ungradable image rates for non-mydriatic digital photography in a predominantly white Caucasian population are of the order of 20–26% (19.7% and 26% being reported in the two studies). Age is the strongest correlate to poor-quality images in non-mydriatic digital photography as shown in the publication by Scanlon[64]. The Health Technology Board for Scotland used data from the Scanlon[62] study in their report[65] and concluded that similar sensitivities and specificities could be achieved by dilating the eyes of those patients with ungradable images. This relies on the ability of the screener to accurately determine an ungradable image at the time of screening and, in the Scottish system, relies on the assumption that the grading of one field will detect referable retinopathy

with the same degree of accuracy as the grading of two fields (giving evidence from Olson's study[47]). Other proponents of digital photography have attempted to capture three fields[66,67] and five fields,[68] and remarkably Shiba[69] excluded the over-70 age group and attempted 9 × overlapping non-mydriatic 450 fields.

Digital camera systems have lower flash intensities than those using Polaroid or 35-mm film. Taylor[56] reported a low flash power of 10 W in one of the earlier digital systems compared to approximately 300 W that was used with the conventional 35-mm film or Polaroid cameras. Modern digital camera backs require more light and this level of 10 W has increased but not to the level of 35-mm film or Polaroid cameras.

Mydriatic digital photography (Fig. 4.5)

Studies of mydriatic digital photography against a recognized reference standard of seven-field stereo photography

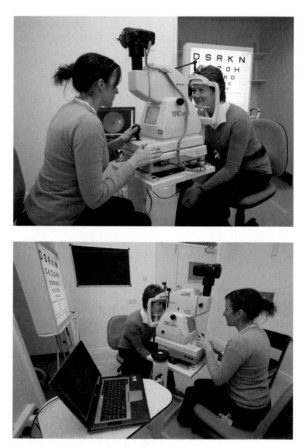

Fig. 4.5 A screening episode being undertaken i.e. a screener photographing a patient's fundi.

or an ophthalmologist using slit-lamp biomicroscopy have shown showed consistently good results by Taylor,[56] Newsom,[70] Razvi,[71] Rudnisky,[72] Olson,[47] Sharp[48] and Scanlon.[62] The study by Olson[47] and Sharp[48] demonstrated in 586 patients that for the detection of sight-threatening retinopathy, manual grading of two-field red-free digital images achieved a sensitivity of 93% (82–98) and a specificity of 87% (84–90). The reference standard was slit-lamp biomicrocopy by retinal specialists. Digital imaging had an ungradable image rate of 4.4% of patients. In 2003, the Gloucestershire Diabetic Eye study[62] demonstrated the effectiveness of mydriatic digital photography against a reference standard of an ophthalmologist's slit-lamp biomicroscopy, which was further validated[73] against seven-field stereophotography. The same study published results on reasons for poor image quality in digital photographic screening programmes[64] and on the effect of the introduction of the screening programme on the workload of the local ophthalmology department.[74] In 2004, Williams produced a report[75] for the American Academy of ophthalmology summarizing the use of single-field fundus photography for diabetic retinopathy screening.

Two review articles from the USA were written in 2006. The first by Chew[76] concluded that, although screening techniques do not replace the eye examination, in populations with poor access to ophthalmic care, screening techniques such as the non-mydriatic camera used in offices of primary care physicians may be useful in identifying lesions of diabetic retinopathy requiring treatment. The second article by Whited,[77] which included very few non-US-based studies, concluded that, based on existing data, teleophthalmology appears to be an accurate and reliable test for detecting diabetic retinopathy and macular oedema.

The evidence that the costs of screening and effective treatment of sight-threatening diabetic retinopathy balanced economically in relation to total expenditure on healthcare – including the consequences of leaving the disease untreated

In 1982, Savolainen[78] reported on the cost-effectiveness of photocoagulation for sight-threatening diabetic retinopathy in the UK. There have been reports of computer simulation models by Javitt,[79–81] Dasbach,[82] Caro[83] and Fendrick[80] based on the health systems in the USA and Sweden.[84] Modelling studies from the Wessex

Institute[85] suggested that there is greater benefit in reducing the screening interval when the screening programme retains patients until they require treatment than when the screening programme detects early, background retinopathy, with prompt referral to specialist services. James et al.[86] reported results for an organized screening programme using 35-mm retinal photography and demonstrated this to be more cost-effective than the previous system of opportunistic screening.

Meads[87] reviewed published studies of the costs of blindness and compared Fould's 1983 estimate[36] inflated to £7433 in 2002 costs, Dasbach's 1991 estimate[82] inflated to £5391 in 2002 costs and Wright's 2000 estimate[88] inflated to £7452 (£4070–£11,250) in 2002 costs. He concluded that much of the uncertainty in any sensitivity analysis of the cost of blindness in older people is associated with the cost of residential care and that the excess admission to care homes caused by poor vision is impossible to quantify at the present time.

Only two studies have assessed the costs of screening using digital photography. Bjorvig[89] assessed the costs of telemedicine screening for diabetic retinopathy in a trial conducted in northern Norway. At low workloads, telemedicine was more expensive than conventional examination. However, at higher workloads, telemedicine was cheaper. The break-even point occurred at a patient workload of 110 per annum. Tu[49] calculated the cost of screening each patient as £23.99 per patient for an optometry model and £29.29 per patient for a digital photographic model. However, in this study there was poor compliance rates in the newly introduced screening programme in both models.

The UK National Screening Committee has recommended digital imaging as the preferred method of retinal photography for screening.[90,91] They have used estimates of costs by Garvican[92] for a theoretical population of 500,000. For a mobile photographic screening service, the cost of the initial screen is estimated as approximately £21 per diabetic patient registered or £24 per attendee at 85–90% uptake.

THE EXETER STANDARDS

The 'Exeter Standards' form the basis for an acceptable method for use in a systematic screening programme for DR in the UK. The Exeter Standards recommended that a screening test for sight-threatening DR should achieve a minimum sensitivity of 80% and a minimum specificity of 95%. In the Liverpool Diabetic Eye study[42] mydriatic 35-mm photography achieved 84% sensitivity and

89% specificity and the Gloucestershire Diabetic Eye study[62] achieved 87.8% sensitivity and 86.1% specificity for mydriatic digital photography with an ungradable image rate of 3.7%. These results suggest that 95% specificity may have been set too high and sensitivity too low, but these have not been challenged and the standard has been maintained for guidance. In some studies the specificity is reported as higher than those quoted, but variations in whether ungradables are counted as positive test results often explains this difference. If the sensitivity and specificity studies were repeated with modern digital cameras the results would be likely to improve because of the higher resolution of the modern cameras.

CASE HISTORY 1
Screening for sight-threatening diabetic retinopathy

A 20-year-old man with type 1 diabetes diagnosed at the age of 7 years attended his local optician for a sight test and was told that he did not have any significant diabetic retinopathy. Two months later he was invited to a local photographic screening service and attended. Photographs were taken (Fig. 4.6a,b).

Laser treatment was commenced to his left eye:
- left 30 burns, 100-micron size, 210–230 mW, 0.1 s, area centralis lens, argon laser.

One year after presentation, the vision deteriorated in the left eye to 6/24 (20/180) and red-free and fluorescein photographs were taken (Fig. 4.6c–e).

Further laser treatment was given to the left macular area:
- left 53 burns, 100-micron size, 180–250 mW, 0.1 s, area centralis lens, argon laser.

The following week, panretinal photocoagulation was commenced to the left eye:
- 1522 burns, 350-micron spot size, power 140–180 mW, transequatorial lens, argon laser split over two sessions 1 week apart;
- a further session of 706 burns, 500-micron spot size, power 170 mW, Karickhoff lens, argon laser.

The vision in the left eye remained at the level of 6/24 (20/180) and a retrohyaloid haemorrhage then developed in the left eye as shown in the red-free and fluorescein photographs (Fig. 4.6f–g). Some exudates and leakage were seen in the right macular area (Fig. 4.6h–j).

A B-scan was performed, which showed an appearance similar to a detachment but was, in this instance, caused by the retrohyaloid haemorrhage (see Fig. 4.6k).

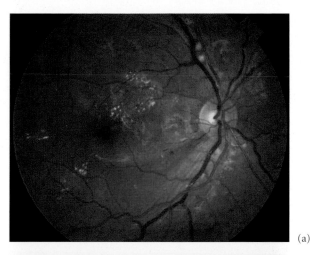

(a)

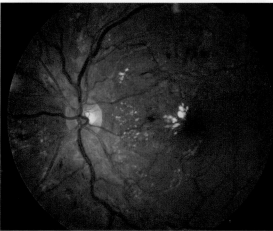

(b)

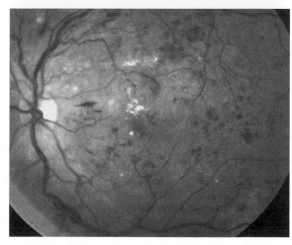

(c)

Fig. 4.6 Case history 1. (a) Year 0: right macula colour. (b) Year 0: left macula colour. (c) Year 1: left macula red free. (*Continued on p. 52*)

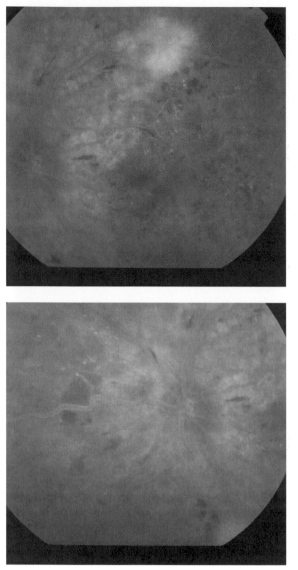

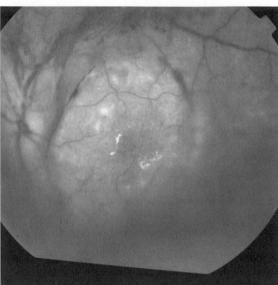

(d)

(f)

(e)

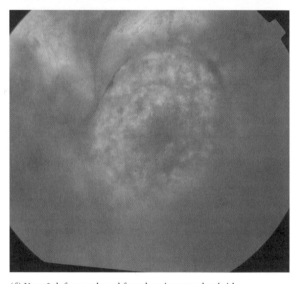

(g)

Fig. 4.6 (*Cont'd*) (d) Year 1: left macula fluorescein showing left macular oedema and leakage from NVE above the left macula. (e) Year 1: left disc/nasal view fluorescein showing extensive leakage and ischaemic area in left nasal retina.

(f) Year 2: left macula red free showing retrohyaloid haemorrhage with sparing around the fovea. (g) Year 2: left macula fluorescein showing retrohyaloid haemorrhage with sparing around the fovea. (*Continued on facing page*)

A left pars plana vitrectomy was performed. Laser treatment was commenced to his right eye:

- right 36 burns, 100-micron size, 190 mW, 0.1 s, area centralis lens, argon laser.

Three years later (age 25 years), the fluorescein angiogram was repeated. At this stage the visual acuity (VA) was right 6/4 (20/14) and left 6/9 (20/30), and further photographs were taken (Fig. 4.6l–o).

At the age of 28 years his vision and the photographic appearances have remained stable.

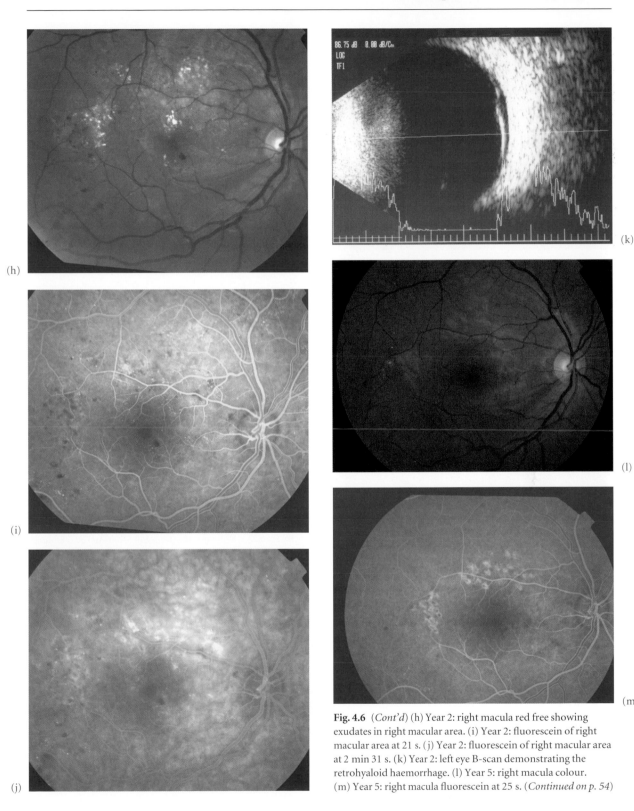

Fig. 4.6 (*Cont'd*) (h) Year 2: right macula red free showing exudates in right macular area. (i) Year 2: fluorescein of right macular area at 21 s. (j) Year 2: fluorescein of right macular area at 2 min 31 s. (k) Year 2: left eye B-scan demonstrating the retrohyaloid haemorrhage. (l) Year 5: right macula colour. (m) Year 5: right macula fluorescein at 25 s. (*Continued on p. 54*)

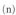
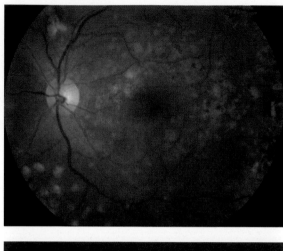

(n)

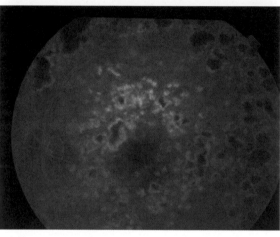

(o)

Fig. 4.6 (*Cont'd*) (n) Year 5: left macula colour. (o) Year 5: left macula fluorescein at 2 min 44 s.

PRACTICE POINTS

- An effective treatment has been available for most patients with diabetic retinopathy since the first reports from the Diabetic Retinopathy Study[14] were published in 1976. It is therefore a tragedy that in healthcare systems where appropriate treatment is readily available, so many patients are presenting so late in the course of the disease that treatment is much more difficult and unnecessary blindness is often the result.
- Systematic screening programmes with good population coverage do reduce the incidence and prevalence of blindness in the population with diabetes and many countries are now looking to introduce these programmes.

REFERENCES

1 Wilson J, Jungner G. The principles and practice of screening for disease. Public Health Papers 34. Geneva: WHO, 1968.

2 Scanlon PH. An evaluation of the effectiveness and cost-effectiveness of screening for diabetic retinopathy by digital imaging photography and technician ophthalmoscopy and the subsequent change in activity, workload and costs of new diabetic ophthalmology referrals. [MD]. London, 2005.

3 Younis N, Broadbent DM, Harding SP, Vora JR. Prevalence of diabetic eye disease in patients entering a systematic primary care-based eye screening programme. *Diabet Med* 2002;**19**(12):1014–21.

4 Evans J. Causes of blindness and partial sight in England and Wales 1990–1991. London: OPCS, 1995:1–29.

5 Kocur I, Resnikoff S. Visual impairment and blindness in Europe and their prevention. *Br J Ophthalmol* 2002;**86**(7): 716–22.

6 Amos AF, McCarty DJ, Zimmet P. The rising global burden of diabetes and its complications: estimates and projections to the year 2010. *Diabet Med* 1997;**14 Suppl 5**:S1–85.

7 Sorensen TI. The changing lifestyle in the world. Body weight and what else? *Diabetes Care* 2000;**23 Suppl 2**:B1–4.

8 Klein R, Klein BE, Moss SE, Cruickshanks KJ. The Wisconsin Epidemiologic Study of Diabetic Retinopathy: XVII. The 14-year incidence and progression of diabetic retinopathy and associated risk factors in type 1 diabetes. *Ophthalmology* 1998;**105**(10):1801–15.

9 Burger W, Hovener G, Dusterhus R, Hartmann R, Weber B. Prevalence and development of retinopathy in children and adolescents with type 1 (insulin-dependent) diabetes mellitus. A longitudinal study. *Diabetologia* 1986;**29**(1):17–22.

10 Early Treatment Diabetic Retinopathy Study Research Group. Fundus photographic risk factors for progression of diabetic retinopathy. ETDRS report number 12. *Ophthalmology* 1991; **98**(5 Suppl):823–33.

11 Stratton IM, Kohner EM, Aldington SJ, Turner RC, Holman RR, Manley SE *et al.* UKPDS 50: risk factors for incidence and progression of retinopathy in Type II diabetes over 6 years from diagnosis. *Diabetologia* 2001;**44**(2):156–63.

12 Younis N, Broadbent DM, Harding SP, Vora JP. Incidence of sight-threatening retinopathy in Type 1 diabetes in a systematic screening programme. *Diabet Med* 2003;**20**(9):758–65.

13 Younis N, Broadbent DM, Vora JP, Harding SP. Incidence of sight-threatening retinopathy in patients with type 2 diabetes in the Liverpool Diabetic Eye Study: a cohort study. *Lancet* 2003;**361**(9353):195–200.

14 The Diabetic Retinopathy Study Research Group. Preliminary report on effects of photocoagulation therapy. *Am J Ophthalmol* 1976;**81**(4):383–96.

15 The Diabetic Retinopathy Study Research Group. Photocoagulation treatment of proliferative diabetic retinopathy: the second report of diabetic retinopathy study findings. *Ophthalmology* 1978;**85**(1):82–106.

16 The Diabetic Retinopathy Study Research Group. Four risk factors for severe visual loss in diabetic retinopathy. The third report from the Diabetic Retinopathy Study. *Arch Ophthalmol* 1979;**97**(4):654–5.

17 Early Treatment Diabetic Retinopathy Study Research Group. Photocoagulation for diabetic macular edema. Early Treatment Diabetic Retinopathy Study report number 1. *Arch Ophthalmol* 1985;**103**(12):1796–806.

18 Early Treatment Diabetic Retinopathy Study Research Group. Treatment techniques and clinical guidelines for photocoagulation of diabetic macular edema. Early Treatment Diabetic Retinopathy Study Report Number 2. *Ophthalmology* 1987; **94**(7):761–74.

19 Early Treatment Diabetic Retinopathy Study Research Group. Photocoagulation for diabetic macular edema: Early Treatment Diabetic Retinopathy Study Report no. 4. *Int Ophthalmol Clin* 1987;**27**(4):265–72.

20 Davies EG, Petty RG, Kohner EM. Long term effectiveness of photocoagulation for diabetic maculopathy. *Eye* 1989;**3 (Pt 6)**:764–7.

21 Blankenship GW. Fifteen-year argon laser and xenon photocoagulation results of Bascom Palmer Eye Institute's patients participating in the diabetic retinopathy study. *Ophthalmology* 1991;**98**(2):125–8.

22 Sullivan P, Caldwell G, Alexander N, Kohner E. Long-term outcome after photocoagulation for proliferative diabetic retinopathy. *Diabet Med* 1990;**7**(9):788–94.

23 Chew EY, Ferris FL 3rd, Csaky KG, Murphy RP, Agron E, Thompson DJ et al. The long-term effects of laser photocoagulation treatment in patients with diabetic retinopathy: the early treatment diabetic retinopathy follow-up study. *Ophthalmology* 2003;**110**(9):1683–9.

24 The Diabetes Control and Complications Trial Research Group. The effect of intensive treatment of diabetes on the development and progression of long-term complications in insulin-dependent diabetes mellitus. *N Engl J Med* 1993; **329**(14):977–86.

25 The Diabetes Control and Complications Trial Research Group. Progression of retinopathy with intensive versus conventional treatment in the Diabetes Control and Complications Trial. *Ophthalmology* 1995;**102**(4):647–61.

26 The Diabetes Control and Complications Trial Research Group. The effect of intensive diabetes treatment on the progression of diabetic retinopathy in insulin-dependent diabetes mellitus. *Arch Ophthalmol* 1995;**113**(1):36–51.

27 Matthews DR, Stratton IM, Aldington SJ, Holman RR, Kohner EM. Risks of progression of retinopathy and vision loss related to tight blood pressure control in type 2 diabetes mellitus: UKPDS 69. *Arch Ophthalmol* 2004;**122**(11):1631–40.

28 UK Prospective Diabetes Study Group. Tight blood pressure control and risk of macrovascular and microvascular complications in type 2 diabetes: UKPDS 38. *BMJ* 1998;**317**(7160): 703–13.

29 UK Prospective Diabetes Study Group. Efficacy of atenolol and captopril in reducing risk of macrovascular and micro-

vascular complications in type 2 diabetes: UKPDS 39. *BMJ* 1998;**317**(7160):713–20.

30 Chase HP, Garg SK, Jackson WE, Thomas MA, Harris S, Marshall G et al. Blood pressure and retinopathy in type I diabetes. *Ophthalmology* 1990;**97**(2):155–9.

31 Estacio RO, Jeffers BW, Gifford N, Schrier RW. Effect of blood pressure control on diabetic microvascular complications in patients with hypertension and type 2 diabetes. *Diabetes Care* 2000;**23 Suppl 2**:B54–64.

32 Chew EY, Klein ML, Ferris FL 3rd, Remaley NA, Murphy RP, Chantry K et al. Association of elevated serum lipid levels with retinal hard exudate in diabetic retinopathy. Early Treatment Diabetic Retinopathy Study (ETDRS) Report 22. *Arch Ophthalmol* 1996;**114**(9):1079–84.

33 Cusick M, Chew EY, Chan CC, Kruth HS, Murphy RP, Ferris FL 3rd. Histopathology and regression of retinal hard exudates in diabetic retinopathy after reduction of elevated serum lipid levels. *Ophthalmology* 2003;**110**(11):2126–33.

34 Palmberg P, Smith M, Waltman S, Krupin T, Singer P, Burgess D et al. The natural history of retinopathy in insulindependent juvenile-onset diabetes. *Ophthalmology* 1981; **88**(7):613–18.

35 Sussman EJ, Tsiaras WG, Soper KA. Diagnosis of diabetic eye disease. *JAMA* 1982;**247**(23):3231–4.

36 Foulds WS, MacCuish ATB. Diabetic Retinopathy in the West of Scotland: Its Detection and Prevalence, and the Cost-effectiveness of a Proposed Screening Programme. *Health Bulletin* 1983;**41**(6):318–26.

37 Moss SE, Klein R, Kessler SD, Richie KA. Comparison between ophthalmoscopy and fundus photography in determining severity of diabetic retinopathy. *Ophthalmology* 1985;**92**(1):62–7.

38 Kleinstein RN, Roseman JM, Herman WH, Holcombe J, Louv WC. Detection of diabetic retinopathy by optometrists. *J Am Optom Assoc* 1987;**58**(11):879–82.

39 Awh CC, Cupples HP, Javitt JC. Improved detection and referral of patients with diabetic retinopathy by primary care physicians. Effectiveness of education. *Arch Intern Med* 1991;**151**(7):1405–8.

40 Nathan DM, Fogel HA, Godine JE, Lou PL, D'Amico DJ, Regan CD et al. Role of diabetologist in evaluating diabetic retinopathy. *Diabetes Care* 1991;**14**(1):26–33.

41 Pugh JA, Jacobson JM, Van Heuven WA, Watters JA, Tuley MR, Lairson DR et al. Screening for diabetic retinopathy. The wide-angle retinal camera. *Diabetes Care* 1993;**16**(6):889–95.

42 Harding SP, Broadbent DM, Neoh C, White MC, Vora J. Sensitivity and specificity of photography and direct ophthalmoscopy in screening for sight threatening eye disease: the Liverpool Diabetic Eye Study. *BMJ* 1995;**311**(7013):1131–5.

43 Hammond CJ, Shackleton J, Flanagan DW, Herrtage J, Wade J. Comparison between an ophthalmic optician and an ophthalmologist in screening for diabetic retinopathy. *Eye* 1996;**10 (Pt 1)**:107–12.

44 Burnett S, Hurwitz B, Davey C, Ray J, Chaturvedi N, Salzmann J et al. The implementation of prompted retinal

screening for diabetic eye disease by accredited optometrists in an inner-city district of North London: a quality of care study. *Diabet Med* 1998;**15 Suppl 3**:S38–43.

45 Prasad S, Kamath GG, Jones K, Clearkin LG, Phillips RP. Effectiveness of optometrist screening for diabetic retinopathy using slit-lamp biomicroscopy. *Eye* 2001;**15**(Pt 5): 595–601.

46 Hulme SA, Tin UA, Hardy KJ, Joyce PW. Evaluation of a district-wide screening programme for diabetic retinopathy utilizing trained optometrists using slit-lamp and Volk lenses. *Diabet Med* 2002;**19**(9):741–5.

47 Olson JA, Strachan FM, Hipwell JH, Goatman KA, McHardy KC, Forrester JV *et al.* A comparative evaluation of digital imaging, retinal photography and optometrist examination in screening for diabetic retinopathy. *Diabet Med* 2003;**20**(7): 528–34.

48 Sharp PF, Olson J, Strachan F, Hipwell J, Ludbrook A, O'Donnell M *et al.* The value of digital imaging in diabetic retinopathy. *Health Technol Assess* 2003;**7**(30):1–119.

49 Tu KL, Palimar P, Sen S, Mathew P, Khaleeli A. Comparison of optometry vs digital photography screening for diabetic retinopathy in a single district. *Eye* 2004;**18**(1):3–8.

50 Warburton TJ, Hale PJ, Dewhurst JA. Evaluation of a local optometric diabetic retinopathy screening service. *Diabet Med* 2004;**21**(6):632–5.

51 Kalm H, Egertsen R, Blohme G. Non-stereo fundus photography as a screening procedure for diabetic retinopathy among patients with type II diabetes. Compared with 60D enhanced slit-lamp examination. *Acta Ophthalmol (Copenh)* 1989;**67**(5):546–53.

52 Lee VS, Kingsley RM, Lee ET, Lu M, Russell D, Asal NR *et al.* The diagnosis of diabetic retinopathy. Ophthalmoscopy versus fundus photography. *Ophthalmology* 1993;**100**(10): 1504–12.

53 Schachat AP, Hyman L, Leske MC, Connell AM, Hiner C, Javornik N *et al.* Comparison of diabetic retinopathy detection by clinical examinations and photograph gradings. Barbados (West Indies) Eye Study Group. *Arch Ophthalmol* 1993;**111**(8):1064–70.

54 Aldington SJ, Kohner EM, Meuer SM, Klein R, Sjolie AK. Methodology for retinal photography and assessment of diabetic retinopathy: the EURODIAB IDDM Complications Study. *Diabetologia* 1995;**38**:437–44.

55 Kiri A, Dyer DS, Bressler NM, Bressler SB, Schachat AP. Detection of diabetic macular edema: Nidek 3Dx stereophotography compared with fundus biomicroscopy. *Am J Ophthalmol* 1996;**122**(5):654–62.

56 Taylor DJ, Fisher J, Jacob J, Tooke JE. The use of digital cameras in a mobile retinal screening environment. *Diabet Med* 1999;**16**(8):680–6.

57 Sensitivity and specificity of detection of diabetic maculopathy by a modified method. European Association for the Study of Diabetic Eye Complications (EASDec); 2000 26–28 May; Copenhagen, Denmark.

58 Moller F, Hansen M, Sjolie AK. Is one 60 degrees fundus photograph sufficient for screening of proliferative diabetic retinopathy? *Diabetes Care* 2001;**24**(12):2083–5.

59 Stellingwerf C, Hardus PL, Hooymans JM. Two-field photography can identify patients with vision-threatening diabetic retinopathy: a screening approach in the primary care setting. *Diabetes Care* 2001;**24**(12):2086–90.

60 Pandit RJ, Taylor R. Quality assurance in screening for sight-threatening diabetic retinopathy. *Diabet Med* 2002;**19**(4): 285–91.

61 Leese GP, Ahmed S, Newton RW, Jung RT, Ellingford A, Baines P *et al.* Use of mobile screening unit for diabetic retinopathy in rural and urban areas. *BMJ* 1993;**306**(6871):187–9.

62 Scanlon PH, Malhotra R, Thomas G, Foy C, Kirkpatrick JN, Lewis-Barned N *et al.* The effectiveness of screening for diabetic retinopathy by digital imaging photography and technician ophthalmoscopy. *Diabet Med* 2003;**20**(6):467–74.

63 Murgatroyd H, Ellingford A, Cox A, Binnie M, Ellis JD, MacEwen CJ *et al.* Effect of mydriasis and different field strategies on digital image screening of diabetic eye disease. *Br J Ophthalmol* 2004;**88**(7):920–4.

64 Scanlon PH, Foy C, Malhotra R, Aldington SJ. The influence of age, duration of diabetes, cataract, and pupil size on image quality in digital photographic retinal screening. *Diabetes Care* 2005;**28**(10):2448–53.

65 Facey K, Cummins E, Macpherson K, Morris A, Reay L, Slattery J. Organisation of Services for Diabetic Retinopathy Screening. Glasgow: Health Technology Board for Scotland, 2002:1–224.

66 Bursell SE, Cavallerano JD, Cavallerano AA, Clermont AC, Birkmire-Peters D, Aiello LP *et al.* Stereo nonmydriatic digital-video color retinal imaging compared with Early Treatment Diabetic Retinopathy Study seven standard field 35-mm stereo color photos for determining level of diabetic retinopathy. *Ophthalmology* 2001;**108**(3):572–85.

67 Lim JI, LaBree L, Nichols T, Cardenas I. A comparison of digital non mydriatic fundus imaging with standard 35-millimeter slides for diabetic retinopathy. *Ophthalmology* 2000;**107**(5):866–70.

68 Massin P, Erginay A, Ben Mehidi A, Vicaut E, Quentel G, Victor Z *et al.* Evaluation of a new non-mydriatic digital camera for detection of diabetic retinopathy. *Diabet Med* 2003;**20**(8):635–41.

69 Shiba T, Yamamoto T, Seki U, Utsugi N, Fujita K, Sato Y *et al.* Screening and follow-up of diabetic retinopathy using a new mosaic 9-field fundus photography system. *Diabetes Res Clin Pract* 2002;**55**(1):49–59.

70 Newsom R, Moate B, Casswell T. Screening for diabetic retinopathy using digital colour photography and oral fluorescein angiography. *Eye* 2000;**14** (Pt 4):579–82.

71 Razvi FM, Kritzinger EE, Tsaloumas MD, Ryder RE. Use of oral fluorescein angiography in the diagnosis of macular oedema within a diabetic retinopathy screening programme. *Diabet Med* 2001;**18**(12):1003–6.

72 Rudnisky CJ, Hinz BJ, Tennant MT, de Leon AR, Greve MD. High-resolution stereoscopic digital fundus photography versus contact lens biomicroscopy for the detection of clinically significant macular edema. *Ophthalmology* 2002;**109**(2): 267–74.

73 Scanlon PH, Malhotra R, Greenwood RH, Aldington SJ, Foy C, Flatman M *et al*. Comparison of two reference standards in validating two field mydriatic digital photography as a method of screening for diabetic retinopathy. *Br J Ophthalmol* 2003;**87**(10):1258–63.

74 Scanlon PH, Carter S, Foy C, Ratiram D, Harney B. An evaluation of the change in activity and workload arising from diabetic ophthalmology referrals following the introduction of a community based digital retinal photographic screening programme. *Br J Ophthalmol* 2005;**89**(8):971–5.

75 Williams GA, Scott IU, Haller JA, Maguire AM, Marcus D, McDonald HR. Single-field fundus photography for diabetic retinopathy screening: a report by the American Academy of Ophthalmology. *Ophthalmology* 2004;**111**(5):1055–62.

76 Chew EY. Screening options for diabetic retinopathy. *Curr Opin Ophthalmol* 2006;**17**(6):519–22.

77 Whited JD. Accuracy and reliability of teleophthalmology for diagnosing diabetic retinopathy and macular edema: a review of the literature. *Diabetes Technol Ther* 2006;**8**(1): 102–11.

78 Savolainen EA, Lee QP. Diabetic retinopathy – need and demand for photocoagulation and its cost-effectiveness: evaluation based on services in the United Kingdom. *Diabetologia* 1982;**23**(2):138–40.

79 Javitt JC, Canner JK, Sommer A. Cost effectiveness of current approaches to the control of retinopathy in type I diabetics. *Ophthalmology* 1989;**96**(2):255–64.

80 Fendrick AM, Javitt JC, Chiang YP. Cost-effectiveness of the screening and treatment of diabetic retinopathy. What are the costs of underutilization? *Int J Technol Assess Health Care* 1992;**8**(4):694–707.

81 Javitt JC, Aiello LP. Cost-effectiveness of detecting and treating diabetic retinopathy. *Ann Intern Med* 1996;**124**(1 Pt 2):164–9.

82 Dasbach EJ, Fryback DG, Newcomb PA, Klein R, Klein BE. Cost-effectiveness of strategies for detecting diabetic retinopathy. *Med Care* 1991;**29**(1):20–39.

83 Caro JJ, Ward AJ, O'Brien JA. Lifetime costs of complications resulting from type 2 diabetes in the U.S. *Diabetes Care* 2002;**25**(3):476–81.

84 Nystrom L, Dahlquist G, Ostman J, Wall S, Arnqvist H, Blohme G *et al*. Risk of developing insulin-dependent diabetes mellitus (IDDM) before 35 years of age: indications of climatological determinants for age at onset. *Int J Epidemiol* 1992;**21**(2):352–8.

85 Mellanby A, Milner R. Reducing the interval for diabetic retinal screening. Development and Evaluation Committee Report No.107. Southampton: Wessex Institue for Health Research and Development, 1999:1–45.

86 James M, Turner DA, Broadbent DM, Vora J, Harding SP. Cost effectiveness analysis of screening for sight threatening diabetic eye disease. *BMJ* 2000;**320**(7250):1627–31.

87 Meads C, Hyde C. What is the cost of blindness? *Br J Ophthalmol* 2003;**87**(10):1201–4.

88 Wright SE, Keeffe JE, Thies LS. Direct costs of blindness in Australia. *Clin Experiment Ophthalmol* 2000;**28**(3):140–2.

89 Bjorvig S, Johansen MA, Fossen K. An economic analysis of screening for diabetic retinopathy. *J Telemed Telecare* 2002;**8**(1):32–5.

90 Garvican L, Clowes J, Gillow T. Preservation of sight in diabetes: developing a national risk reduction programme. *Diabet Med* 2000;**17**(9):627–34.

91 Gillow JT, Gray JA. The National Screening Committee review of diabetic retinopathy screening. *Eye* 2001;**15**(Pt 1): 1–2.

92 Garvican L. Resources required for a local service in the national diabetic retinopathy screening programme: English National Screening Programme. http://www.nscretinopathy.org.uk, 2004.

Stage R0: the normal eye

Stephen J. Aldington

THE RELEVANT ANATOMY OF THE EYE

The human eye is an organ which is an extension of the brain. Its function is to convert light stimulations which occur at wavelengths (colours) that humans can detect into electrical neurological impulses and to transmit these to specialized portions of the brain so as to generate an 'image'. Of course most people have two eyes, generally pointing forwards, so in good health the two eyes work together to form a single full-colour detailed image comprising elements of shape, pattern, colour, tone and movement with which we are all, as adults, familiar. Our two eyes also give us the ability to 'see' depth and work out distances; essential in so many aspects of our daily lives. The eye is, however, a delicate organ. Whilst it is generally well protected, to essentially operate it has to protrude slightly out from the safety of the human body and so present its own beautiful manifestation, visible to the world at large. As such it also affords us, the viewer, an opportunity to look in onto the actual workings of the eye and indeed onto a representation of the workings of the body in health and disease.

The eye is an approximate globe, averaging 23 mm in horizontal and vertical diameters and 22–24 mm in axial length in emmetropes (normal-sighted persons). Long-sighted persons (hypermetropes) have slightly shorter eyeballs, whilst those with short-sightedness (myopes) are correspondingly slightly longer. As a primary function of the eye is to bring light rays into sharp focus onto the retina (the inside surface of the eye), short- or long-sighted people usually need the help of a pair of spectacles to achieve this. With the assistance of spectacles if required, most of us can see perfectly well and clearly.

A Practical Manual of Diabetic Retinopathy Management.
Peter H Scanlon, Charles P Wilkinson, Stephen J Aldington and David R Matthews. Published 2009 by Blackwell Publishing, ISBN 978-1-4051-7035-2.

The eyeball basically consists of three concentric major layers of tissue which in their anterior aspect are transparent like a window to allow the passage of light through them. The posterior, by far the major portion of the globe, is filled with a normally transparent collagen jelly, the vitreous humour. This also permits the passage of light. The innermost surface of the eye, the retina, contains specialized photoreceptor cells which when light falls onto them, encode and transmit signals to the brain to convert the complex light stimuli into recognizable images (Fig. 5.1).

The outermost layer of most of the eye is the tough protective 'white' of the eye, the sclera. At the front of the eye this outermost layer has developed to be completely transparent (in health) and forms the cornea. Inside the sclera and hence not visible from the outside is the uveal layer which posteriorly comprises the choroid, a large and highly vascular bed, and anteriorly the ciliary body and iris (which is visible from outside). Within the choroid is the innermost major layer, the retina, containing the actual photoreceptors. Lying between the choroid and the retina are the very thin Bruch's membrane and the pigment epithelium, both essential for normal retinal function. The choroid itself contains three vascular layers, the vessels in which get progressively smaller as the retina is approached. The retina also actually comprises several discrete layers, the details of which will be discussed later as they have relevance to many aspects of the development and presentation of diabetic eye disease.

Moving anteriorly, the ciliary body and its processes responsible for production of aqueous humour, lies with its inner surface in contact with the vitreous humour, its outer surface contacting the sclera and forming a ring encircling the iris. The iris is internally separated from the cornea by the anterior chamber and from the lens of the eye immediately behind it by the much shallower posterior chamber. The iris edge effectively rests on the anterior surface of the lens capsule. Both chambers are filled with aqueous humour, balanced through posterior outflow

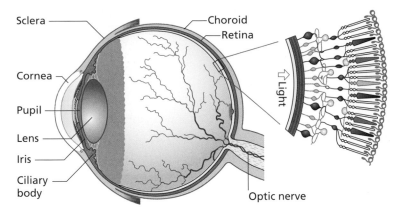

Fig. 5.1 Cross-section of the eye and major structures.

from the anterior chamber, through the trabecular mesh-work and canal of Schlemm to connect to the aqueous and scleral veins.

Through contraction of the circular and relaxation of the radial elements of the ciliary muscles, the eye causes the iris to expand and advance inwards towards the centre, diminishing the size of or constricting the apparent central pupil. This has the joint effect of limiting the amount of light falling on the retina and of increasing the depth of field of the optical viewing system (equivalent to 'stopping down' a camera lens). Conversely, through contraction of radial and relaxation of circular elements, the iris recedes outwards, enlarging or dilating the central pupil. This can be achieved either through normal reflex reaction in reduced light levels, or through pharmacological intervention, intentionally when desired or accidentally.

Moving backwards again but on the visual axis, the crystalline lens, lying within an elastic capsule, is situated between the iris elements and the vitreous body and is suspended on a series of radial suspensory ligaments (the zonule), which through contraction or relaxation control the shape and thickness of the lens they encircle. This affords the ability to finely focus light entering the eye onto the retina.

Moving further backwards along the visual axis through the vitreous, we encounter the retina. The retina is in intimate contact with and surrounds the vitreous outer surface layer, the posterior hyaloid (or internal limiting) membrane, and represents over 70% of the inside of the globe's surface. Normally largely transparent, the retina contains the light-sensitive photoreceptor elements of the eye along with an active blood supply clearly visible by means of investigative techniques which illuminate and view the inside of the globe. The retina varies in thickness

from approximately 0.1 mm (100 μm) in the periphery to over 0.6 mm (600 μm) at its thickest in the central regions of the posterior pole.

On viewing the retina through the central pupil formed by the iris, the most apparent object is the yellow head of the optic nerve, the optic disc. This slightly off-centred feature with its associated pattern of radiating arteries and veins represents the point at which the major retinal blood supply enters and leaves the eye and provides the termination point for the eye's neurosensory nerve fibres to coalesce and leave the eye for communication with the brain (Fig. 5.2a).

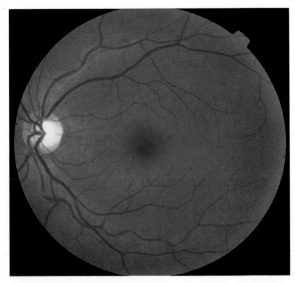

(a)

Fig. 5.2 (a) Basic retinal appearance on examination of the left macula. (*Continued on p. 60*)

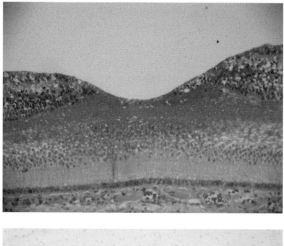

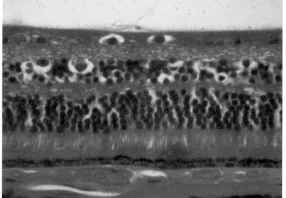

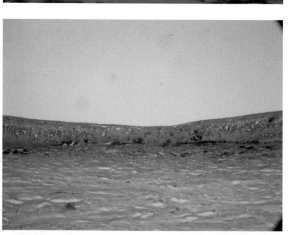

Fig. 5.2 (*Cont'd*) (b) Normal human fovea. This slide shows the inner and outer nuclear cell layers at the edge of the fovea and the concentration of cones centrally. (c) The receptive retina. This slide shows the ganglion cell layer, the bipolar layer, the nuclei of the cones and rods, the pigment epithelium and the choroid. (d) Gliosis of the retina following laser treatment.

Lying approximately 3.5 mm temporal to the optic disc and close to the optical axis of the eye and exactly on its visual axis is the fovea and the surrounding macular region. The macula, about 1.5–2 mm across, represents the area containing (yellow) macular luteine pigment. The <1 mm foveal region is characterized by its high concentration of cone photoreceptors and much lower concentrations of rod receptors as compared to the retinal periphery (correspondingly where cones are less frequent). Cones provide the colour vision capabilities of the human eye and increasing acuity capability as the visual axis is approached.

Within the central foveola, 200–250 μm in diameter and devoid of rods, the cones themselves within this region are narrower and tightly packed into a complex hexagonal pattern (Fig. 5.2b–d).

The majority of the retina, excepting the central foveal region, is provided with nourishment, oxygen and its waste-product removal system by means of the retinal vascular circulation. The central retinal artery, branching into the major and more minor arterioles, leads to a capillary network (invisible to the naked eye), then through the minor and then more major venules and veins eventually to the central retinal vein which leaves the eye down the centre of the optic nerve and provides the major retinal circulation.

In the foveal region, however, where high acuity and accurate colour perception are required, no extraneous objects such as blood vessels exist within the retinal layers. The foveola is responsible for the highest acuity capabilities associated with reading, detailed working, driving etc. The central foveal region is thinner (approximately 150–250 μm thick) and importantly and uniquely is devoid of retinal blood supply, essential supply being provided through diffusion from the capillaries of the innermost vascular layer of underlying choroid through the intimate contact with the retinal pigment epithelium. By this means, light being 'focused' at or around the fovea will not be adversely affected by any retinal structures or blood vessels before its presentation to the densely packed foveal cone photoreceptors.

The blood vessels in the retina, like those in the brain and much of the central nervous system, exhibit tight junctions between adjacent cells. This is important, as it largely prevents leakage of blood components, fluids, chemicals or drugs (endogenous or exogenous) through the retinal blood vessel wall and hence maintains the aptly termed *blood–retinal barrier* formed by both the tight junctions in retinal cell walls and those in the unilayer retinal pigment epithelium (RPE) immediately outside the retina. The RPE is itself supported by the adjacent layer of Bruch's membrane; damage to which is frequently manifest as (amongst other things) drusen and ultimately as age-related macular degeneration (ARMD) with its associated visual loss.

The cells of the choroidal circulation, however, are quite different from those in the retina in that they are essentially designed to have small gaps (fenestrations) between the cells in the walls of smaller choroidal vessels. These fenestrations allow transport of essential nutrients and other small molecules and hence support the nutrition and oxygenation of the foveal region by the underlying choriocapillaris through the RPE (Fig. 5.3).

THE PHOTOGRAPHIC APPEARANCE

On examination the normal adult human retina appears as an orange-red (Caucasian) or green-red (Indian Asian and Caribbean) mottled layer bearing a series of branching retinal blood vessels which originate from the near-circular yellow-white head of the optic nerve or optic disc as it enters/leaves the eye and spread across the entire visible retinal surface (Fig. 5.4).

Retinal examination in juveniles and young adults frequently shows there to be a very distinct and bright reflection across and surrounding the entire macular

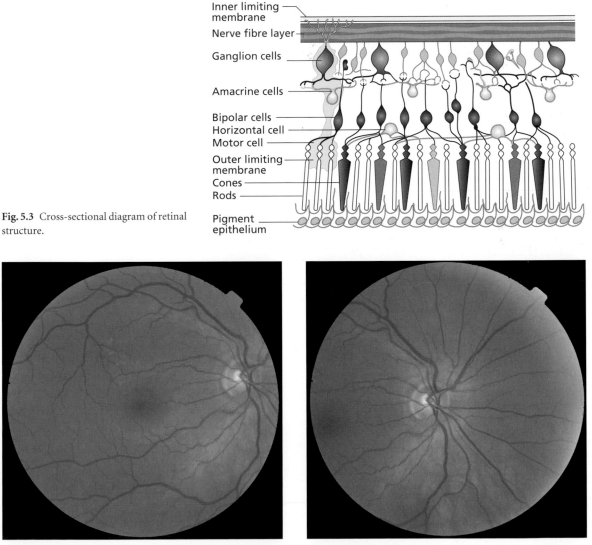

Fig. 5.3 Cross-sectional diagram of retinal structure.

Inner limiting membrane
Nerve fibre layer
Ganglion cells
Amacrine cells
Bipolar cells
Horizontal cell
Motor cell
Outer limiting membrane
Cones
Rods
Pigment epithelium

(a)

(b)

Fig. 5.4 (a) Normal Caucasian retinal appearance: right macular view. (b) Normal Caucasian retinal appearance: right nasal view (disc centred). (*Continued on p. 62*)

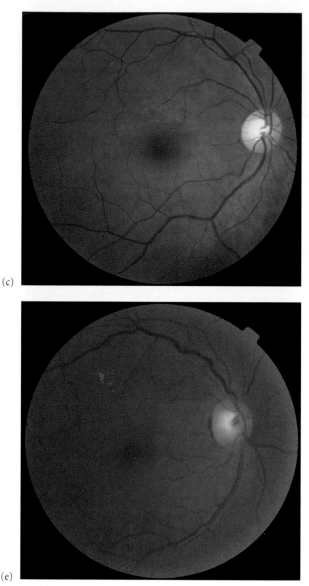

(c)

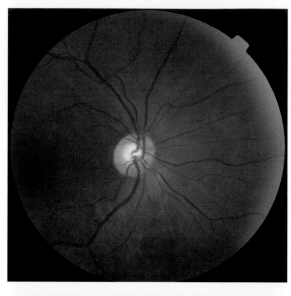

(d)

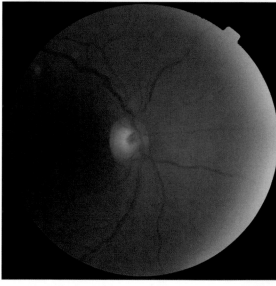

(e)

(f)

Fig. 5.4 (*Cont'd*) (c) Normal Asian Indian retinal appearance: right macular view. (d) Normal Asian Indian retinal appearance: right nasal view (disc centred). (e) Normal Caribbean retinal appearance: right macular view. (f) Normal Caribbean retinal appearance: right nasal view (disc centred).

region (Fig. 5.5). This is a feature of light from the examination equipment (usually a fundus camera) hitting the highly reflective interface between the back surface of the vitreous body (the posterior hyaloid) and the inner surface of the retina which then bounces straight back to the viewer/recording medium. This often makes accurate assessment of the macular region in these people quite difficult as the high reflectivity masks much of the underlying pathology. In such cases multiple images, taken with slightly different angles onto the macula, are recommended.

Examination of the right eye shows the yellow-white or sometimes pinkish coloured optic disc as lying to the right of (i.e. nasal to) the darker coloured macular region, itself demarcated by the superior and inferior retinal vessel 'arcades' curving respectively above and below the macula. The centre of the macula is slightly darker still

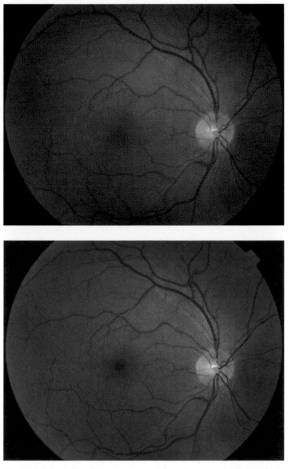

(a)

(b)

Fig. 5.6 Nerve fibre layer patterns: (a) right macular view colour photograph; (b) right macular view, red-free photograph.

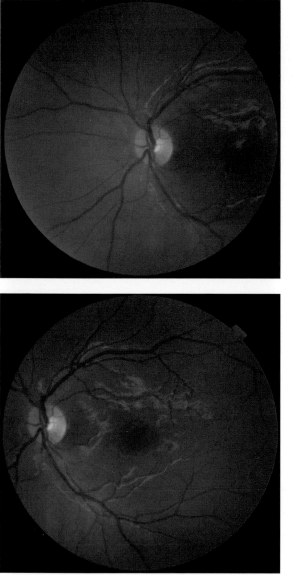

(a)

(b)

Fig. 5.5 Image of young person's retina showing posterior hyaloid reflections – there are also some mild changes of diabetic retinopathy. (a) left nasal view; (b) left macular view.

in colour, often appearing dark grey and represents the foveal region in which pigmentation is densest.

The temporal vessel arcades meet lateral to the macular region at a point on the horizontal meridian of the globe. Whilst the retinal blood vessels supplying the temporal aspect of the eye are formed as curving arcades, vessels supplying the nasal portions of the eye leave the optic disc and traverse the retina in straighter, less deviating patterns.

The overall pattern of the visible retinal vessels is the same as that for the usually invisible retinal nerve fibres; temporally the nerve fibres follow the curved arcades to meet laterally beyond the macular region whilst nasally they radiate straight out towards the periphery (Figs 5.6 & 5.7).

The major retinal artery and vein usually enter and leave the eye at a point which lies slightly towards the nasal aspect of the optic disc, i.e. slightly further away from the fovea than the centre of the disc. At or around the surface of the optic disc, the central retinal artery bifurcates into two branches, and then before reaching the outer margin of the optic disc each again branches to form the four major retinal artery branches serving the superior temporal, superior nasal, inferior nasal and inferior temporal quadrants of the retina. These are usually geographically followed by the retinal veins, which, as they return from

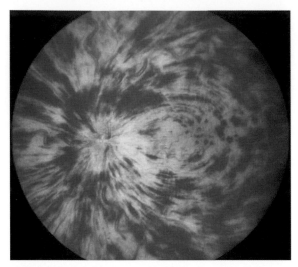

Fig. 5.7 Nerve fibre layer patterns. This image from a patient who has had a left central retinal vein thrombosis with haemorrhages under the nerve fibre layer clearly shows the pattern of the nerve fibre layer.

the retinal periphery to the optic disc, sequentially join to form the four retinal quadrant venous branches before finally forming the central retinal vein leaving the eye.

Retinal veins and arteries generally alternate around the circumference of the optic disc, veins generally having larger diameters than the corresponding retinal artery at that point and are slightly darker in colour. Whilst both veins and arteries can display a central light 'reflex' along their length, constant or interrupted, which is literally a reflection of the illuminating light source from the top-most surface of the circular vessel, this is more usually apparent from arteries. It is important to note that this normal light reflex from vessels is quite common and must not be confused with threading or white-lining of vessels, which is a feature of vessel occlusion in advanced disease states.

Normal, non-diseased retinal blood vessels can be seen to evenly and gradually reduce in diameter as they are followed away from the optic nerve head and out towards the retinal periphery. This is a typical form of vascular bed with decreasing diameters of arterioles down to the level of the capillary bed, followed by increasing diameters of venules and veins. Assessment of changes in vessel calibre, locally or generally, can be a crucial indicator of advanced or progressing retinal vascular disease and damage.

The areas of retina lying between retinal vessels are, in the absence of disease, generally relatively featureless and are reasonably homogenous in colour and pattern. It is not common to see individual vessels within these areas, as capillaries in the normal eye are too fine to be seen on colour images or by direct examination of the retina.

It is, however, quite normal and common to see variously sized predominantly greenish or darker-coloured striations within the areas between major vessels. These are vessels of the underlying and major choroidal circulation, visible as indistinct 'shapes' through the pigment epithelium and retina. The lighter skinned the patient, and hence the lighter the retinal pigment epithelium, the more apparent can be the choroidal vessels when viewing the retina. Albino and even blond patients can have extremely apparent choroidal vessels. It tends not to be possible to see the choroidal vessels of dark-skinned and heavily pigmented individuals. Very highly myopic patients usually have thin retinae and RPE, and in these cases it is sometimes possible to clearly see the white sclera.

Historically, permanent photographic recording of retinal appearance was carried out by means of colour transparency (diapositive) films. During the late 1990s and into the 21st century, colour film recording has been almost if not entirely replaced by digital image recording. Amongst the many advantages of digital imaging (discussions on which are largely beyond the remit of this publication), a most significant aspect relates to the ability to simply select and view individual colour 'channels' of the image. This allows examination of the 'normal' retinal appearance across differential 'slices' of the colour spectrum generated by the retinal camera illumination flash source and recorded by the digital imaging sensor. As such, the 'red-free' and 'green' image, which potentially provide much useful additional information, are routinely available without additional image recording.

FLUORESCEIN ANGIOGRAPHY

Fluorescein principles and techniques

Whilst the apparently disease-free or complication-free retina, when clinically examined or investigated using colour imaging may display no or few visible defects, dynamic fluorescein angiography can yield significant and at times dramatic and crucial additional information. Retinal fluorescein angiography, though invasive and not without risk,[1] remains a vitally important investigative tool in assessment[2] of diabetic retinal (and other) disease. For retinal angiography the patient being studied should ideally have well fixed and dilated pupils, and they must consent to having a needle inserted into a suitable superficial arm vein around the antecubital fossa, through which a 5, 10 or 20% dilute solution of sodium fluorescein in aqueous suspension will be injected. Whilst injection techniques vary, for investigating diabetic retinopathy it is usual to deliver the 2–5 mL injection as a quick or relatively quick (2–6 s) bolus to allow generation of a sufficiently strong 'dye front' to facilitate enhanced viewing of the early and mid-phases of the angiogram.

Fluorescein angiography is carried out using a retinal fundus camera producing monochromatic (filtered) light of around 490 nm (blue) wavelength as the retinal illumination source and a green 520–530 nm passing filter to block all extraneous blue light and only pass the fluorescent emission element. As such, it is normal practice to record and present the results of fluorescein angiography as black-and-white images. These have the added advantage (generally) of also being higher contrast and resolution than full-colour images.

The injected fluorescein sodium salt preparation is water soluble (unlike fluorescein itself) and also quickly starts to bind to and be absorbed by plasma proteins. Eventually it is almost totally metabolized[3] to fluorescein glucuronide, so as to be suitable for urinary excretion. It thereby loses its ability to fluoresce over time both through natural extinction and due to the lower (12–15%) fluorescence of the glucuronide than that of the unmetabolized sodium salt. This gives rise to the normally observed phenomenon of intense fluorescein 'activity' at the start of the investigation, steadily reducing in intensity as the investigation progresses, to a point where only those remaining non-quenched and unbound sodium fluorescein molecules which have caused staining to any abnormal retinal and vessel structures remain visible. Whilst the patient's skin, sclera and most vital bodily fluids are after 30–60 min completely and intensely stained with the residual yellow fluorescein metabolites, the structures of the normal eye are free of fluorescent markers or staining. Any that remain visible are due to diseased or damaged structures.

A summary of the normal course of timing of fluorescein events is:

0 s	injection of fluorescein into arm
6–10 s	choroidal flush (prearterial phase)
8–12 s	arterial stage
12–15 s	maximum capillary transition stage
15–20 s	early venous stage (lamellar or early arteriovenous stage)
20–40 s	venous stage (late arteriovenous stage)
3–10 min	late staining
30–60 min	little residual retinal appearance (except in disease).

These figures presume that the 5 mL 10–20% fluorescein injection is delivered as a bolus (less than 5 s) into the antecubital fossa site and that the patient has no significant circulatory disease preventing free and normal flow. Use of a more peripheral and hence smaller arm or a hand vein will cause a prolongation of arm-to-eye transit time, as will impaired cardiac output and any form of constriction of the arm (such as pressing against the camera structures), or any constrictions to the ocular blood supply.

Angiography images are less susceptible than are colour images to errors caused by camera artefacts and to confusion caused by variations in retinal pigmentation (with provisos). In general, the darker the patient's skin and RPE pigmentation, the higher the contrast displayed in the fluorescein angiogram, as light from the choroidal circulation is effectively masked by the RPE. Fair-skinned and fair-haired patients with little pigmentation have considerable choroidal show-through on angiography.

Normal fluorescein appearance

High-quality fluorescein angiography will not only reveal the vascular system visible in colour images but also delineate and permit the examination of ocular vessels as small as individual retinal capillaries. No other currently available truly objective external imaging system affords this opportunity. The closest alternative is the so-called *blue-field (or light) entoptic*[4] technique or Scheerer's phenomenon[5] wherein a person can visualize a shadowgraphic appearance of their own pulsatile leukocytes as they traverse the perifoveal capillary network. This is however highly subjective, rather non-reproducible and is not independently recordable or verifiable.

For capillaries to be visible on an angiogram:

1 the imaging system must have sufficient resolution and power
2 the patient's ocular media must be sufficiently clear and it must be possible to achieve accurate focus on retinal structures
3 the imaging technique and methodology must be exemplary
4 the fluorescein injection must be given so as to provide a sufficient dye-front
5 darker pigmentation means better capillary contrast.

The fluorescein angiogram shown in Figs 5.8–5.15 is from a non-diabetic patient and shows a midcapillary phase image. Arteries remain filled, veins have recently filled and the contrast between the perifoveal capillaries and the underlying RPE is at its greatest. The foveal

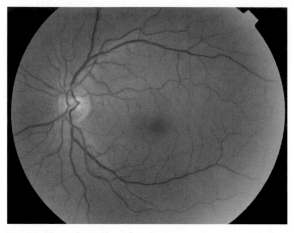

Fig. 5.8 Normal macular colour image.

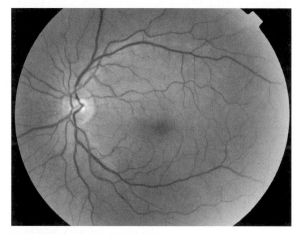

Fig. 5.9 Normal macular red-free image.

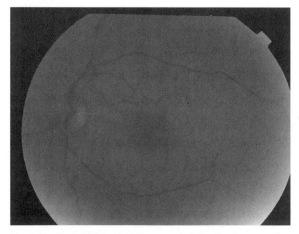

Fig. 5.10 Choroidal flush with very early filling in arteries at 13 s after injection.

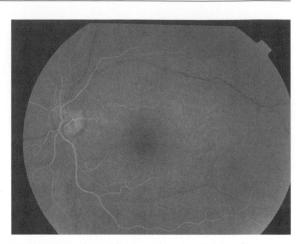

Fig. 5.11 Retinal arterial stage with very early signs of fluorescein in veins at 16 s after injection.

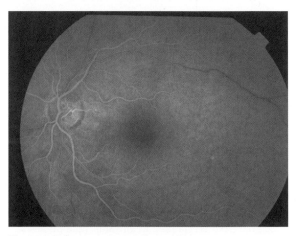

Fig. 5.12 Early arteriovenous phase at 20 s.

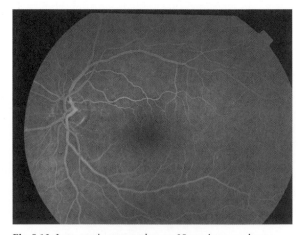

Fig. 5.13 Late arteriovenous phase at 25 s: veins now almost completely full.

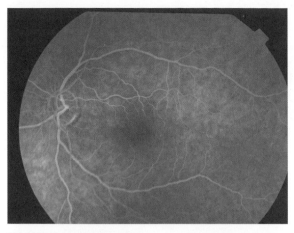

Fig. 5.14 Venous phase at 53 s.

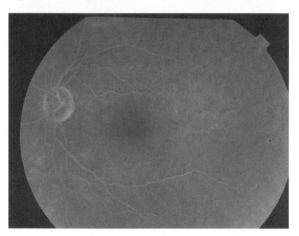

Fig. 5.15 Late venous phase at 4 min.

avascular zone (FAZ) can clearly be seen in the centre of the image, showing the slight diffuse central mottling in the fovea, associated with the masked choroidal fluorescence, the clearly delineated capillary encircling the FAZ and a normal capillary network distribution outside of this.

Abnormal fluorescein distribution

Hypofluorescence
- Transmission defect (retinal or preretinal blood, pigment, hard exudates etc.).
- Filling defect (circulation abnormality).

Hyperfluorescence
- Window defect (RPE defect).
- Leakage of dye (retinal new vessels or subretinal neovascular membrane).
- Staining of retinal structures (damaged blood vessels, drusen).
- Fluorescein pooling (retinal or RPE detachments).
- Autofluorescence (disc drusen).

NORMAL OCT APPEARANCE

Optical coherence tomography (OCT) has provided ophthalmologists with depth resolution in imaging the diabetic retina only previously possible in post-mortem histological slides (Figs 5.16–5.19). This technique is described in the Introduction and in the section on technological advances in imaging in Chapter 15.

(a)

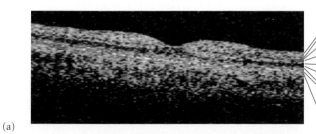 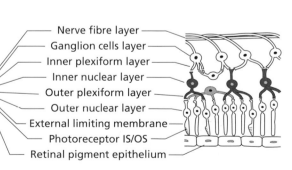

Nerve fibre layer
Ganglion cells layer
Inner plexiform layer
Inner nuclear layer
Outer plexiform layer
Outer nuclear layer
External limiting membrane
Photoreceptor IS/OS
Retinal pigment epithelium

Fig. 5.16 (a) Diagram to show the OCT layers. (*Continued on p. 68*)

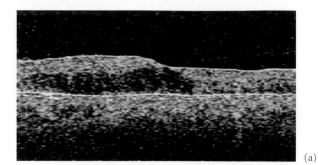

(b)

(a)

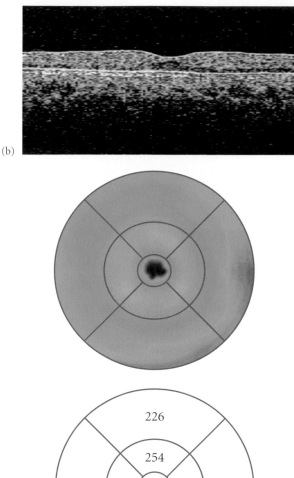

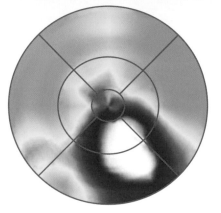

(c)

268

305

274 310 382 357 282

461

397

Microns

(b)

226

254

227 254 201 248 210

251

212

Microns

Fig. 5.16 (*Cont'd*) (b) Normal OCT appearance. (c) Topographical map of normal eye.

Fig. 5.18 (a) OCT appearance of diabetic macular oedema. (b) Topographical map of same patient with clinically significant macular oedema.

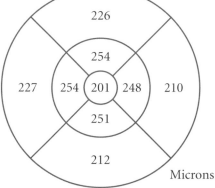

Fig. 5.17 OCT appearance of macular hole.

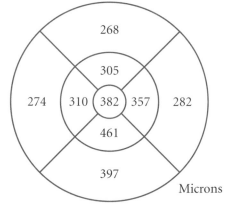

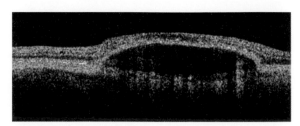

Fig. 5.19 OCT appearance of pigment epithelial detachment.

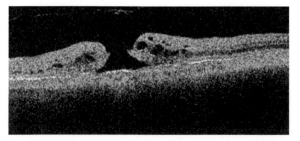

ELECTRORETINOGRAPHY

A review by Parisi[6] reported that people with type 1 diabetes show electrophysiological abnormalities of the visual system which are revealed by methods such as flash electroretinogram (FERG), oscillatory potentials (OPs), pattern electroretinogram (PERG), focal electroretinogram (focal ERG) and visual evoked potentials (VEPs) in basal condition and after photostress.

Multifocal electroretinography (mfERG) is an imaging technique that is based on the principle of electroretinography (or VEPs), which involves stimulating areas of the retina using an electrical signal and mapping the response. The resulting images are of higher resolution than electroretinography and stimulation of multiple spots simultaneously is possible, hence producing a changing pattern which gives greater diagnostic information.

Multifocal ERG is currently used as a research tool and is not in general clinical use. Bearse[7] has described the use of multifocal ERG to predict, quantitatively, the retinal locations of new nonproliferative diabetic retinopathy development over a 1-year period.

PRACTICE POINT

- The uniqueness of appearance and layout of each individual's retinal vasculature is both a blessing and a curse. Whilst it certainly affords opportunities for high-level biometric security systems based on retinal vascular pattern analysis, it also indicates the immensely wide range of parameters which must be taken into account when defining an eye as being 'normal'. As such, more correctly, the term normal eye (or patient) should be considered to be that which is not displaying or manifesting the particular characteristic or disease under study or investigation.

REFERENCES

1 Morris P. Fluorescein sodium and indocyanine green: uses and side-effects. In: Saine P, Tyler M, eds. *Ophthalmic Photography: a Textbook of Retinal Photography, Angiography and Electronic Imaging.* Boston: Butterworth-Heinemann, 1997: 117–46.

2 Saine P, Tyler M. (eds) Fluorescein angiography: instrumentation and technique. In: *Ophthalmic Photography: a Textbook of Retinal Photography, Angiography and Electronic Imaging.* Boston: Butterworth-Heinemann, 1997: 147–67.

3 Chahal PS, Neal MJ, Kohner EM. Metabolism of fluorescein after intravenous administration. *Invest Ophthalmol Vis Sci* 1985; **26**(5): 764–8.

4 Sinclair SH, Azar-Cavanagh M, Soper KA, Tuma RF, Mayrovitz HN. Investigation of the source of the blue field entoptic phenomenon. *Invest Ophthalmol Vis Sci* 1989; **30**(4): 668–73.

5 Scheerer R. Die entoptische Sichtbarkeit der Blutbewegungen im Auge und ihre klinische Bedeutung (in German). *Klinisches Monatsblatt Augenheilkunde* 1924; **73**: 67–107.

6 Parisi V, Uccioli L. Visual electrophysiological responses in persons with type 1 diabetes. *Diabetes Metab Res Rev* 2001; **17**(1): 12–18.

7 Bearse MAJ, Adams AJ, Han Y, Schneck ME, Ng J, Bronson-Castain K *et al.* A multifocal electroretinogram model predicting the development of diabetic retinopathy. *Prog Retin Eye Res* 2006; **25**(5): 425–48.

Stage M1: maculopathy

Peter H. Scanlon

Diabetic maculopathy may be classified into focal (sub-divided into focal exudates and focal/multifocal oedema), diffuse and ischaemic types.

FOCAL MACULOPATHY (Figs 6.1–6.3)

In focal maculopathy, focal leakage tends to occur from microaneurysms, often with extravascular lipoprotein in a circinate pattern around the focal leakage.[1]

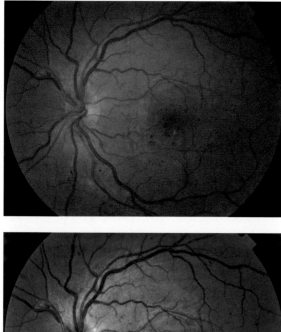

(a)

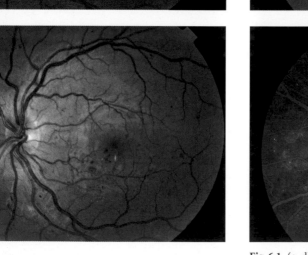

(b)

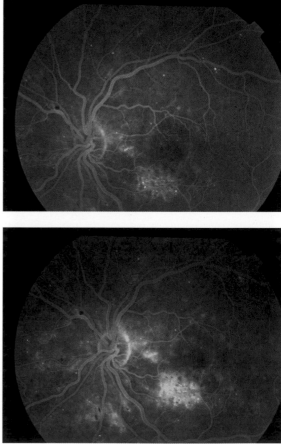

(c)

(d)

Fig. 6.1 (a–d) Focal maculopathy: colour and fluorescein photographs.

A Practical Manual of Diabetic Retinopathy Management.
Peter H Scanlon, Charles P Wilkinson, Stephen J Aldington and David R Matthews. Published 2009 by Blackwell Publishing, ISBN 978-1-4051-7035-2.

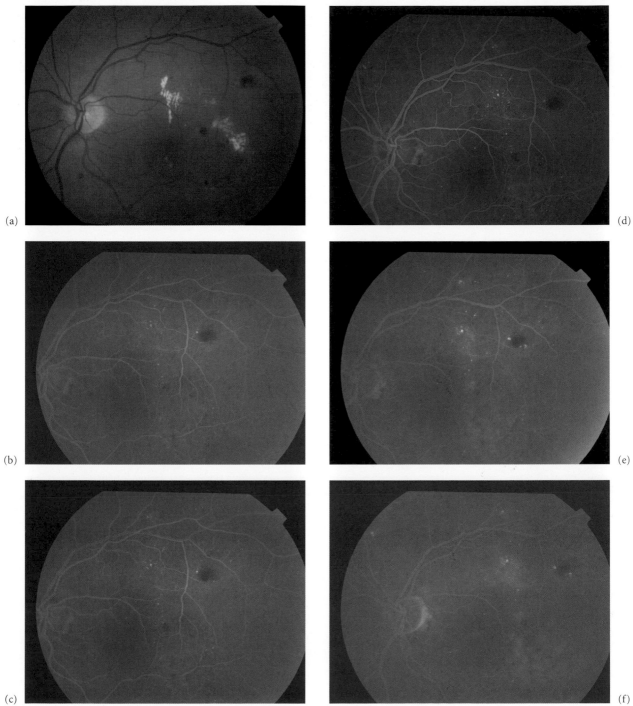

Fig. 6.2 (a–f) Focal maculopathy: colour and fluorescein photographs.

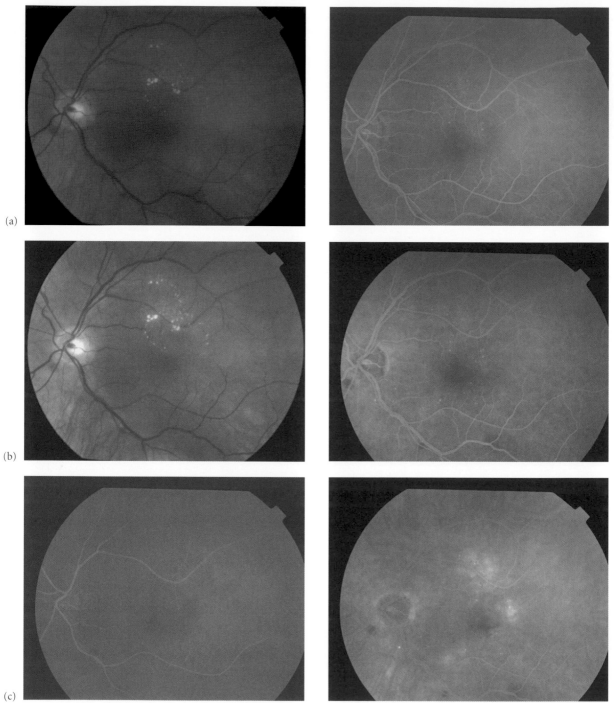

Fig. 6.3 (a–f) Focal maculopathy: colour and fluorescein photographs.

DIFFUSE MACULOPATHY (Fig. 6.4)

In the diffuse variety there is a generalized breakdown of the blood–retina barrier and profuse early leakage from the entire capillary bed of the posterior pole[2] often accompanied by cystoid macular changes.[1] As well as considering laser treatment it is important to consider correction of systemic abnormalities such as hypertension and severe fluid retention.

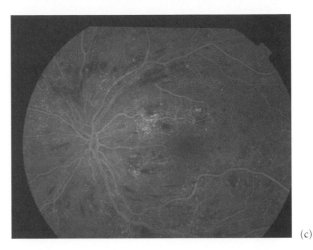

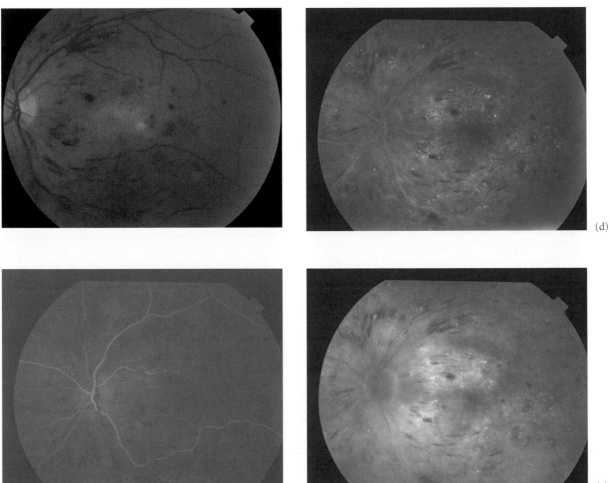

Fig. 6.4 (a–e) Diffuse maculopathy: colour and fluorescein photographs.

ISCHAEMIC MACULOPATHY (Fig. 6.5)

In ischaemic maculopathy, enlargement of the foveal avascular zone (FAZ) due to capillary closure is found but may not have any visual consequences. Extensive capillary and arteriolar closure is more serious and more commonly associated with visual loss. In ischaemic maculopathy it is particularly important to treat systemic hypertension.

OPTICAL COHERENCE TOMOGRAPHY

Optical coherence tomography (OCT) has an increasing role to play in the assessment and monitoring of patients with diabetic macular oedema. The development of OCT has been described in the Introduction. Examples are shown in Figs 6.6 and 6.7(a,b).

Macular traction can also occur from contracture of fibrotic proliferations, particularly as new vessels regress after panretinal photocoagulation, and also from a taut posterior hyaloid. If macular traction is severe, surgical intervention is required (see Fig. 6.7c,d).

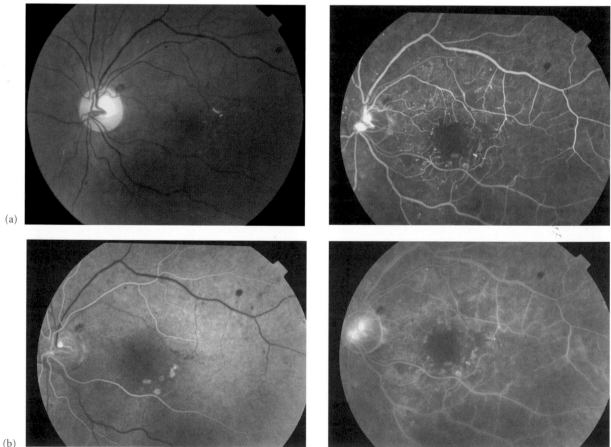

(a)

(b)

(c)

(d)

Fig. 6.5 (a–d) Ischaemic maculopathy: colour and fluorescein photographs.

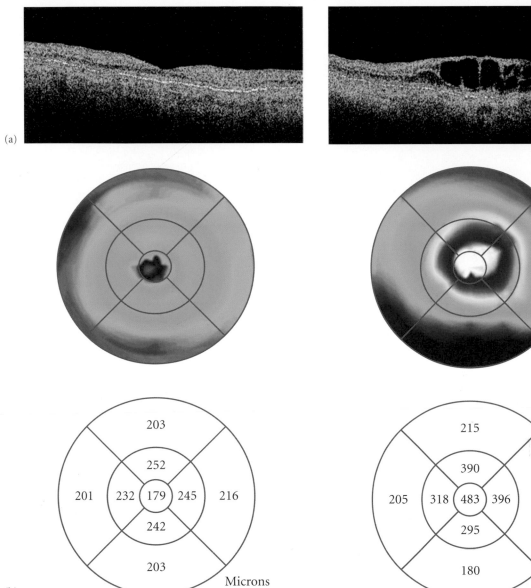

(a)

(a)

(b)

Fig. 6.6 (a) Normal OCT. (b) Normal tomographic map.

Fig. 6.7 (a) OCT of clinically significant macular oedema (CSMO). (b) Tomographic map of CSMO. (*Continued on p. 76*)

(*Continued on p. 76*)

(b)

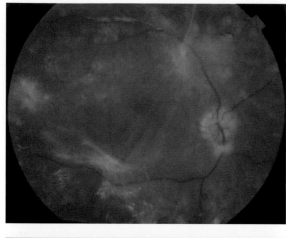

(c)

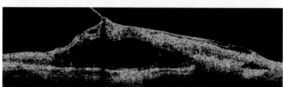

(d)

Fig. 6.7 (*Cont'd*) (c) Colour photograph of regressed fibrous proliferations following PRP causing macular traction. (d) OCT of macular traction.

TREATMENT OF ASSOCIATED RISK FACTORS

Systemic hypertension

The importance of good blood pressure control on the progression of diabetic retinopathy is explained in the diabetes section of this book (Chapter 2).

CASE HISTORY 1
Hypertension in diabetic maculopathy

This 39-year-old man (BMI 21) presented as an emergency admission under the physicians with symptoms of tiredness, weight loss and blurring of vision. On admission his blood glucose was 20.7 mmol/L, HbA1c 13.7% and blood pressure 220/109. He gave a 1-year history of symptoms including neuropathic symptoms in his feet, which made it more likely that he had type 2 diabetes. He had a strong family history of diabetes in his father, maternal grandmother and two maternal uncles. He was commenced on insulin during this admission. When he was seen in the eye department his visual acuity (VA) was

found to be right 6/36 (20/180), left 6/18 (20/60). Red-free photographs and a fluorescein angiogram show haemorrhages and extensive signs of ischaemia in both macular areas, but also ischaemic signs in the peripheral retinal areas, particularly the left nasal retina where signs of severe IRMA are shown (Fig. 6.8a–i).

The hypertension was treated with ramipril 10 mg daily, and lacidipine 4 mg and furosemide 20 mg and dixasocin MR 4 mg were subsequently added. His other medications were actrapid 10 + 10 + 12 units, insulatard 18 units, simvastatin 40 mg and aspirin 75 mg.

Six months after presentation, his blood pressure had improved to 122/75 and HbA1c to 6.8%, but his VA had remained the same in his right eye at 6/36 (20/120) and deteriorated in his left to 6/60 (20/200). A decision was made to treat both eyes with panretinal photocoagulation.

The left eye was treated first:
- 2518 burns of 350-micron size, power 250–290 mW, duration 0.1 s, transequatorial lens (magnification factor 1.44), argon laser.

The right eye was then treated:
- 2331 burns of 350-micron size, power 210–260 mW, duration 0.1 s, transequatorial lens (magnification factor 1.44), argon laser.
- One year after presentation, a small area of leakage in the left macular area was treated with 16 burns, 100-micron size, 230 mW, 0.1 s, area centralis lens, argon laser.

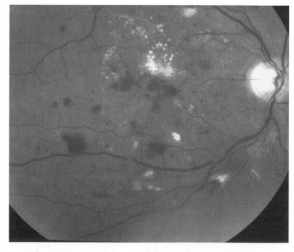

(a)

Fig. 6.8 Case history 1. (a–m) Hypertension and diabetic maculopathy. (*Continued on facing page*)

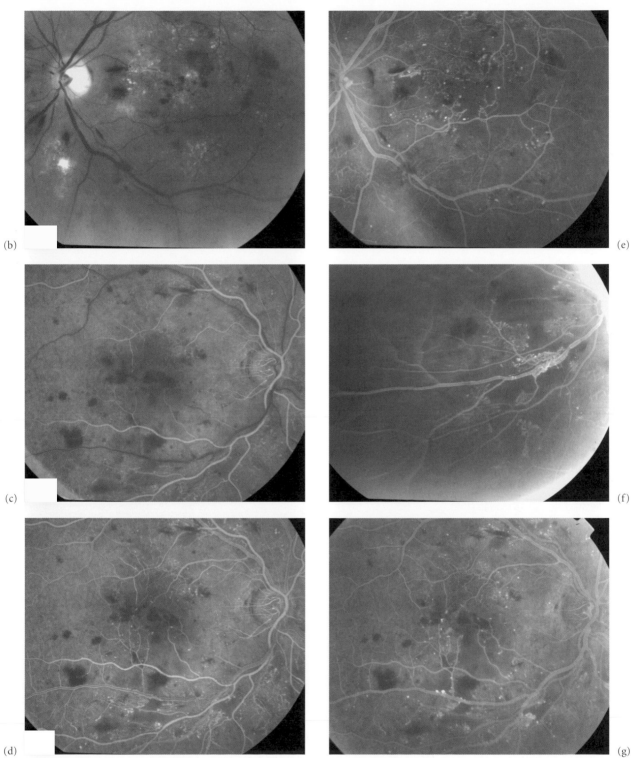

(b)

(e)

(c)

(f)

(d)

(g)

Fig. 6.8 (*Cont'd*) (*Continued on p. 78*)

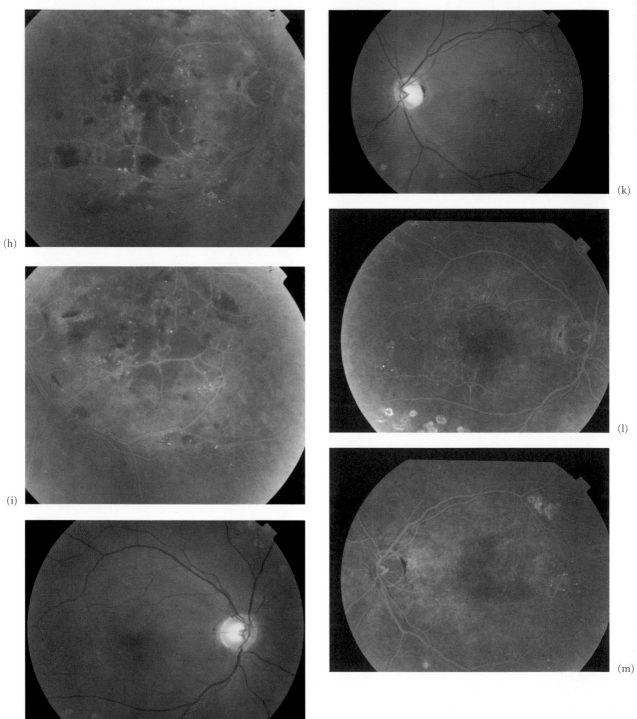

Fig. 6.8 (*Cont'd*)

- 18 months after presentation the VA had improved to right 6/18 (20/60), left 6/36 (20/120).
- 2 years after presentation, the VA had improved to right 6/12 (20/40), left 6/24 (20/80).
- 3 years after presentation, the VA had improved to right 6/9 (20/30), left 6/18 (20/60).
- 4 years after presentation, the VA had improved to right 6/9 (20/30), left 6/12 (20/40). Fig. 6.8(j–m) shows photographs taken at the year 4 visit.

We believe that the primary reason for the improvement in appearance of the macular areas and the improvement in VAs was the control of the blood pressure. The following blood pressure readings had been recorded over this 4 year period – 122/75, 165/72, 132/80 and 154/87. The corresponding HbA1c results were 6.7%, 7.4%, 6.6% and 6.8%.

Glucose control

The importance of good blood glucose control on the progression of diabetic retinopathy is explained in the Diabetes section of this book (Chapter 2).

Blood lipids

The importance of good blood lipid control on the progression of diabetic retinopathy is explained in the Diabetes section of this book (Chapter 2).

LASER FOR MACULOPATHY

Spalter[3] first described the photocoagulation of circinate maculopathy in diabetic retinopathy in 1971 and subsequent reports appeared by Whitelocke[4] in 1979 and a British Multicentre Study Group[5] in 1983.

However, it was in 1985 that the Early Treatment Diabetic Retinopathy Study[6] (ETDRS) demonstrated that focal (direct/grid) laser photocoagulation reduces moderate vision loss caused by diabetic macular oedema (DME) by 50% or more and described 'clinically significant macular oedema', which defined the parameters for treatment.

The ETDRS reported the results of 754 eyes that were randomly assigned to focal argon laser and 1490 eyes to deferral, which showed that focal photocoagulation of 'clinically significant' diabetic macular oedema (CSMO) substantially reduced the risk of visual loss. Clinically significant macular oedema was defined in a further report from the ETDRS[7] study group as:

1 thickening of the retina at or within 500 microns of the centre of the macula
2 hard exudates at or within 500 microns of the centre of the fovea, if associated with thickening of the adjacent retina (not residual hard exudates remaining after disappearance of retinal thickening)
3 a zone or zones of retinal thickening 1 disc area or larger, any part of which is within 1 disc diameter of the centre of the macula.

Focal and grid treatment were used singly or in combination as was considered appropriate for each treated eye and were not compared with one another.

Focal treatment was recommended for focal lesions located between 500 and 3000 microns from the centre of the macula and believed to be causing retinal thickening or hard exudates.

The majority of focally treated lesions were microaneurysms, treated with 50–100-micron burns of moderate intensity, preferably to produce a whitening or darkening of the larger microaneurysms (≥40 microns) or mild to moderate whitening of the adjacent retinal for smaller microaneurysms (<40 microns), and 0.05–0.1 s duration.

Grid treatment was recommended for areas of thickened retina that showed diffuse fluorescein leakage or capillary dropout. Burns of 50–200-micron spot size were placed one burn width apart in areas of intense leakage and more widely spaced in areas of less intense leakage. Grid treatment was not recommended within 500 microns of the centre of the macula or within 500 microns of the disc margin but could be placed in the papillomacular bundle. Grid treatment could extend in all directions up to 2 disc diameters from the centre of the macula.

Follow-up treatment was recommended at the 6-week follow-up visit if obvious treatable lesions had been missed during the initial treatment and at subsequent 4-monthly follow-up visits if macular oedema persisted.

ETDRS results

Among eyes with clinically significant macular oedema not involving the centre of the macula approximately 8% of control group eyes had visual loss at the 1-year visit, and 16% at the 2-year visit. Treatment reduced these percentages to 1% and 6% respectively.

When the centre of the macula was involved, visual loss was more frequent, reaching 33% in the control group after 3 years. Treatment reduced this frequency by approximately 60%, to 13%.

After 5 years of this 9-year study, the accumulating data showed that focal photocoagulation was effective in reducing moderate visual loss and the protocol was therefore changed to allow focal photocoagulation for clinically significant macular oedema whenever it occurred. Moderate visual loss was defined as the loss of 15 or more letters between baseline and follow-up visit, equivalent to doubling of the visual angle.

The 'early worsening' phenomenon

In 1998 the Diabetes Control and Complications Trial[8] (DCCT) described the effect of early worsening of diabetic retinopathy at the 6- and/or 12-month visit in 13.1% of 711 patients assigned to intensive treatment. Early worsening led to clinically significant macular oedema in three patients in the DCCT. The most important risk factors for early worsening were higher haemoglobin A1c level at screening and reduction of this level during the first 6 months after randomization.

CASE HISTORY 2
The early worsening phenomenon soon after commencing insulin treatment

This man with type 2 diabetes (BMI 39) was diagnosed at the age of 41 years. He was initially treated with diet. His blood glucose levels were between 6 and 10 mmol/L in the first 2 years but in the subsequent 5 years were recorded at levels between 10 and 12 mmol/L and he was therefore started on glibenclamide 2.5 mg o.d. at the age of 48 years. Over the next 13 years the glibenclamide was gradually increased to 15 mg and at the age of 51 years metformin 500 mg b.d. was added. Six months later, the blood glucose was varying between 10 and 14 mmol/L during the day, the HbA1c was 10.5, a foot ulcer had formed on his right foot and a decision was made to commence insulin, stop the glibenclamide and continue the metformin. At that time, he had had some laser treatment for circinate areas of maculopathy but the VA was 6/9 before commencement of insulin. Within a few days of starting insulin the VA dropped to right 6/18, left 6/24, and slit-lamp biomicroscopy confirmed that both macular areas had developed a cystoid type of macular oedema. The HbA1c improved over the next 3 months to a reading of 7.5 and has subsequently remained at a level below 8.5. Red-free photographs taken at the time are shown (Fig. 6.9a,b).

The vision gradually returned to a level of 6/9 (20/30) in each eye over the next 7 months as the cystoid macular oedema subsequently resolved spontaneously. Figure 6.9(c,d) shows NVDs developing at both discs 18 months later.

Despite panretinal photocoagulation to both eyes, vitrectomies were required for both eyes at the age of 66 years. Following the vitrectomies, the VAs have stabilized at right 6/9 (20/30), left 6/60 (20/200). The left vision is reduced due to an ischaemic maculopathy (Fig. 6.9e,f).

Key points

Control of glycaemia has been shown to be linked to microvascular complications. If a person has had poor control for years and is placed on insulin to control the glycaemia well, there is a risk of early worsening of VA, particularly due to an effect on the macular area. However the long-term benefits outweigh any short-term disadvantages of improving control. Good communication between the diabetologist and ophthalmologist is essential for this group of patients.

Other studies

In 1986, Olk[9] reported results of modified grid photocoagulation for eyes with diffuse macular oedema (defined as at least two disc areas of retinal thickening with the involvement of the centre of the macula) and VA of 20/32 to 20/200. Mild burns 100–200 microns in diameter were scattered throughout the posterior pole, one burn diameter apart, except for the foveal avascular zone. Focal areas of leakage were treated. Treatment was repeated at least once in approximately 70% of cases. After 1 and 2 years of follow-up, losses of VA were less frequent in treated than in untreated eyes. Patients complained of annoying scotomas and those with VA of 20/63 or better in each eye before treatment generally favoured the untreated eye until its VA fell to 20/80 or worse.

In 1989, Davies[10] reported a 10-year follow-up of 62 eyes of 40 patients treated with focal photocoagulation for 'clinically significant' diabetic macular oedema. Of those eyes with baseline VA ≥6/12, 60% maintained this level of acuity at 10 years.

In 2003, Chew[11] described a follow-up study of 214 surviving patients enrolled at the Johns Hopkins Clinical Centre for the ETDRS. Of the 71 who were examined 42% had VA ≥20/20 and 84% had VA ≥20/40 in the better eye.

In 1997, Fong[12] described the characteristics of and risk factors for subretinal fibrosis (SRF) in patients with diabetic macular oedema. The strongest risk factor for the development of SRF was very severe hard exudates.

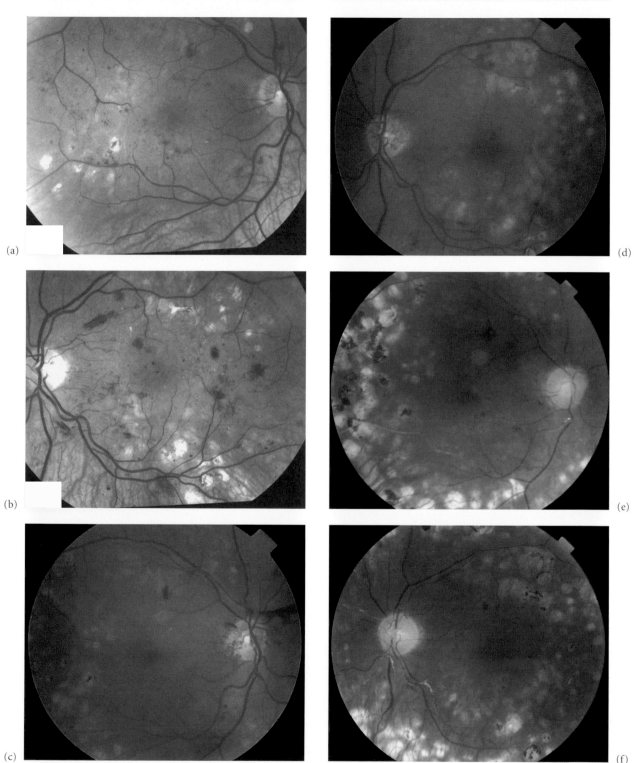

Fig. 6.9 (a–f) Case history 2.

In 1998, Bailey[13,14] reported the results of the UK National Diabetic Retinopathy Laser Treatment Audit of 546 patients undergoing their first photocoagulation treatment for maculopathy with 9-month follow-up. Improvement in the macular oedema occurred in 64.6% and exudates in 77.3%; 9.2% had deterioration in VA equivalent to a doubling of the visual angle; 3.3% of eyes had a VA <6/60 at follow-up.

In 2002, Gogi[15] described retinal microaneurysmal closure following focal laser photocoagulation in diabetic macular oedema. The mean microaneurysm count reduced by 35% at 1 week, 50% at 3 weeks, 61% at 6 weeks, and 75% at 12 weeks.

In 2005, Bandello[16] reported the results of a prospective randomized pilot clinical trial in which 29 eyes of 24 diabetic patients with mild to moderate non-proliferative diabetic retinopathy (NPDR) and CSMO were randomized to either 'classic' or 'light' Nd : YAG 532-nm (frequency-doubled) green laser. 'Light' laser treatment differed from conventional ('classic') photocoagulation in that the energy employed was the lowest capable to produce barely visible burns at the level of the retinal pigment epithelium. This study suggests that 'light' photocoagulation for CSMO may be as effective as 'classic' laser treatment, thus supporting the rationale for a larger equivalence trial.

In 2007, Fong[17] reported a comparison of two laser photocoagulation techniques for treatment of diabetic macular oedema: the modified Early Treatment Diabetic Retinopathy Study (ETDRS) direct/grid photocoagulation technique and a potentially milder (but potentially more extensive) mild macular grid (MMG) laser technique in which microaneurysms are not treated directly and small mild burns are placed throughout the macula, whether or not oedema is present. Two hundred and sixty-three subjects (mean age, 59 years) with previously untreated diabetic macular oedema were randomly assigned to receive laser photocoagulation by either the modified ETDRS (162 eyes) or MMG (161 eyes) technique. At 12 months after treatment, the MMG technique was less effective at reducing optical coherence tomography-measured retinal thickening than the more extensively evaluated current modified ETDRS laser photocoagulation approach. However, the VA outcome with both approaches is not substantially different. The article concluded that modified ETDRS focal photocoagulation should continue to be a standard approach for treating diabetic macular oedema.

CASE HISTORY 3
Focal maculopathy left eye

This 25-year-old man (BMI 25) with type 1 diabetes from the age of 3 years was referred from the retinal screening service. His HbA1c levels had improved from 10.8 to 7.8 over the previous 5 years and his blood pressure was normal at levels averaging 133/67. He was found to have clinically significant macular oedema in his left eye as shown in the colour photograph (Fig. 6.10a).

A colour photograph (Fig. 6.10b) taken within a few minutes of the laser treatment shows the pale spots produced by the laser from blanching of the retina. A colour photograph taken 4 months after the laser treatment shows clearing of the exudates and of the clinically significant macular oedema (Fig. 6.10c).

CASE HISTORY 4
Focal maculopathy left eye

This 49-year-old woman (BMI 28) with type 2 diabetes for 10 years, controlled on insulin for the previous 8 years, presented with signs of bilateral maculopathy and VAs of right 6/9 (20/30), left 6/9 (20/30), and extensive exudates in both macular regions. Her HbA1c results have varied between 9.5 and 10.4 and blood pressure results have varied between 130/80 and 140/70.

Her photographs on presentation are shown in Fig. 6.11(a,b).

Treatment was given to the right macular area:
• right 77 burns, 100-micron size, 180 mW, 0.1 s, area centralis lens, argon laser.

Treatment was given to the left macular area:
• left 46 burns, 100-micron size, 160 mW, 0.1 s, area centralis lens, argon laser.

Twelve months after presentation, this resulted in some clearing in the right macular area but the left macular area had not improved (Fig. 6.11c). Further treatment was given to the left macular area:
• left 76 burns, 100-micron size, 180 mW, 0.1 s, area centralis lens, argon laser.

Further treatment was given to the right macular area:
• left 76 burns, 100-micron size, 180 mW, 0.1 s, area centralis lens, argon laser.

Eighteen months after presentation, this resulted in clearing of exudates and thickening in both macular areas but there was some concerning leakage and exudates close to the central fovea in both eyes, more marked in the left (Fig. 6.11d,e). Further treatment was given to the right macular area:

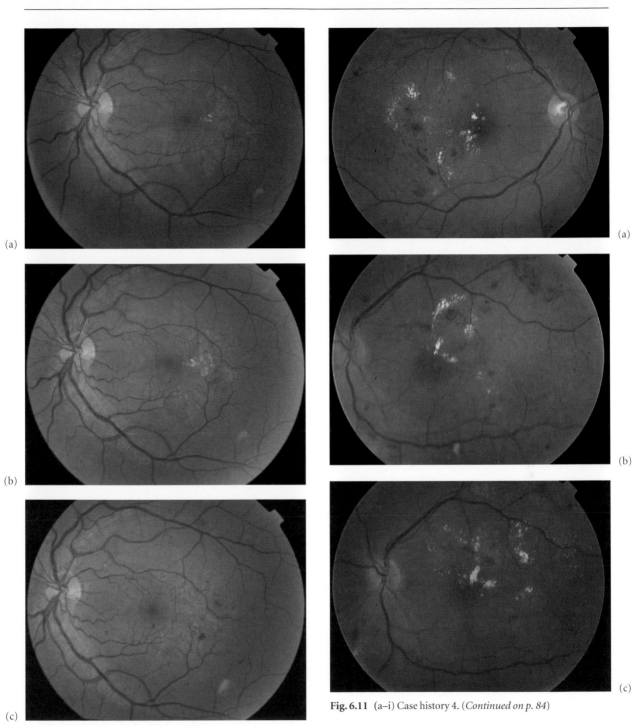

(a)

(b)

(c)

(a)

(b)

(c)

Fig. 6.11 (a–i) Case history 4. (*Continued on p. 84*)

Fig. 6.10 (a–c) Case history 3.

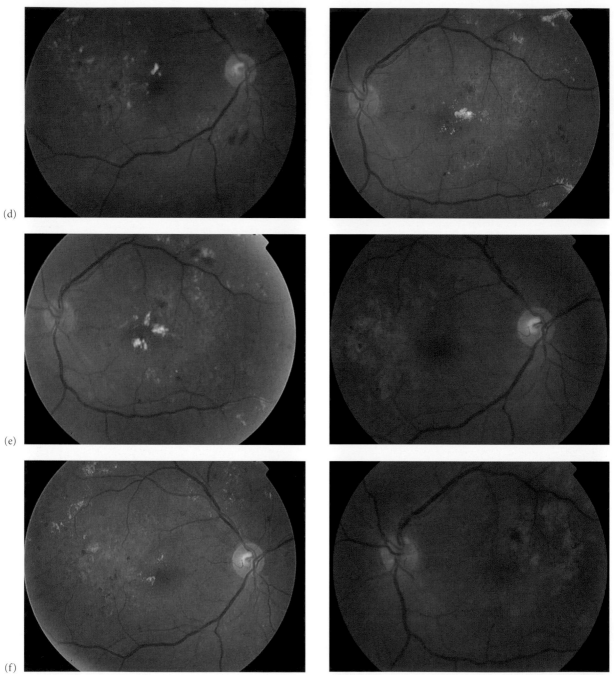

(d)

(g)

(e)

(h)

(f)

(i)

Fig. 6.11 (*Cont'd*)

- left 11 burns, 100-micron size, 150 mW, 0.1 s, area centralis lens, argon laser.

  Further treatment was given to the left macular area:

- left 15 burns, 100-micron size, 180 mW, 0.1 s, area centralis lens, argon laser.

Two years after presentation, this resulted in clearing of exudates and thickening in the right macular area and below the left macular area but there was still some leakage and exudates temporal to the left central fovea (Fig. 6.11f,g). Further treatment was given to the left macular area:

- left 27 burns, 100-micron size, 160 mW, 0.1 s, area centralis lens, argon laser.

This resulted in clearing of exudates and thickening in both macular areas 3 years after presentation, and remaining clear of exudates in the photographs taken 8 years after presentation (Fig. 6.11h,i). Her visual acuity remains stable at right 6/9 (20/30), left 6/9 (20/30).

CASE HISTORY 5
Focal maculopathy left eye

This 58-year-old man (BMI 29) with type 2 diabetes diagnosed 15 years ago controlled on metformin 500 mg b.d. presented with a left maculopathy as shown in the colour photograph and the fluorescein angiogram shown below (Fig. 6.12a–f).

Over the last 7 years he has managed a progressive improvement in HbA1c from 9.1 to 6.4 and his blood pressure readings have averaged 144/83. His cholesterol is 4.0 and Ch : HDL ratio 4.4.

Treatment was given to the left macular area:
- left 75 burns, 100-micron size, 230 mW, 0.1 s, area centralis lens, argon laser.

This resulted in some clearing of the exudates and thickening as shown in Fig. 6.12(g).

Further treatment was given to the left macular area:
- left 25 burns, 100-micron size, 210 mW, 0.1 s, area centralis lens, argon laser.

This resulted in further clearing of the exudates and thickening as shown in Fig. 6.12(h). Further treatment was given to the left macular area:
- left 30 burns, 100-micron size, 290 mW, 0.1 s, area centralis lens, argon laser.

This resulted in further clearing of the exudates and thickening as shown in Fig. 6.12(i).

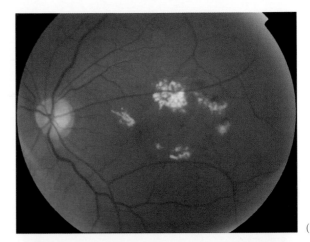

(a)

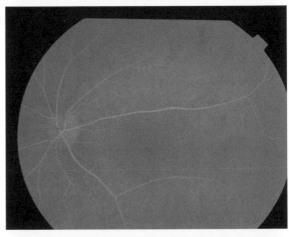

(b)

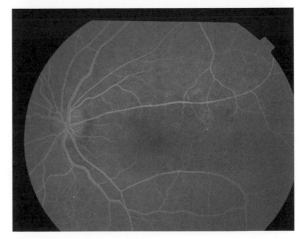

(c)

Fig. 6.12 Case history 5. (a) Presentation: left macula colour. (b) Fluorescein: left macula 17 s. (c) Fluorescein: left macula 24 s. (*Continued on p. 86*)

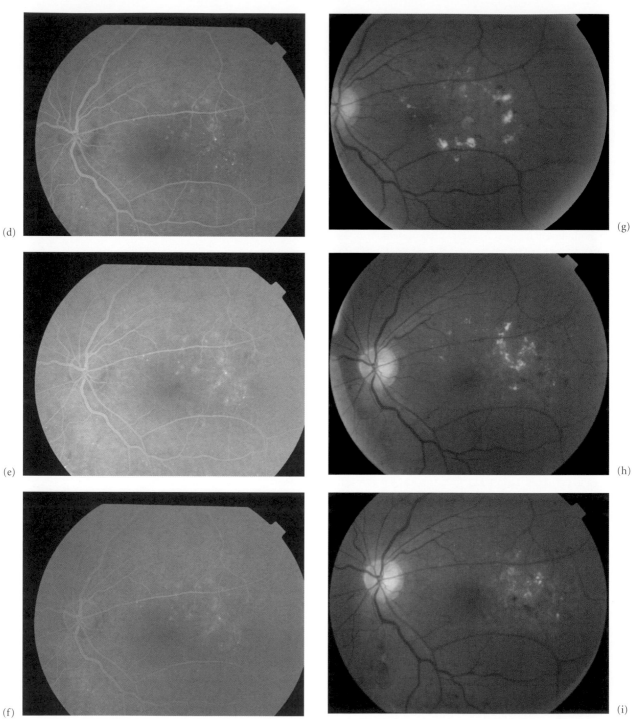

Fig. 6.12 (*Cont'd*) (d) Fluorescein: left macula 44 s. (e) Fluorescein: left macula 2 min 22 s. (f) Fluorescein: left macula 3 min 44 s. (g) Colour: left macula after first laser treatment. (h) Colour: left macula after second laser treatment. (i) Colour: left macula after third laser treatment.

CASE HISTORY 6
Diffuse maculopathy

This 55-year-old man presented with visual symptoms and was diagnosed with type 2 diabetes following a blood glucose reading of 17.1 mmol/L and a history of weight loss of 14.1 kg (31 lb) over 2 years. His VA at presentation was right 6/36 (20/180), left 6/9 (20/30). Retinal photography was more difficult because of old posterior synechiae in his right eye, due to a previous episode of anterior uveitis (Fig. 6.13a).

Colour photography and fluorescein angiography showed diffuse leakage in both macular areas, more marked in his right eye (Fig. 6.13b–i).

An OCT scan demonstrated leakage in the right macular area and less leakage in the left macular area (Fig. 6.13j–m). Treatment was given to the right macular area:
- right 41 burns, 100-micron size, 210–290 mW, 0.1 s, area centralis lens, argon laser.

Treatment was given to the left macular area:
- right 52 burns, 100-micron size, 220–250 mW, 0.1 s, area centralis lens, argon laser.

Four months later, a subsequent treatment was given to the right macular area:
- right 32 burns, 100-micron size, 260 mW, 0.1 s, area centralis lens, argon laser.

Following this second treatment, over the subsequent 4 months the VA in the right eye improved from right 6/36 (20/180) to 6/9 (20/30), and the left vision improved from 6/9 (20/30) to 6/6 (20/20).

At year 2 after presentation both the colour and red-free images (Fig. 6.13n–q) and the OCT images (Fig. 6.13r–u) showed an improvement.

During this 2-year period, his HbA1c improved from 14.5 to 5.9, and his blood pressure had remained satisfactory with readings of 111/64, 147/73, 147/84 and 131/60. His cholesterol was 3.2 and Ch:HDL ratio 2.7.

The improvement in his glycaemia is likely to have contributed significantly (as well as the laser treatment) to the improvement in the macular appearance.

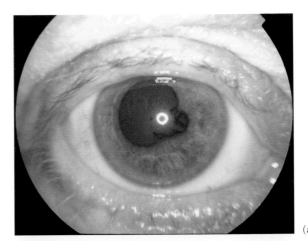

(a)

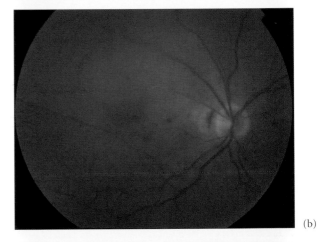

(b)

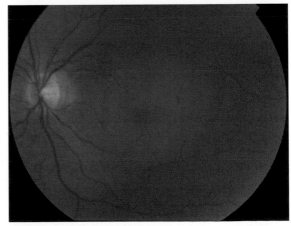

(c)

Fig. 6.13 Case history 6. Presentation: (a) right anterior segment colour showing old posterior synechiae; (b) right macula colour making fundus photography more difficult; (c) left macula colour; (*Continued on p. 88*)

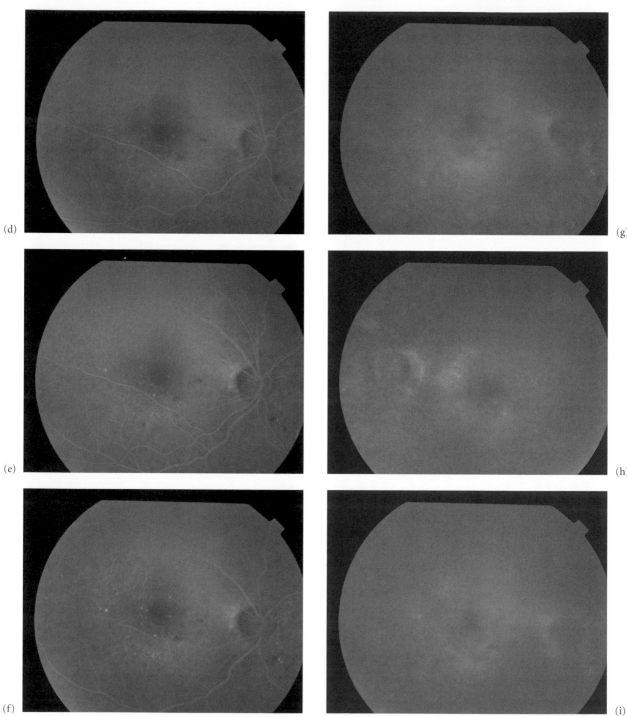

(d)

(e)

(f)

(g)

(h)

(i)

Fig. 6.13 (*Cont'd*) (d) right macula fluorescein 25 s; (e) right macula fluorescein 34 s; (f) right macula fluorescein 1 min 46 s; (g) right macula fluorescein 2 min 29 s; (h) left macula fluorescein 3 min 26 s; (i) right macula fluorescein 2 min 29 s; (*Continued on facing page*)

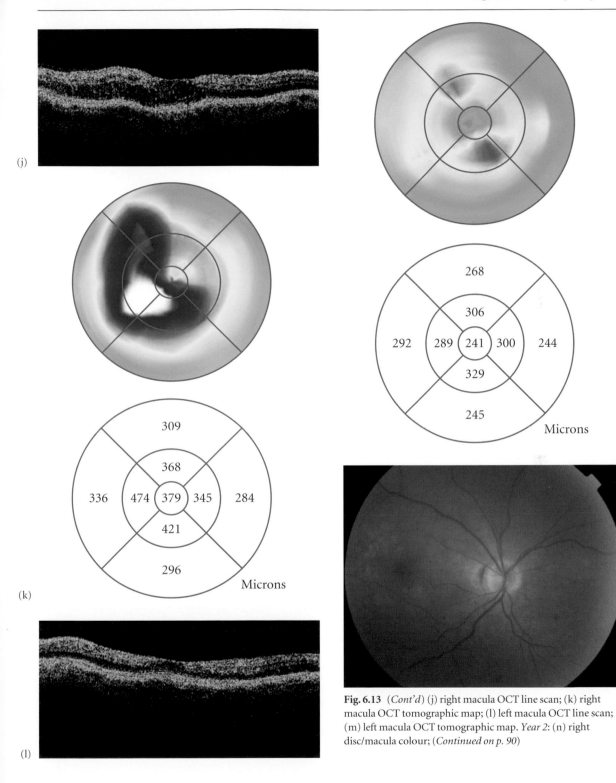

Fig. 6.13 (*Cont'd*) (j) right macula OCT line scan; (k) right macula OCT tomographic map; (l) left macula OCT line scan; (m) left macula OCT tomographic map. *Year 2*: (n) right disc/macula colour; (*Continued on p. 90*)

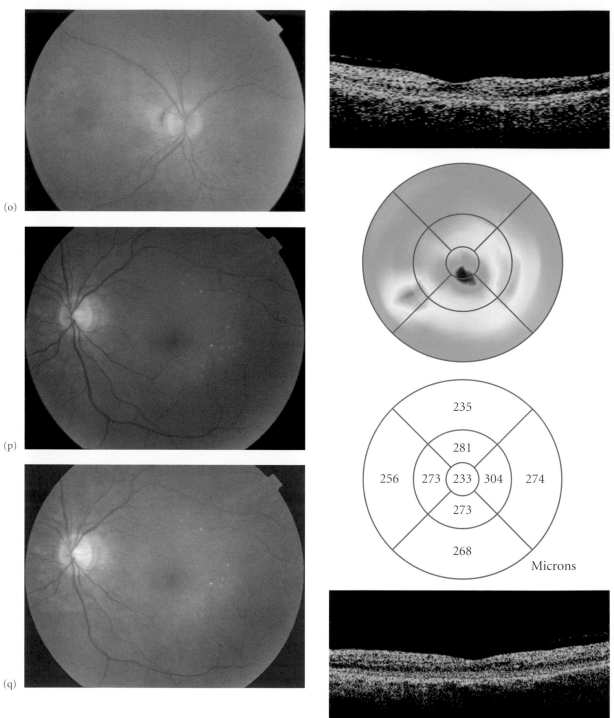

(o)

(p)

(q)

(r)

235

281

256 273 233 304 274

273

268

Microns

(s)

(t)

Fig. 6.13 (*Cont'd*) (o) right macula red free; (p) left macula colour; (q) left macula red free; (r) right macula OCT line scan; (s) right macula OCT tomographic map; (t) left macula OCT line scan; (*Continued on facing page*)

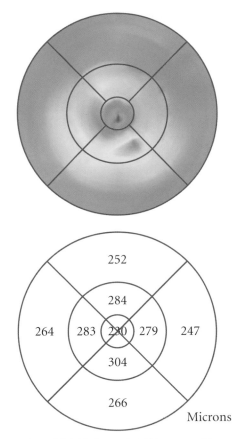

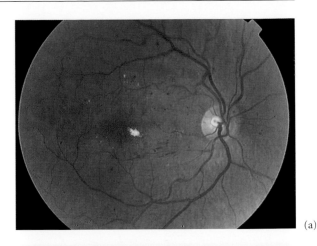

(a)

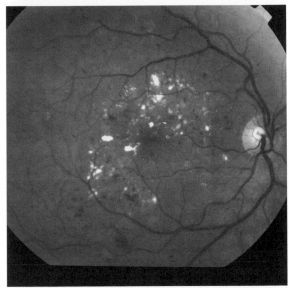

(b)

252

284

264   283   230   279   247

304

266

Microns

(u)

Fig. 6.13 (*Cont'd*) (u) left macula OCT tomographic map.

CASE HISTORY 7
Mixed focal and diffuse maculopathy

This 39-year-old man (BMI 25) with type 2 diabetes for 10 years controlled on insulin presented with a maculopathy in his right eye and VA of 6/9 (20/30) (Fig. 6.14a).

Treatment was given to the right macular area:
- right 44 burns 100-micron size, 180 mW, 0.1 s, area centralis lens, argon laser.

This resulted in some initial clearing in the right macular area but there was a subsequent increase in leakage and a drop in his right VA to 6/18 (20/60); Fig. 6.14(b) shows a photograph taken 7 months later.

Treatment was given to the right macular area:
- right 45 burns 100-micron size, 170 mW, 0.1 s, area centralis lens, argon laser.

Subsequently treatment was given to the right macular area:
- right 27 burns 100-micron size, 220 mW, 0.1 s, area centralis lens, argon laser.

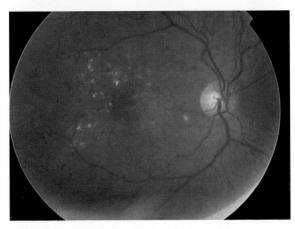

(c)

Fig. 6.14 (a–f) Case history 7. (*Continued on p. 92*)

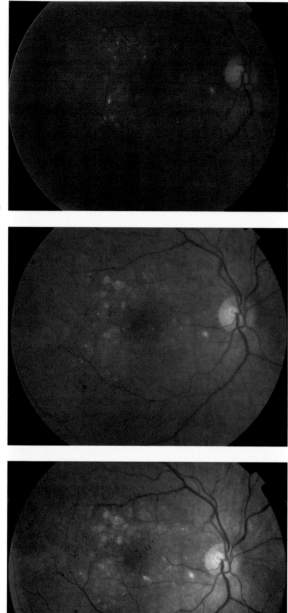

(d)

(e)

(f)

Fig. 6.14 (*Cont'd*)

This resulted in an improvement in VA to 6/12 (20/40) and clearing of much of the exudates and thickening as shown in Figs 6.14(c–e) and this improvement was maintained in the photograph taken 8 years after the initial presentation (Fig. 6.14f).

During the last 9 years, over which the laser treatment has been applied, his HbA1c has fluctuated between 8.5% and 9.5%, with his most recent result being 8.9%. His blood pressure has been difficult to control, running at 152/88 at the beginning of the period and the most recent recording is 167/71. His cholesterol is 3.6 mmol/L and Ch : HDL ratio 4.5.

Mechanisms of action of laser for macular oedema

The effectiveness of focal laser treatment may be due, in part, to the closure of leaky microaneurysms, but the specific mechanisms by which focal photocoagulation reduces macular oedema is not known. Studies have shown histopathological changes[18] and biochemical changes,[19,20] which have been suggested as mechanisms for improvement in macular oedema although some investigators have suggested alternative mechanisms for clearance of the oedema such as the application of Starling's law and improved oxygenation.[21]

Adverse effects of macular laser treatment

Adverse effects of laser treatment have been principally covered in the section on panretinal photocoagulation in the treatment of proliferative diabetic retinopathy (Chapter 9).

However, potential side-effects specific to macular laser are as follows.

1 Laser close to the central fovea – resulting in a drop in VA immediately after laser treatment or a visible scotoma or laser scars increasing in size over time to involve a more central area of fovea than the original lasered area. Laser burns may be associated with paracentral scotomas and may become larger than the original spot size[22] and encroach on fixation. In an attempt to reduce adverse effects, many retinal specialists now treat patients using burns that are lighter and less intense than originally specified in the ETDRS.

2 Choroidal neovascular membrane developing in an area that has received laser treatment – this complication is extremely rare and in fact people with diabetic maculopathy do seem to get fewer choroidal neovascular membranes than one might expect.

The pattern argon laser and the evidence behind the recommendations for this laser in treatment of macular oedema

With conventional methods of retinal laser photocoagulation, the ophthalmologist uses a mechanical joystick and foot pedal to deliver single 50- or 100-millisecond laser pulses to the macular area.

Optimedia Corporation introduced the PASCAL (Pattern Scan Laser) photocoagulator in June 2006, which is a frequency-doubled Nd : YAG diode-pumped solid state laser producing a wavelength of 532 nm. The operator can select different arcs, circular grid patterns or sectors of grids for treatment, or use a rectangular array. Once the pattern is selected, a separate red beam is used for aiming and visualization of the placement before delivery.

With patterned scanning laser photocoagulation, the laser pulse time can be reduced from 100 ms to just 10–30 ms and automated multiple spots are produced with each depression of the foot pedal. Higher power is required where burns of shorter duration are applied.

The long-term results of focal/grid laser treatment using short-duration burns (10–30 ms) with higher power as recommended for the PASCAL laser is unknown and studies comparing this to the currently recommended modified ETDRS technique for macular laser treatment need to be undertaken (Table 6.1).

The authors would advise caution in using the grid patterns with four concentric rings in one treatment session as this could potentially drop vision in a macula that has extensive capillary or arteriolar closure and had hitherto maintained a reasonable VA, or could produce annoying scotomas as was found by patients in the study reported by Olk[9].

Subthreshold micropulse diode laser

There are some proponents of this technique for treatment of clinically significant macular oedema. However, the studies that have currently been reported have been small case series[23,24] (25 eyes and 23 eyes) or retrospective[25] (95 eyes). The technique does have the disadvantage that there is no ophthalmoscopically visible endpoint to confirm the effect of treatment.

MEDICAL THERAPIES

Current attempts to manage patients with diabetic maculopathy are aimed at preserving vision and reducing progression of the disease by appropriate management of glucose, blood pressure, weight and lipids, and laser treatment at the appropriate stage in the disease process. Ongoing studies on the use of ACE inhibitors, angiotensin receptor blockers, fenofibrate and PKC inhibitors are discussed in Chapter 15.

OTHER TREATMENT OPTIONS AND EVIDENCE FOR THESE TREATMENTS

Anti-VEGF treatments

Increased vascular permeability has been associated with vascular endothelial growth factor (VEGF). However, there is a concern that VEGF does have a neuroprotective effect

Table 6.1 Recommended modified ETDRS treatment technique (focal/grid photocoagulation).

Direct treatment	Directly treat all leaking microaneurysms in areas of retinal thickening 500–3000 microns from the centre of the macula (but not within 500 microns of the disc)
Change in microaneurysm colour	Not required, but at least a mild grey-white burn should be evident beneath all microaneurysms
Burn size for direct treatment	50–100 microns
Burn duration for direct treatment	0.05–0.10 s
Grid treatment	Applied to all areas of diffuse leakage or non-perfusion within the area considered for grid treatment
Area considered for grid treatment	500–3000 microns superiorly, nasally and inferiorly from centre of the macula 500–3500 microns temporally from the macular centre. No burns are placed within 500 microns of the disc
Burn size for grid treatment	50–100 microns
Burn duration for grid treatment	0.05–0.10 s
Burn intensity for grid treatment	Barely visible (light grey)
Burn separation for grid treatment	Two visible burn widths apart
Wavelength (grid and focal treatment)	Green to yellow

and that there might be neurological adverse effects if there is significant systemic absorption of these substances.

There are three potential VEGF inhibitors:

- pegaptanib (Macugen)
- ranibizumab (Lucentis)
- bevacizumab (Avastin).

Ranibizumab (Lucentis) is an antibody fragment derived from bevacizumab (Avastin), which is a full-length humanized monoclonal antibody against human VEGF currently used for treatment of several solid organ tumours (colorectal etc.). These drugs have not been extensively studied in diabetic eye disease and there are only early reports of their use in diabetic retinopathy without any randomized controlled trials (RCTs).

There are reports of reduction in macular thickness using intravitreal injections of these agents. However, the effect does not last and therefore repeated injections would be required to sustain any beneficial effects.

In 2007, Kumar[26] reported the results of a prospective, interventional case series study of 20 eyes given two intravitreal injections of bevacizumab 1.25 mg in 0.05 mL 6 weeks apart. This resulted in a significant decrease in macular thickness (p = 0.001) and improvement in VA (p = 0.008) at 3 months but the effect was somewhat blunted, though still statistically significant, at the end of 6 months.

In 2007, Yanyali[27] reported a retrospective, non-comparative, interventional case series of 11 eyes of 10 patients who underwent intravitreal bevacizumab injection for persistent diabetic macular oedema (DME). No change in VA and foveal thickness was observed in the short term after intravitreal bevacizumab for DME in previously vitrectomized eyes.

In 2006, Haritoglou[28] reported the results of 51 consecutive patients (26 females and 25 males; mean age, 64 years) with diffuse DME treated with a 0.05-mL injection containing 1.25 mg of bevacizumab. All patients completed 6 weeks of follow-up; 23 (45%) completed 12 weeks of follow-up. Their results suggested that improvement of VA and decrease of retinal thickness could be observed after intravitreal injection of bevacizumab.

In 2006, the Pan-American Collaborative Retina Study Group reported a 6-month study[29] on primary intravitreal bevacizumab (Avastin) in patients with DME. They reviewed the clinical records of 88 consecutive patients (110 eyes) with DME. Seventy-eight eyes of 64 consecutive patients with a minimum follow-up of 6 months and mean age of 59.7 +/– 9.3 years were included in this analysis. It was concluded that primary intravitreal bevacizumab at doses of 1.2–2.5 mg seem to provide stability or improvement in VA, OCT and fluorescein angiography in DME at 6 months. However they acknowledged that follow-up is still too short to make any specific treatment recommendations. Evaluation in a multicentre RCT with longer follow-up is needed.

In a 2006 multicentre RCT evaluating pegaptanib for treatment of diabetic macular oedema, Starita[30] compared eyes of patients receiving sham injections to those receiving 0.3 mg intravitreous pegaptanib. The latter eyes displayed superior VA (p = 0.04) as well as a reduction in retinal thickness of 68 micrometers compared to a slight increase under sham treatment (p = 0.021).

In view of the potential complications from intravitreal injections, extreme caution is advised in the use of this technique. RCTs utilizing varying doses of the VEGF inhibitors are now required to assess the long-term efficacy and safety and to define optimum treatment regimens.

Intravitreal triamcinolone

Promising results in the short term for improving the vision in eyes with chronic diabetic macular oedema unresponsive to conventional laser treatment, reducing macular thickness and inducing reabsorption of hard exudates have been described in the following studies: Ciardella,[31] Jonas,[32,33] Lam,[34] Massin,[35] Micelli Ferrari,[36] Ozkiris,[37] Sutter,[38] Chieh,[39] Er,[40] Islam,[41] Khairallah,[42] Negi,[43] Ozdemir,[44] Patelli,[45] Zacks[46] and Avci.[47] One case study did report regression of NVD in addition to the decrease in macular oedema.

The effects are reported to last for 3–8 months. This may be partially dependent on the dose given: doses as low as 1 mg have been reported by Chieh; 4 mg is the commonest dose used by Ciardella,[31] Lam,[34] Massin,[35] Er,[40] Islam,[41] Negi,[43] Ozdemir,[44] Patelli[45] and Avci;[47] 8 mg by Ozkiris,[37] 13 mg by Spandau[48] and 20–25 mg by Jonas.[32,33]

Garcia-Arumi[49] recommended that one should reduce the concentration of the solvent agent benzyl alcohol (9.9 mg/mL) from a commercially prepared triamcinolone acetonide (TA) suspension by centrifugation before administering the drug. Oishi[50] developed a new TA injection made of pure TA suspended in 0.5% sodium hyaluronate.

A further study[51] described an interventional case series of nine patients with bilateral proliferative diabetic retinopathy one eye ascribed to intravitreal triamcinolone before PRP and suggested that this may be useful in improving the effects of PRP in eyes with proliferative diabetic retinopathy by reducing neovascularization and macular thickening.

One of the proponents of intravitreal triamcinolone in diabetic retinopathy (Jonas) has written a review article[52] on the subject.

However, the following complications have been reported:

- posterior subcapsular cataract[31,39,47,53]
- vitreous haemorrhage[28]
- transient rise in intraocular pressure[34,35,37,40,42,43,48]
- early rapid increases in intraocular pressure requiring surgical intervention[54]
- severe subconjunctival haemorrhage[55]
- culture-negative sterile endophthalmitis[39,40]
- infectious endophthalmitis.[38]

In view of these reported complications, extreme caution is advised in the use of this technique. RCTs utilizing varying doses of steroid are now required to assess the long-term efficacy and safety and to define optimum treatment regimens.

CASE HISTORY 8
Use of intravitreal triamcinolone

This 45-year-old man with type 2 diabetes controlled with insulin (diagnosed at the age of 32 years), presented with blurred vision in his left eye and a left VA reduced to 6/18 (20/60). A colour photograph and fluorescein angiogram of the left macular area is shown (Fig. 6.15).

An OCT showed thickening in the left central foveal region.

He was treated with an intravitreal injection of triamcinolone and this was followed by focal laser treatment to

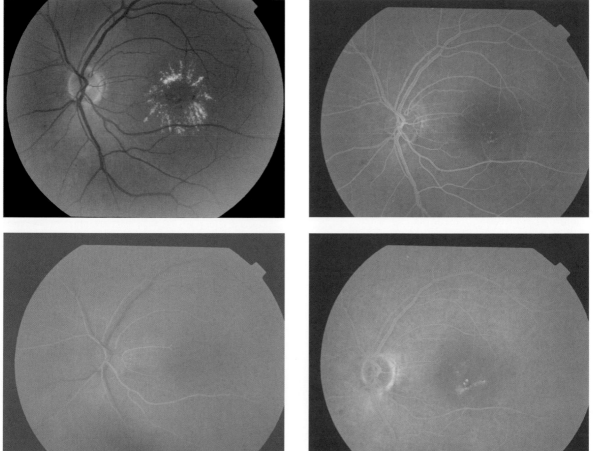

(a)

(b)

(c)

(d)

Fig. 6.15 Case history 8. Presentation: (a) left macula colour; (b) fluorescein left macula 25 s; (c) fluorescein left macula 36 s; (d) fluorescein left macula 3 min 01 s; (*Continued on p. 96*)

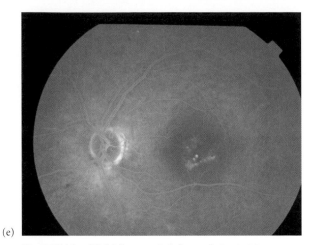

(e)

Fig. 6.15 (*Cont'd*) (e) fluorescein left macula 3 min 26 s.

the microaneurysms on the edge of the foveal avascular zone. Clearly the central microaneurysms could not be treated with laser.

Treatment given was:

- 15 burns 110-micron size, 30–130 mW, area centralis lens, argon laser.

The central foveal thickness has reduced but not cleared and the VA has improved to 6/9 (20/30).

PRACTICE POINTS

- Modified Early Treatment Diabetic Retinopathy Study focal photocoagulation to areas of clinically significant macular oedema should continue to be the standard approach for treating diabetic macular oedema.
- Anti-VEGF treatments should only be used routinely in the context of clinical trials so that their place in the treatment of diabetic maculopathy can be established.
- Modern investigative techniques such as optical coherence tomography (OCT) have an increasing role to play in the assessment and monitoring of patients with diabetic macular oedema.
- Following laser treatment, prognosis for the maculopathy and vision will depend on control of systemic factors such as glucose[53,54], hypertension[55] and lipids.[56]

REFERENCES

1 Bresnick GH. Diabetic macular edema. A review. *Ophthalmology* 1986; **93**(7): 989–97.

2 Kearns M, Hamilton AM, Kohner EM. Excessive permeability in diabetic maculopathy. *Br J Ophthalmol* 1979; **63**(7): 489–97.

3 Spalter HF. Photocoagulation of circinate maculopathy in diabetic retinopathy. *Am J Ophthalmol* 1971; **1**(1 Part 2): 242–50.

4 Whitelocke RA, Kearns M, Blach RK, Hamilton AM. The diabetic maculopathies. *Trans Ophthalmol Soc UK* 1979; **99**(2): 314–20.

5 Photocoagulation for diabetic maculopathy. A randomized controlled clinical trial using the xenon arc. British Multicentre Study Group. *Diabetes* 1983; **32**(11): 1010–16.

6 Early Treatment Diabetic Retinopathy Study Research Group. Photocoagulation for diabetic macular edema. Early Treatment Diabetic Retinopathy Study report number 1. *Arch Ophthalmol* 1985; **103**(12): 1796–806.

7 Early Treatment Diabetic Retinopathy Study Research Group. Treatment techniques and clinical guidelines for photocoagulation of diabetic macular edema. Early Treatment Diabetic Retinopathy Study Report Number 2. *Ophthalmology* 1987; **94**(7): 761–74.

8 Early worsening of diabetic retinopathy in the Diabetes Control and Complications Trial. *Arch Ophthalmol* 1998; **116**(7): 874–86.

9 Olk RJ. Modified grid argon (blue-green) laser photocoagulation for diffuse diabetic macular edema. *Ophthalmology* 1986; **93**(7): 938–50.

10 Davies EG, Petty RG, Kohner EM. Long term effectiveness of photocoagulation for diabetic maculopathy. *Eye* 1989; **3**(Pt 6): 764–7.

11 Chew EY, Ferris FL 3rd, Csaky KG, Murphy RP, Agron E, Thompson DJ *et al.* The long-term effects of laser photocoagulation treatment in patients with diabetic retinopathy: the early treatment diabetic retinopathy follow-up study. *Ophthalmology* 2003; **110**(9): 1683–9.

12 Fong DS, Segal PP, Myers F, Ferris FL, Hubbard LD, Davis MD. Subretinal fibrosis in diabetic macular edema. ETDRS report 23. Early Treatment Diabetic Retinopathy Study Research Group. *Arch Ophthalmol* 1997; **115**(7): 873–7.

13 Bailey CC, Sparrow JM, Grey RH, Cheng H. The National Diabetic Retinopathy Laser Treatment Audit. I. Maculopathy. *Eye* 1998; **12**(Pt 1): 69–76.

14 Bailey CC, Sparrow JM, Grey RH, Cheng H. The National Diabetic Retinopathy Laser Treatment Audit. III. Clinical outcomes. *Eye* 1999; **13**(Pt 2): 151–9.

15 Gogi D, Gupta A, Gupta V, Pandav SS, Dogra MR. Retinal microaneurysmal closure following focal laser photocoagulation in diabetic macular edema. *Ophthalmic Surg Lasers* 2002; **33**(5): 362–7.

16 Bandello F, Polito A, Del Borrello M, Zemella N, Isola M. 'Light' versus 'classic' laser treatment for clinically significant diabetic macular oedema. *Br J Ophthalmol* 2005; **89**(7): 864–70.

17 Writing Committee for the Diabetic Retinopathy Clinical Research Network. Comparison of the modified Early Treatment Diabetic Retinopathy Study and mild macular grid laser photocoagulation strategies for diabetic macular edema. *Arch Ophthalmol* 2007; **125**(4): 469–80.

18 Apple DJ, Goldberg MF, Wyhinny G. Histopathology and ultrastructure of the argon laser lesion in human retinal and choroidal vasculatures. *Am J Ophthalmol* 1973; **75**(4): 595–609.

19 Ogata N, Tombran-Tink J, Jo N, Mrazek D, Matsumura M. Upregulation of pigment epithelium-derived factor after laser photocoagulation. *Am J Ophthalmol* 2001; **132**(3): 427–9.

20 Xiao M, McLeod D, Cranley J, Williams G, Boulton M. Growth factor staining patterns in the pig retina following retinal laser photocoagulation. *Br J Ophthalmol* 1999; **83**(6): 728–36.

21 Arnarsson A, Stefansson E. Laser treatment and the mechanism of edema reduction in branch retinal vein occlusion. *Invest Ophthalmol Vis Sci* 2000; **41**(3): 877–9.

22 Schatz H, Madeira D, McDonald HR, Johnson RN. Progressive enlargement of laser scars following grid laser photocoagulation for diffuse diabetic macular edema. *Arch Ophthalmol* 1991; **109**(11): 1549–51.

23 Sivaprasad S, Sandhu R, Tandon A, Sayed-Ahmed K, McHugh DA. Subthreshold micropulse diode laser photocoagulation for clinically significant diabetic macular oedema: a three-year follow up. *Clin Experiment Ophthalmol* 2007; **35**(7): 640–4.

24 Laursen ML, Moeller F, Sander B, Sjoelie AK. Subthreshold micropulse diode laser treatment in diabetic macular oedema. *Br J Ophthalmol* 2004; **88**(9): 1173–9.

25 Luttrull JK, Musch DC, Mainster MA. Subthreshold diode micropulse photocoagulation for the treatment of clinically significant diabetic macular oedema. *Br J Ophthalmol* 2005; **89**(1): 74–80.

26 Kumar A, Sinha S. Intravitreal bevacizumab (Avastin) treatment of diffuse diabetic macular edema in an Indian population. *Indian J Ophthalmol* 2007; **55**(6): 451–5.

27 Yanyali A, Aytug B, Horozoglu F, Nohutcu AF. Bevacizumab (Avastin) for diabetic macular edema in previously vitrectomized eyes. *Am J Ophthalmol* 2007; **144**(1): 124–6.

28 Haritoglou C, Kook D, Neubauer A, Wolf A, Priglinger S, Strauss R *et al.* Intravitreal bevacizumab (Avastin) therapy for persistent diffuse diabetic macular edema. *Retina* 2006; **26**(9): 999–1005.

29 Arevalo JF, Fromow-Guerra J, Quiroz-Mercado H, Sanchez JG, Wu L, Maia M *et al.* Primary intravitreal bevacizumab (Avastin) for diabetic macular edema: results from the Pan-American Collaborative Retina Study Group at 6-month follow-up. *Ophthalmology* 2007; **114**(4): 743–50.

30 Starita C, Patel M, Katz B, Adamis AP. Vascular endothelial growth factor and the potential therapeutic use of pegaptanib (macugen) in diabetic retinopathy. *Dev Ophthalmol* 2007; **39**: 122–48.

31 Ciardella AP, Klancnik J, Schiff W, Barile G, Langton K, Chang S. Intravitreal triamcinolone for the treatment of refractory diabetic macular oedema with hard exudates: an optical coherence tomography study. *Br J Ophthalmol* 2004; **88**(9): 1131–6.

32 Jonas JB, Degenring RF, Kamppeter BA, Kreissig I, Akkoyun I. Duration of the effect of intravitreal triamcinolone ace-

tonide as treatment for diffuse diabetic macular edema. *Am J Ophthalmol* 2004; **138**(1): 158–60.

33 Jonas JB, Martus P, Degenring RF, Kreissig I, Akkoyun I. Predictive factors for visual acuity after intravitreal triamcinolone treatment for diabetic macular edema. *Arch Ophthalmol* 2005; **123**(10): 1338–43.

34 Lam DS, Chan CK, Tang EW, Li KK, Fan DS, Chan WM. Intravitreal triamcinolone for diabetic macular oedema in Chinese patients: six-month prospective longitudinal pilot study. *Clin Experiment Ophthalmol* 2004; **32**(6): 569–72.

35 Massin P, Audren F, Haouchine B, Erginay A, Bergmann JF, Benosman R *et al.* Intravitreal triamcinolone acetonide for diabetic diffuse macular edema: preliminary results of a prospective controlled trial. *Ophthalmology* 2004; **111**(2): 218–24; discussion 224–5.

36 Micelli Ferrari T, Sborgia L, Furino C, Cardascia N, Ferreri P, Besozzi G *et al.* Intravitreal triamcinolone acetonide: valuation of retinal thickness changes measured by optical coherence tomography in diffuse diabetic macular edema. *Eur J Ophthalmol* 2004; **14**(4): 321–4.

37 Ozkiris A, Evereklioglu C, Erkilic K, Tamcelik N, Mirza E. Intravitreal triamcinolone acetonide injection as primary treatment for diabetic macular edema. *Eur J Ophthalmol* 2004; **14**(6): 543–9.

38 Sutter FK, Simpson JM, Gillies MC. Intravitreal triamcinolone for diabetic macular edema that persists after laser treatment: three-month efficacy and safety results of a prospective, randomized, double-masked, placebo-controlled clinical trial. *Ophthalmology* 2004; **111**(11): 2044–9.

39 Chieh JJ, Roth DB, Liu M, Belmont J, Nelson M, Regillo C *et al.* Intravitreal triamcinolone acetonide for diabetic macular edema. *Retina* 2005; **25**(7): 828–34.

40 Er H, Yilmaz H. Intravitreal cortisone injection for refractory diffuse diabetic macular edema. *Ophthalmologica* 2005; **219**(6): 394–400.

41 Islam MS, Negi A, Vernon SA. Improved visual acuity and macular thickness 1 week after intravitreal triamcinolone for diabetic macular oedema. *Eye* 2005; **19**(12): 1325–7.

42 Khairallah M, Zeghidi H, Ladjimi A, Yahia SB, Attia S, Zaouali S *et al.* Primary intravitreal triamcinolone acetonide for diabetic massive macular hard exudates. *Retina* 2005; **25**(7): 835–9.

43 Negi AK, Vernon SA, Lim CS, Owen-Armstrong K. Intravitreal triamcinolone improves vision in eyes with chronic diabetic macular oedema refractory to laser photocoagulation. *Eye* 2005; **19**(7): 747–51.

44 Ozdemir H, Karacorlu M, Karacorlu SA. Regression of serous macular detachment after intravitreal triamcinolone acetonide in patients with diabetic macular edema. *Am J Ophthalmol* 2005; **140**(2): 251–5.

45 Patelli F, Fasolino G, Radice P, Russo S, Zumbo G, FM DIT *et al.* Time course of changes in retinal thickness and visual acuity after intravitreal triamcinolone acetonide for diffuse diabetic macular edema with and without previous macular laser treatment. *Retina* 2005; **25**(7): 840–5.

46 Zacks DN, Johnson MW. Combined intravitreal injection of triamcinolone acetonide and panretinal photocoagulation for concomitant diabetic macular edema and proliferative diabetic retinopathy. *Retina* 2005; **25**(2): 135–40.

47 Avci R, Kaderli B, Akalp FD. Intravitreal triamcinolone injection for chronic diffuse diabetic macular oedema. *Clin Experiment Ophthalmol* 2006; **34**(1): 27–32.

48 Spandau UH, Derse M, Schmitz-Valckenberg P, Papoulis C, Jonas JB. Dosage dependency of intravitreal triamcinolone acetonide as treatment for diabetic macular oedema. *Br J Ophthalmol* 2005; **89**(8): 999–1003.

49 Garcia-Arumi J, Boixadera A, Giralt J, Martinez-Castillo V, Gomez-Ulla F, Corcostegui B *et al.* Comparison of different techniques for purification of triamcinolone acetonide suspension for intravitreal use. *Br J Ophthalmol* 2005; **89**(9): 1112–14.

50 Oishi M, Maeda S, Nakamura A, Kurokawa N, Ohguro N, Tano Y. Examination of purification methods and development of intravitreal injection of triamcinolone acetonide. *Jpn J Ophthalmol* 2005; **49**(5): 384–7.

51 Bandello F, Polito A, Pognuz DR, Monaco P, Dimastrogiovanni A, Paissios J. Triamcinolone as adjunctive treatment to laser panretinal photocoagulation for proliferative diabetic retinopathy. *Arch Ophthalmol* 2006; **124**(5): 643–50.

52 Jonas JB. Intravitreal triamcinolone acetonide for diabetic retinopathy. *Dev Ophthalmol* 2007; **39**: 96–110.

53 Jonas JB, Kreissig I, Degenring RF. Cataract surgery after intravitreal injection of triamcinolone acetonide. *Eye* 2004; **18**(4): 361–4.

54 Singh IP, Ahmad SI, Yeh D, Challa P, Herndon LW, Allingham RR *et al.* Early rapid rise in intraocular pressure after intravitreal triamcinolone acetonide injection. *Am J Ophthalmol* 2004; **138**(2): 286–7.

55 Gupta R, Negi A, Vernon SA. Severe sub conjunctival haemorrhage following intravitreal triamcinolone for refractory diabetic oedema. *Eye* 2005; **19**(5): 590–1.

56 Stratton IM, Kohner EM, Aldington SJ, Turner RC, Holman RR, Manley SE *et al.* UKPDS 50: risk factors for incidence and progression of retinopathy in Type II diabetes over 6 years from diagnosis. *Diabetologia* 2001; **44**(2): 156–63.

57 The Diabetes Control and Complications Trial Research Group. The effect of intensive treatment of diabetes on the development and progression of long-term complications in insulin-dependent diabetes mellitus. *N Engl J Med* 1993; **329**(14): 977–86.

58 Matthews DR, Stratton IM, Aldington SJ, Holman RR, Kohner EM. Risks of progression of retinopathy and vision loss related to tight blood pressure control in type 2 diabetes mellitus: UKPDS 69. *Arch Ophthalmol* 2004; **122**(11): 1631–40.

59 Lyons TJ, Jenkins AJ, Zheng D, Lackland DT, McGee D, Garvey WT *et al.* Diabetic retinopathy and serum lipoprotein subclasses in the DCCT/EDIC cohort. *Invest Ophthalmol Vis Sci* 2004; **45**(3): 910–18.

7 Stage R1: mild non-proliferative diabetic retinopathy (background diabetic retinopathy)

Peter H. Scanlon

Optimum control of glycaemia, hypertension and lipids is recommended for all patients with diabetes.

MICROANEURYSMS

The *earliest sign* of mild non-proliferative diabetic retinopathy (mild NPDR) or background DR is microaneurysms (Table 7.1).

Patients with no DR and microaneurysms only were not included in the ETDRS study.

In the Wisconsin Epidemiological Study of Diabetic Retinopathy, the rate of progression to proliferative retinopathy 4 years after the initial evaluation showed 'no DR' was 0.4% for young insulin-dependent patients <30 years, 0% for older patients ≥30 years with diabetes taking insulin and 0.6% for those not using insulin.

For those with microaneurysms or one haemorrhage in one eye only, the rate of progression to proliferative retinopathy 4 years after the initial evaluation was 3.0% for young insulin-dependent people <30, 0% for older patients ≥30 with diabetes taking insulin, and 1.5% for those not using insulin (Fig. 7.1).

The *other signs* of mild NPDR are one or more of the following:
- retinal haemorrhages
- exudates (termed hard exudates in ETDRS)
- cotton wool spots (termed soft exudates in ETDRS)
- a single venous loop (in ETDRS definition of mild NPDR but not included in UK definition of background DR).

A Practical Manual of Diabetic Retinopathy Management.
Peter H Scanlon, Charles P Wilkinson, Stephen J Aldington and David R Matthews. Published 2009 by Blackwell Publishing, ISBN 978-1-4051-7035-2.

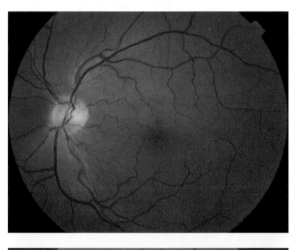

(a)

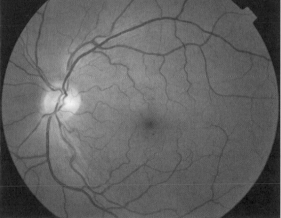

(b)

Fig. 7.1 Microaneurysms in mild NPDR. (a) Colour photograph (b) Red-free photograph. (*Continued on p. 100*)

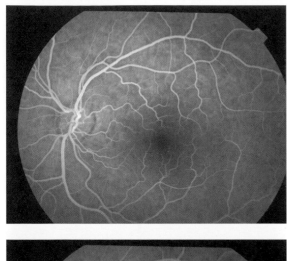

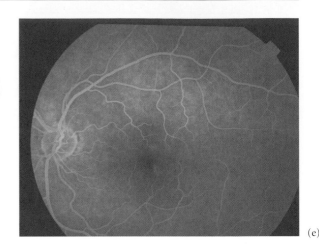

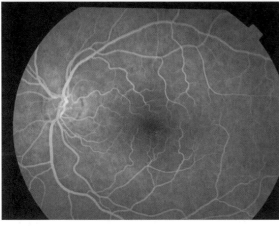

Fig. 7.1 (*Cont'd*) (c) Fluorescein angiogram at 44 s showing fluorescence from microaneurysms but no signs of leakage. (d) Fluorescein angiogram at 1 min 30 s showing fluorescence from microaneurysms but no signs of leakage. (e) Fluorescein angiogram at 4 min 20 s showing a small amount of leakage from microaneurysms.

Table 7.1 Mild NPDR (ETDRS and International) and background DR (UK screening).

ETDRS final retinopathy severity scale[1]	ETDRS (final) grade	Lesions	Risk of progression to PDR in 1 year (ETDRS interim)	Background DR (UK screening)
Mild NPDR	20	Microaneurysms only		Microaneurysm(s)
	35	One or more of the following:	ETDRS level	Retinal haemorrhage(s)
	a	venous loops ≥definite in 1 field	30 = 6.2% risk of	± any exudate
	b	SE, IRMA or VB questionable	progression to	
	c	retinal haemorrhages present	proliferative in	
	d	HE ≥definite in 1 field	1 year	
	e	SE ≥definite in 1 field		

RETINAL HAEMORRHAGES

In mild NPDR, retinal haemorrhages are usually small dot haemorrhages or flame-shaped haemorrhages. Because small retinal haemorrhages can be difficult to differentiate from microaneurysms they are commonly referred to as HMa.

Flame-shaped haemorrhages are present just under the superficial nerve fibre layer. Blot haemorrhages are usually in a deeper retinal layer and denote a sign of ischaemia. Hence multiple blot haemorrhages would not be considered mild NPDR (Fig. 7.2).

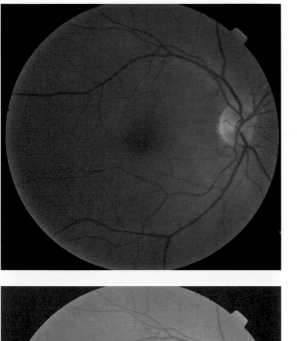

(a)

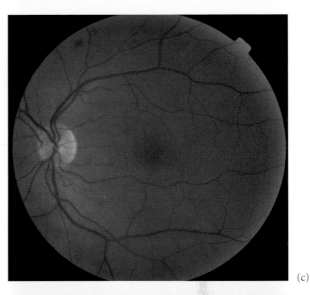

(c)

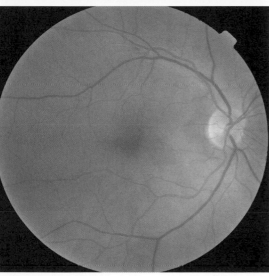

(b)

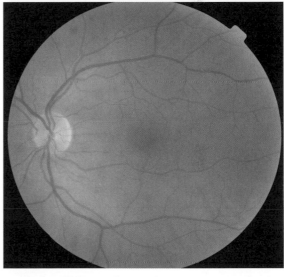

(d)

Fig. 7.2 Haemorrhages, microaneurysms, occasional cotton wool spots (CWS) and hard exudates in mild NPDR. (a) Haemorrhages and microaneurysms in mild NPDR: colour photograph right macula view. (b) Haemorrhages and microaneurysms in mild NPDR: red-free photograph right

macula view. (c) Haemorrhages, microaneurysms, occasional CWS and hard exudates in mild NPDR: colour photograph left macula view. (d) Haemorrhages, microaneurysms, occasional CWS and hard exudates in mild NPDR: red-free photograph left macula view.

EXUDATES (OR HARD EXUDATES)

Exudates (or hard exudates) are a feature of mild NPDR. They are small white or yellowish-white deposits with sharp margins, located typically in the outer layers of the retina, but they may be more superficial, particularly when retinal oedema is present. In mild NPDR, exudates

may develop in the macular area and be a photographic marker of clinically significant macular oedema (Fig. 7.3).

COTTON WOOL SPOTS

Cotton wool spots are fluffy white opaque areas caused by an accumulation of axoplasm in the nerve fibre layer

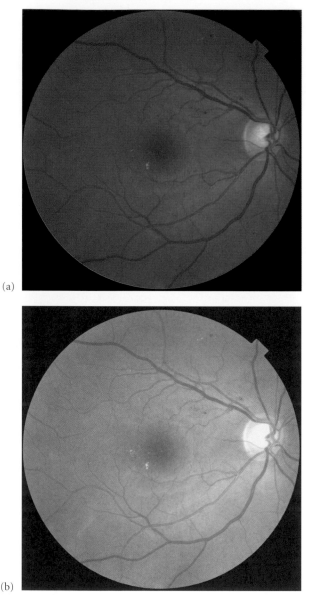

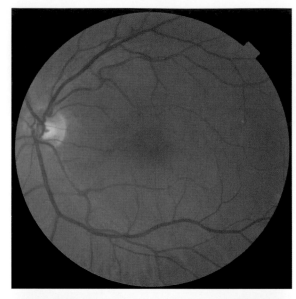

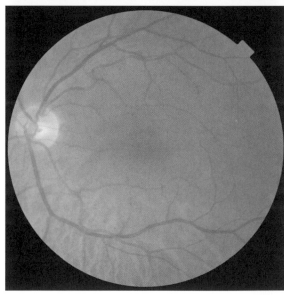

(a)

(b)

(c)

(d)

Fig. 7.3 Exudates in mild NPDR developing in right macular area. (a) Colour photograph right macular view. (b) Red-free photograph right macular view. (c) Colour photograph left macular view showing exudates in superotemporal retina. (d) Red-free photograph left macular view showing exudates in superotemporal retina.

of the retina. They may be present in mild NPDR or background DR and are caused by an arteriolar occlusion in that area of retina, but despite this being the underlying cause they are not a good sign of increasing retinal ischaemia. They are often associated with hypertension. When several are present one needs to look closely at the level of blood pressure and for signs of ischaemia that are more closely associated with progression of diabetic retinopathy such as venous beading, intraretinal microvascular abnormalities and multiple blot haemorrhages, which would classify the retinopathy into a more severe grade (Fig. 7.4).

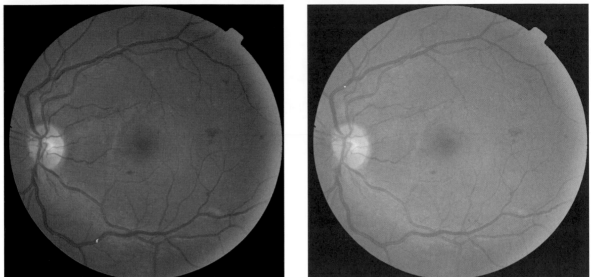

(a)   (b)

Fig. 7.4 (a) Cotton wool spots in mild NPDR. (b) Red-free version of (a) showing cotton wool spots, exudates, haemorrhages and microaneurysms.

A SINGLE VENOUS LOOP

A venous loop is an abrupt curving deviation of a vein from its normal path and the ETDRS included a single venous loop in their classification of mild NPDR. However, this rarely occurs in isolation without other significant signs of retinal ischaemia and a venous loop is therefore not a feature of the English screening definition of background diabetic retinopathy.

PRACTICE POINTS

- For mild non-proliferative diabetic retinopathy there is a 6.2% risk of progression to proliferative in 1 year.
- The International Classification[2] of diabetic retinopathy recommends that anyone who has more than just microaneurysms is referred to an ophthalmologist.
- In the UK, patients who are screened and who show signs of background diabetic retinopathy only are

rescreened annually. For the purposes of the National Screening Programme, background DR is defined[3] by the following lesions:

- microaneurysm(s)
- retinal haemorrhage(s) ± any exudate.

REFERENCES

1 Early Treatment Diabetic Retinopathy Study Research Group. Fundus photographic risk factors for progression of diabetic retinopathy. ETDRS report number 12. *Ophthalmology* 1991; **98**(5 Suppl): 823–33.

2 Wilkinson CP, Ferris FL 3rd, Klein RE, Lee PP, Agardh CD, Davis M *et al.* Proposed international clinical diabetic retinopathy and diabetic macular edema disease severity scales. *Ophthalmology* 2003; **110**(9): 1677–82.

3 Harding S, Greenwood R, Aldington S, Gibson J, Owens D, Taylor R *et al.* Grading and disease management in national screening for diabetic retinopathy in England and Wales. *Diabet Med* 2003; **20**(12): 965–71.

8

Stage R2: moderate and severe non-proliferative diabetic retinopathy (preproliferative diabetic retinopathy)

Peter H. Scanlon

MODERATE AND SEVERE NPDR (ETDRS AND INTERNATIONAL)[1] AND PREPROLIFERATIVE DR (UK SCREENING)[2]

Optimum control of glycaemia, hypertension and lipids is recommended for all patients with diabetes. Definitions of moderate and severe non-proliferative DR based on lesion detection in the ETDRS fields is shown in Table 8.1.

Microaneurysms in increasing numbers have been shown to be an important early measure of progression of diabetic retinopathy.[4,5] Hard exudates (sometimes now just referred to as exudates) are not a good marker of retinal ischaemia. Cotton wool spots (referred to as soft exudates in the ETDRS, a term that is now rarely used) are fluffy white opaque areas caused by an arteriolar occlusion in an area of retina resulting in an accumulation of axoplasm in the nerve fibre layer. Despite this being the underlying cause they are not a good sign of increasing retinal ischaemia. They are often associated with hypertension. When several are present one needs to look closely for raised blood pressure and for signs of increasing ischaemia that are more closely associated with progression such as venous beading, intraretinal microvascular abnormalities and multiple blot haemorrhages, which would classify the retinopathy into moderate or severe diabetic retinopathy.

A Practical Manual of Diabetic Retinopathy Management.
Peter H Scanlon, Charles P Wilkinson, Stephen J Aldington and David R Matthews. Published 2009 by Blackwell Publishing, ISBN 978-1-4051-7035-2.

The main features that warrant classifying a diabetic retinopathy level into the higher levels of moderate and severe NPDR (or preproliferative DR) are increasing signs of retinal ischaemia.

Lesions associated with increasing retinal ischaemia are retinal haemorrhages, intraretinal microvascular abnormality and venous beading.

RETINAL HAEMORRHAGES

Increasing numbers of haemorrhages, particularly when the pattern of haemorrhages includes an increasing number of blot haemorrhages, denotes increasing retinal ischaemia and progression of DR. Blot haemorrhages are usually in a deeper retinal layer than more superficial dot haemorrhages and flame haemorrhages (Fig. 8.1).

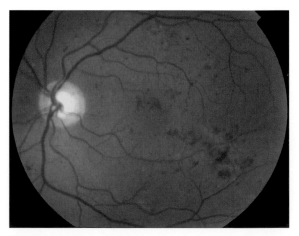

Fig. 8.1 Retinal haemorrhages.

Table 8.1 Lesion classification of moderate to severe NPDR.

ETDRS final retinopathy severity scale[3]	ETDRS (final) grade	Lesions	Risk of progression to PDR in 1 year (ETDRS interim)	Practical clinic follow-up intervals (not ETDRS)
Moderate NPDR	43a	HMa moderate in 4–5 fields or severe in 1 field or	Level 41 = 11.3%	6 months
	b	IRMA definite in 1–3 fields		
Moderately severe NPDR	47 a	Both level 43 characteristics: HMa moderate in 4–5 fields or severe in 1 field and IRMA definite in 1–3 fields **or** any one of the following:	Level 45 = 20.7%	4 months
	b	IRMA in 4–5 fields		
	c	HMa severe in 2–3 fields		
	d	VB definite in 1 field		
Severe NPDR	53	One or more of the following:	Level 51 = 44.2%	3 months
	a	≥2 of the 3 level 47 characteristics	Level 55 = 54.8%	
	b	HMa severe in 4–5 fields		
	c	IRMA ≥ moderate in 1 field		
	d	VB ≥ definite in 2–3 fields		

INTRARETINAL MICROVASCULAR ABNORMALITY

Intraretinal microvascular abnormalities (IRMAs) are defined as tortuous intraretinal vascular segments varying in calibre. By definition, IRMAs are not on the surface of the retina and do not break through the internal limiting membrane. IRMAs are derived from remodelling of the retinal capillaries and small collateral vessels in areas of microvascular occlusion. They are usually found on the borders of areas of non-perfused retina. They are, therefore, a sign of retinal ischaemia (Fig. 8.2).

VENOUS BEADING

In the ETDRS venous beading (VB) was described as a localized increase in calibre of the vein and the severity was dependent on the increase in calibre and the length of vein involved.

VB was found to be associated with retinal ischaemia and is used for assessment of severity of diabetic retinopathy (Fig. 8.3).

With increasing ischaemia, there is an increasing risk of progression to proliferative in 1 year. The risk increases from approximately 11.3% in the lower levels of moderate NPDR to 54.8% progression to proliferative in 1 year in the most severe non-proliferative DR level.

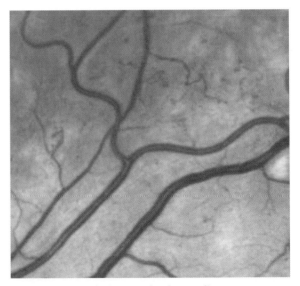

Fig. 8.2 Intraretinal microvascular abnormality.

ETDRS definitions have been simplified to make them easier for everyday clinical use both in the International Classification and in the UK classification for screening.

The ETDRS '4:2:1 rule' indicates that the presence of severe haemorrhages in 4 quadrants (≥20), or VB in 2 quadrants, or IRMA in a single quadrant represents severe non-proliferative DR.

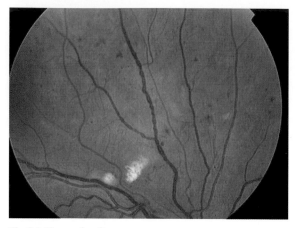

Fig. 8.3 Venous beading.

Hence in the **International Classification**, severe NPDR is defined by any of the following:
- extensive intraretinal haemorrhages (>20) in 4 quadrants
- definite venous beading in 2+ quadrants
- prominent IRMA in 1+ quadrant

<u>and</u> no signs of PDR.

Moderate NPDR is classified in the International Classification as:
- more than 'microaneurysms only'
- and less severe than the 4:2:1 rule.

In the **UK Screening Classification** preproliferative DR is defined by any of the following:
- venous beading
- venous loop or reduplication
- intraretinal microvascular abnormality
- multiple deep, round or blot haemorrhages.

CASE HISTORY 1
Severe non-proliferative DR/early proliferative DR just at the stage when tiny NVDs and NVE are beginning to form

A 59-year-old woman (BMI 30) with type 2 diabetes of 17 years' duration controlled by insulin was referred from retinal screening with multiple haemorrhages in both eyes and followed up within the eye department for the subsequent 4 years. Poorly controlled blood pressure has been a consistent feature; despite determined efforts to control this over the 4 years the blood pressure has only improved from 220/110 to 150/84. HbA1c has improved from 11.3% to 8.6% during this time. She complained of blurriness of vision in her left eye, the visual acuity (VA) having reduced to 6/18 (20/60). The fluorescein angiogram shows multiple haemorrhages, some very early NVD, ischaemic areas, particularly in the superotemporal retina and some NVE adjacent to the superotemporal ischaemia. There is leakage below the left macula (Fig. 8.4).

The left eye was treated with focal laser treatment to the area of leakage below the left macula:
- 31 burns, 100-micron size, 180 mW, 0.1 s, area centralis lens, argon laser.

After 3 months the left vision had improved to 6/9 (20/30) and panretinal photocoagulation was commenced.
- A total of 1552 burns were given in two sessions, 750 using 350-micron spot size and the Transequator lens (magnification factor 1.44), and 802 using the SuperQuad 160 lens (magnification factor 2) and 200-micron spot size. The average power used was 240 mW and the duration 0.1 s.

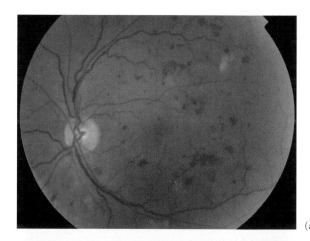

(a)

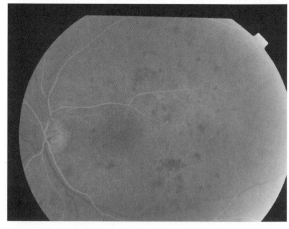

(b)

Fig. 8.4 Case history 1. (a) Left macula colour; (b) fluorescein 33 s; (*Continued on facing page*)

This has resulted in control of the neovascularization over the subsequent 2-year period since this treatment. Her left VA has improved to a level of 6/9 (20/30).

CASE HISTORY 2
Severe non-proliferative DR with maculopathy

A 69-year-old woman (BMI 28) with type 2 diabetes controlled by metformin 1000 mg t.d.s. of 16 years' duration had previously received some laser treatment for clinically significant macular oedema and is now showing increasing leakage in her right macular area and increasing signs of ischaemia. Her HBA1c is 9.3%, blood pressure 140/60, cholesterol 5.7 mmol/L and Ch : HDL ratio 4.4. The colour photograph and fluorescein angiogram in Fig. 8.5 show patches of significant ischaemia in the temporal retina with poor vascular supply and irregularity of the

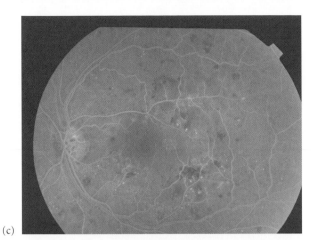

(c)

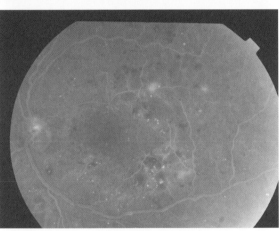

(d)

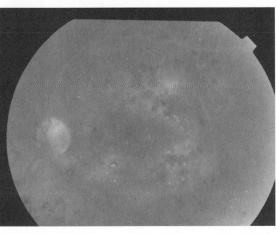

(e)

Fig. 8.4 (*Cont'd*) (c) fluorescein 42 s; (d) fluorescein 1 min 03 s; (e) fluorescein 4 min 00 s.

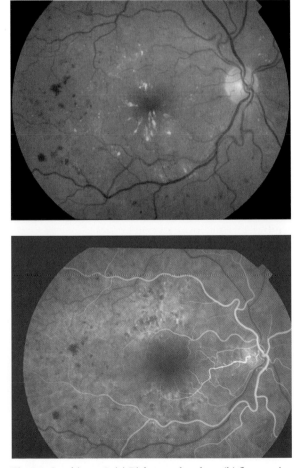

(a)

(b)

Fig. 8.5 Case history 2. (a) Right macula colour; (b) fluorescein 17 s; (*Continued on p. 108*)

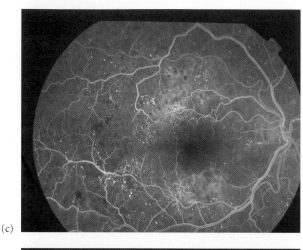

(c)

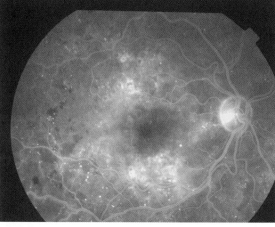

(d)

Fig. 8.5 (*Cont'd*) (c) fluorescein 17 s; (d) fluorescein 3 min 44 s.

vessels on the edge of this area. There is also leakage in the right macular area, which required further laser treatment to the areas of retinal thickening. In addition, moderate IRMA were present in the nasal retina not shown in these macular fields.

PRACTICE POINTS

- The higher levels of moderate and severe NPDR (or preproliferative DR) show increasing signs of retinal ischaemia, which carries an increasing risk of development of proliferative DR.
- Treatment of high blood pressure and hyperglycaemia is important to reduce the combined effects, which further increases the risks of progression.

REFERENCES

1 Wilkinson CP, Ferris FL 3rd, Klein RE, Lee PP, Agardh CD, Davis M *et al.* Proposed international clinical diabetic retinopathy and diabetic macular edema disease severity scales. *Ophthalmology* 2003; **110**(9): 1677–82.

2 Harding S, Greenwood R, Aldington S, Gibson J, Owens D, Taylor R *et al.* Grading and disease management in national screening for diabetic retinopathy in England and Wales. *Diabet Med* 2003; **20**(12): 965–71.

3 Fundus photographic risk factors for progression of diabetic retinopathy. ETDRS report number 12. Early Treatment Diabetic Retinopathy Study Research Group. *Ophthalmology* 1991; **98**(5 Suppl): 823–33.

4 Klein R, Meuer SM, Moss SE, Klein BE. Retinal microaneurysm counts and 10-year progression of diabetic retinopathy. *Arch Ophthalmol* 1995; **113**(11): 1386–91.

5 Kohner EM, Stratton IM, Aldington SJ, Turner RC, Matthews DR. Microaneurysms in the development of diabetic retinopathy (UKPDS 42). UK Prospective Diabetes Study Group. *Diabetologia* 1999; **42**(9): 1107–12.

9

Stage R3: proliferative diabetic retinopathy and advanced diabetic retinopathy

Peter H. Scanlon

THE RELEVANT ANATOMY

New vessels developing in diabetic retinopathy are characterized according to whether they develop at or near the optic disc or elsewhere in the retina. They can develop from the venous or arterial circulation and grow forwards in the vitreous gel. Over time they may fibrose and retract causing traction on the underlying retina or they may haemorrhage. If a patient has a posterior vitreous detachment, this removes the structure that new vessels use to grow forwards into the vitreous gel and although this may cause a haemorrhage if a patient already has new vessels, subsequent haemorrhages are less common as the base of the vessel has often been sheared off.

New vessels on the disc (NVD) are defined as any new vessel developing at the optic disc or within 1 disc diameter (1 DD) of the edge of the optic disc. New vessels on the disc usually occur as a result of generalized retinal ischaemia.

New vessels elsewhere (NVE) are defined as any new vessel developing more than 1 DD away from the edge of the optic disc. New vessels elsewhere usually occur on the edge of an area of retinal ischaemia peripheral to the NVE.

Abortive neovascular outgrowths is a term that has been used in the past to describe small raspberry-like NVE, which usually lie in an area temporal to the fovea and which, like most NVE, lie adjacent to areas of capillary non-perfusion.

A Practical Manual of Diabetic Retinopathy Management.
Peter H Scanlon, Charles P Wilkinson, Stephen J Aldington and David R Matthews. Published 2009 by Blackwell Publishing, ISBN 978-1-4051-7035-2.

Another consequence of generalized retinal ischaemia can be neovascularization in the anterior chamber. If this neovascularization involves the angle of the anterior chamber, neovascular glaucoma may result.

THE PHOTOGRAPHIC APPEARANCE

New vessels appear as fronds appearing either at the disc or elsewhere in the retina. As they develop they grow forwards into the vitreous gel and this is shown on stereo photographs. On a two-dimensional photograph the forward development of these new vessels can be interpreted by the structures that they overlie.

FLUORESCEIN ANGIOGRAPHIC APPEARANCE

The characteristic appearance of new vessels on the fluorescein angiogram, once they have penetrated the internal limiting membrane, is leakage appearing in the arteriovenous phase of the angiogram and increasing through the angiogram (Fig. 9.1a–d).

Abortive neovascular outgrowths are shown leaking in the venous phase of this angiogram (Fig. 9.1e).

Leakage can be variable but very little leakage from a small NVE usually means that these have not yet penetrated the internal limiting membrane (Fig. 9.2a,b).

PRESENTATION

In an ideal world, patients with diabetes would receive annual screening for diabetic retinopathy and more frequent assessments once signs of diabetic retinopathy develop and new vessels are detected at an early stage. At the other end of the spectrum, some patients who have not had their eyes examined for years, and who have

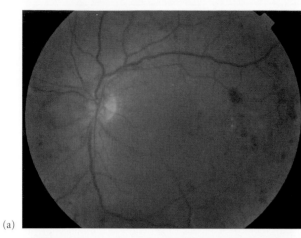

(a)

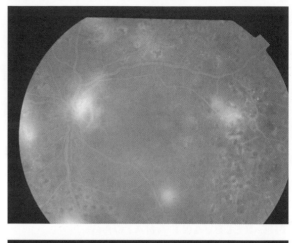

(d)

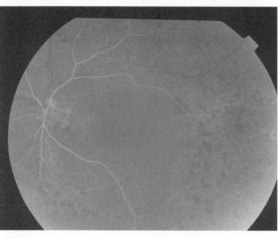

(b)

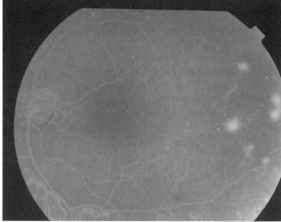

(e)

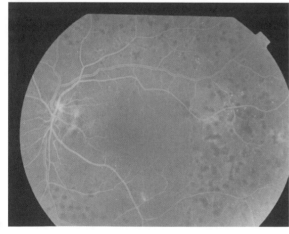

(c)

Fig. 9.1 (a) NVD and NVE colour photograph in patient who has previously received scatter laser treatment. (b) Fluorescein angiogram in early arteriovenous phase from the same patient showing no obvious leakage. (c) Fluorescein angiogram in mid-arteriovenous phase from the same patient showing leakage appearing from NVD and NVE. (d) Fluorescein angiogram in the late venous phase from the same patient showing leakage from NVD and NVE. (e) Fluorescein angiogram showing leakage from raspberry-like NVE (abortive neovascular outgrowths) in the temporal retina in the venous phase. From a patient with ischaemia in the adjacent peripheral retina.

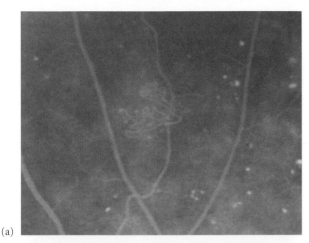

(a)

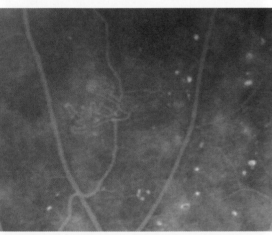

(b)

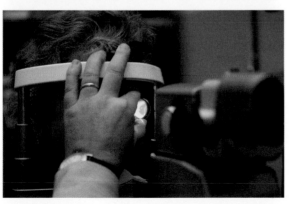

(c)

Fig. 9.2 NVE in superior retina showing minimal or no leakage that have not yet penetrated the internal limiting membrane in (a) midvenous phase and (b) late venous phase. (c) Laser treatment being performed.

advanced changes of diabetic retinopathy, present with a sudden onset of visual loss from a vitreous haemorrhage occurring from bleeding from large new vessels. The initial sight loss from a vitreous haemorrhage will depend on the amount of haemorrhage and the visual prognosis will depend on the level of the underlying diabetic retinopathy and the degree of retinal ischaemia and any associated maculopathy.

THE 'EARLY WORSENING' PHENOMENON

In 1998 the Diabetes Control and Complications Trial[1] (DCCT) described the effect of early worsening of diabetic retinopathy at the 6- and/or 12-month visit in 13.1% of 711 patients assigned to intensive treatment. Early worsening led to high risk proliferative retinopathy in two patients in the DCCT. The most important risk factors for early worsening were higher HbA1c level at screening and reduction of this level during the first 6 months after randomization.

MULTIDISCIPLINARY APPROACH AND TREATMENT OF ASSOCIATED RISK FACTORS

Many patients who end up with severe diabetic eye disease have suboptimal control of blood glucose, blood pressure and lipid levels. It is important to have a multidisciplinary approach to these patients so that the eye is not treated in isolation. Hence it is important that proper attention is paid to the management of:
- systemic hypertension
- glucose control
- blood lipids.

LASER TREATMENT FOR PROLIFERATIVE DIABETIC RETINOPATHY (see Fig. 9.2c)

The Diabetic Retinopathy Study

In 1976, the Diabetic Retinopathy Study[2] (DRS) reported their preliminary results. A total of 1727 patients who could be treated according to the study protocol had been enrolled. The eligibility criteria were: (a) diabetic retinopathy in both eyes, either proliferative changes in at least one eye or severe non-proliferative changes in both eyes and (b) a visual acuity (VA) of 20/100 or better in both eyes.

One eye of each patient was randomly selected for treatment with xenon or argon laser and the control eye observed without treatment. The principal endpoint was the occurrence of VA of less than 5/200 at one or more of the monthly follow-up visits. Visual acuity of less than 5/200 occurred in 129 untreated eyes and 56 treated eyes. This amounted to a reduction in 57% in the occurrence of severe visual loss in treated eyes. The organizers of the DRS modified the trial protocol and recommended treatment for control eyes with 'high risk characteristics'.

Important outcomes of the Diabetic Retinopathy Study

The DRS[3,4] recommended prompt treatment in the presence of DRS high risk characteristics, which reduced the 2-year risk of severe visual loss by 50% or more and were defined by:

- the presence of preretinal or vitreous haemorrhage (Figs 9.3–9.5)
- eyes with NVD equalling or exceeding one-quarter to one-third disc area in extent with no haemorrhage (Fig. 9.6)

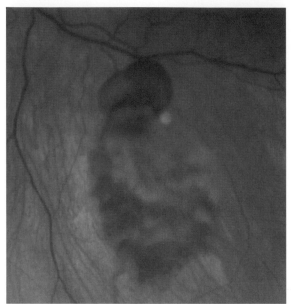

(a)

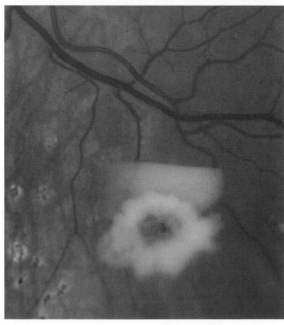

(b)

Fig. 9.4 (a) Preretinal haemorrhage. (b) Preretinal haemorrhage organizing.

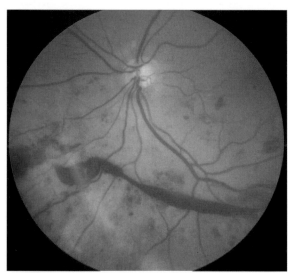

(a)

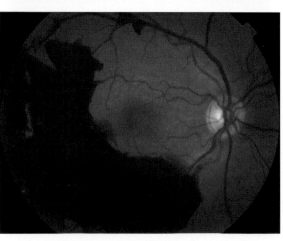

(b)

Fig. 9.3 (a,b) Preretinal haemorrhage.

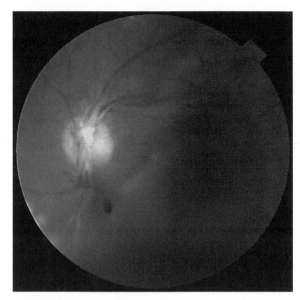

Fig. 9.5 A larger vitreous haemorrhage.

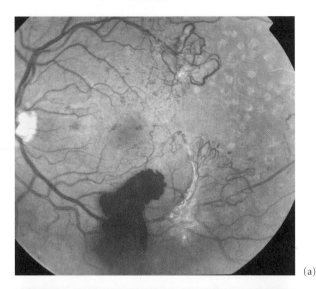

(a)

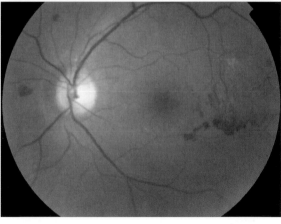

(b)

Fig. 9.7 (a,b) NVE equalling more than half disc area with haemorrhage.

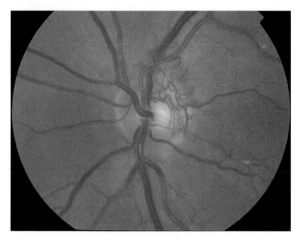

Fig. 9.6 NVD greater than one-third disc area.

- NVE equalling more than a half disc area with haemorrhage (Fig. 9.7).

Untreated, eyes with high risk characteristics had between a 25.6% and 36.9% chance of severe visual loss within 2 years, depending on the size and location of the new vessels and whether or not haemorrhage was present.

The risks for patients without high risk characteristics in the DRS and ETDRS

In eyes with high risk characteristics, the 2-year risk of severe visual loss (25–35%) clearly outweighed the risks of treatment (small reduction in VA or visual field in approximately 15% of eyes).

The risks of severe visual loss in eyes without high risk characteristics did show a benefit from treatment as shown below but, as the difference was not as great as for those with high risk characteristics, the risks of harmful effects of treatment need to be taken into consideration (Fig. 9.8).

For patients with proliferative DR without high risk characteristics and severe NPDR, the DRS findings did not provide a clear choice for these patients between prompt treatment and careful follow-up with deferral of treatment until high risk characteristics develop, and other factors need to be considered in these patients.

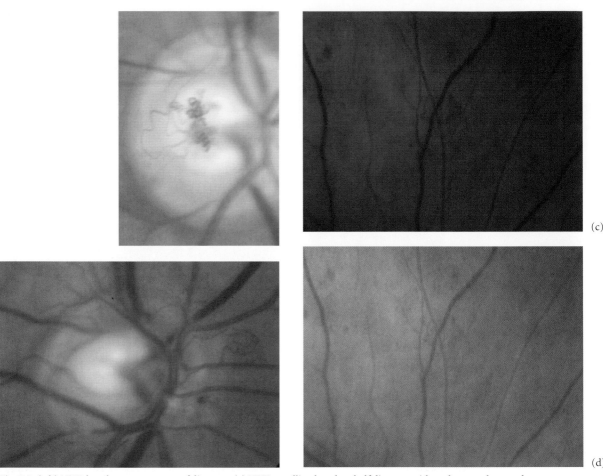

(a)

(b)

(c)

(d)

Fig. 9.8 (a,b) NVD less than one-quarter of disc area. (c) NVE equalling less than half disc area without haemorrhage: colour photograph. (d) NVE equalling less than half disc area without haemorrhage: red-free photograph.

Eyes with low risk characteristics had the following risks of severe visual loss.
- Non-proliferative control group:
  - untreated 2-year 3.2%; 4-year 12.8%
  - treated 2-year 2.8%; 4-year 4.3%.
- Proliferative without high risk characteristics control group:
  - untreated 2-year 7.0%; 4-year 20.9%
  - treated 2-year 3.2%; 4-year 7.4%.

The ETDRS[5] attempted to alter the treatment protocol to reduce harmful effects (division of scatter treatment between two or more sittings or reduction of the number of burns). In the ETDRS only 50% of eyes assigned to deferral had developed high risk proliferative retinopathy. For eyes with very severe non-proliferative retinopathy or moderate proliferative retinopathy, the benefits and risks of early photocoagulation were roughly equal. Very few eyes in the ETDRS had more than 2 disc areas of neovascularization elsewhere and the possibility that for these eyes there might be an advantage of prompt scatter photocoagulation could not be ruled out. For eyes with macular oedema and more severe retinopathy the risk of severe visual loss in eyes assigned to deferral of photocoagulation was relatively high (6.5% at the 5-year visit). This risk was reduced to between 3.8% and 4.7% in the eyes assigned to early photocoagulation. The ETDRS did not include evaluation of a strategy that consisted of prompt focal photocoagulation with delayed scatter in eyes with clinically significant macular oedema and eyes that are approaching the high risk category, which would be the current recommendation.

Adverse effects of laser treatment in the DRS and other studies

The potential adverse effects of panretinal photocoagulation treatment were described in 1987 by the DRS[4] Research Group.

Loss of peripheral areas of visual field

Loss of peripheral areas of visual field was attributed to argon laser in approximately 10% of eyes and field loss was nearly three times more common in the xenon arc-treated group.

Visual acuity loss

Visual acuity loss at the 6-week follow-up visit was assumed to be due to treatment. Among eyes with non-proliferative diabetic retinopathy: 14.3% more argon-treated and 29.7% more xenon-treated eyes than controls had an early persistent loss of one or more lines.

For decreases of more than two lines the comparable percentages were 2.5% (argon-treated) and 10.6% (xenon-treated) and for decreases of 5 or more lines, they were 1.3% (argon-treated) and 1.8% (xenon-treated).

McDonald and Schatz[6] reviewed the results of 175 eyes of 134 patients with proliferative diabetic retinopathy treated with panretinal photocoagulation: 75 (43%) of the treated eyes developed increased macular oedema 6–10 weeks following laser treatment with a median follow-up of 15 months. Fluorescein angiography revealed that the post-laser increase in macular oedema persisted in 47 of the 175 eyes (27%). Fourteen eyes (8%) treated with laser developed chronic macular oedema and visual loss of two or more lines. Patients were treated with argon laser photocoagulation (0.05 s, 500-micron spot size, in two or more sessions with an average of 2300 burns). Although 47 eyes developed a persistent increase in macular oedema following treatment, only 16 lost vision. Thirty-one eyes therefore developed increased oedema (demonstrated on fluorescein angiography) and did not lose vision (Fig. 9.9).

Clearly the disease process itself can have an adverse effect on VA and field and will be more pronounced in those patients with more severe disease. The following studies reported the effect of the disease process, panretinal photocoagulation and vitrectomy on the minimum VA and field for the British driving standard.

In 1994, Mackie[7] reported on the results of the Esterman binocular visual field test and VAs in 100 consecutive patients who had received bilateral panretinal photocoagulation (PRP):

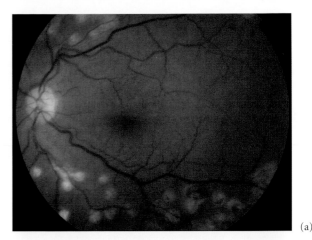

(a)

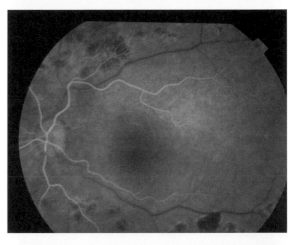

(b)

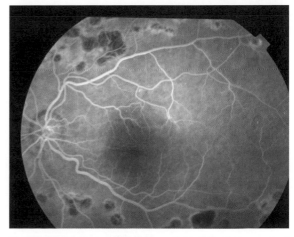

(c)

Fig. 9.9 Persistent cystoid macular oedema following panretinal laser treatment: (a) colour photograph; (b) fluorescein photograph 20 s after injection; (c) fluorescein photograph 31 s after injection; (*Continued on p. 116*)

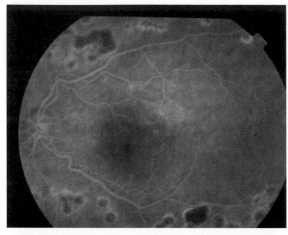

(d)

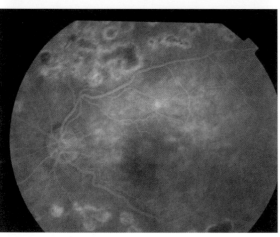

(e)

Fig. 9.9 (*Cont'd*) (d) fluorescein photograph 1 min 31 s after injection; (e) fluorescein photograph 4 min 14 s after injection.

- 4% failed to achieve the VA requirements but met field requirements
- 9% failed to achieve the field requirements but met the VA requirements
- 17% failed to achieve both the field and the VA requirements
- 74% retained the minimum field for the British driving standard.

Of those who failed it was estimated that approximately one-third was due to laser treatment. The remainder failed from a combination of treatment and maculopathy or complications directly related to the disease process.

This compares to a prospective study in 2006 of ETDRS acuity and Humphrey binocular Esterman visual field testing by Barsam[8] in 20 patients who underwent vitrec-

tomy for complications of diabetic retinopathy. Seventy per cent of patients had sufficient binocular acuity to drive and of these 71.4% were shown not to have a minimum visual field for safe driving on binocular Esterman field analysis. Patients who have had a vitrectomy are more likely to have a restricted visual field because their disease is more severe, there is more peripheral retinal ischaemia and they may have received more laser treatment.

CASE HISTORY 1
Driving field difficulties following extensive laser and vitrectomy for very ischaemic retinae

A 48-year-old man (BMI 33) with type 2 diabetes of 24 years' duration controlled by insulin had extensive laser treatment to both eyes before left pars plana vitrectomy and endolaser. During the period of treatment the HBA1c has varied between 7.8% and 8.6% and his blood pressure has been well controlled, averaging 125/75. His corrected VA level is right 6/9 (20/30), left 6/18 (20/60), which would meet the UK visual standard, but the Esterman field shown in Fig. 9.10(a) would not.

For the Esterman field, one needs to be able to see the points in the area 120° horizontally and 40° vertically and this field clearly misses many points in this area. Colour and fluorescein photographs show the underlying retinal ischaemia that has contributed to the reduced field in this patient (Fig. 9.10b–g).

Other possible adverse effects of panretinal laser treatment

Unintended laser absorption
This can occur in the lens of the eye in the presence of lens opacities and from intraretinal haemorrhages. In the latter example, uptake of laser from a flame-shaped haemorrhage, this may result in a burn and destruction of the nerve fibre layer that lies on its surface.

Inadvertent coagulation
Clearly, unintended photocoagulation to the fovea when performing panretinal photocoagulation is the area of most concern and the laser technique employed should allow one to be aware at all times of where the fovea is in relation to the area being lasered.

Choroidal detachment
When a choroidal detachment occurs this is usually as a result of a large dose of laser treatment being applied in a single session. This may result in the precipitation of

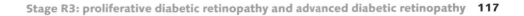

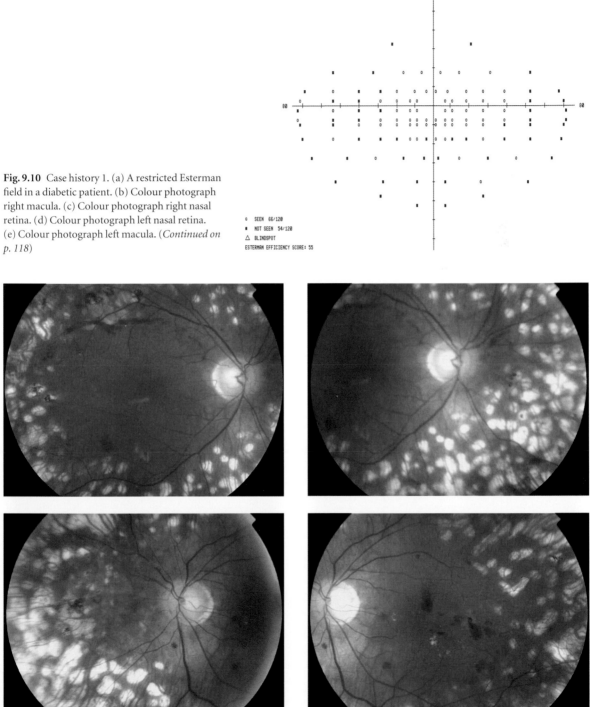

Fig. 9.10 Case history 1. (a) A restricted Esterman field in a diabetic patient. (b) Colour photograph right macula. (c) Colour photograph right nasal retina. (d) Colour photograph left nasal retina. (e) Colour photograph left macula. (*Continued on p. 118*)

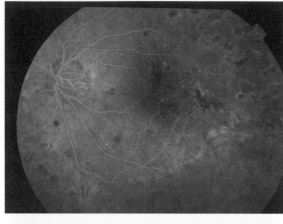

(f)

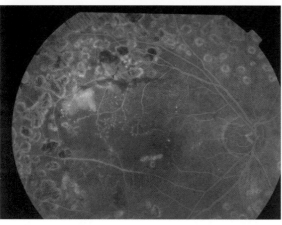

(g)

Fig. 9.10 (*Cont'd*) (f) Fluorescein left macular area 45 s after injection showing ischaemia and IRMA in the area around the left macula. (g) Fluorescein right macular area 1 min 10 s after injection showing ischaemia and IRMA in the area around the left macula.

angle closure glaucoma if a patient has a shallow anterior chamber. The choroidal detachment usually resolves spontaneously within 10 days.

Risks to the ophthalmologist

There has been some concern in the past that the ophthalmologist is exposed to excessive amounts of reflected light, particularly blue light. However, modern technology with appropriate filters has significantly reduced this risk.

Risks to an observer

The risk to an observer is extremely small because they are very unlikely to be exposed to a sufficient dose of reflected

or direct laser light to produce any adverse consequences. However, as a precaution it is advised that any observer wears the appropriate spectacle protection.

Factors other than high risk characteristics influencing the decision to laser

Anterior segment neovascularization

Extensive neovascularization in the anterior chamber angle is an urgent indication for scatter laser photocoagulation, if it is feasible, whether or not high risk characteristics are present.

CASE HISTORY 2
Iris neovascularization

This 68-year-old man with type 2 diabetes, diagnosed at the age of 34 years and treated with oral gliclazide and metformin, had received panretinal and focal laser treatment to his right eye 7 years previously and his right vision had stabilized at 6/36 (20/120). His left eye had been injured as a child and there was a large linear scar on the temporal side of his left macula from an old commotion retinae. the vision in his left eye had also been about 6/36 (20/120) at his previous clinic attendance, which was 20 months before his current presentation.

His present appointment had been delayed and this man presented with a sore eye, which was found to have an intraocular pressure of 58 mmHg due to a rubeotic glaucoma, a hyphaema in the anterior chamber and extensive neovascularization on the iris and in the angle of the anterior chamber. Photographs were taken (Fig. 9.11a).

He was treated with left pars plana vitrectomy and endolaser. One month later, he was given a cyclodiode treatment because the intraocular pressure was still elevated at a level of 50. This brought his left intraocular pressure down to a level of 24 but his VA had dropped to perception of light only in that eye.

Signs of ischaemia

Venous beading in more than one quadrant, extensive retinal haemorrhages and opaque small arteriolar branches are signs suggesting severe retinal ischaemia, which suggests that these eyes are at greater risk of neovascularization (Fig. 9.11b).

Macular oedema

McDonald[6] showed that 43% of the treated eyes in his study developed increased macular oedema 6–10 weeks following laser treatment. It is therefore recommended

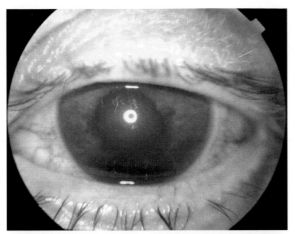

(a)

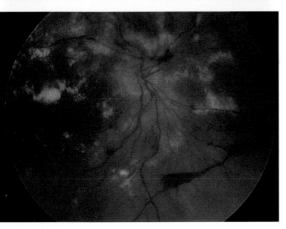

(b)

Fig. 9.11 Case history 2. (a) Iris neovascularization and secondary hyphaema. (b) Ischaemic eye with venous beading, preretinal haemorrhage, NVE and extensive exudation.

that eyes needing scatter laser treatment and also having macular oedema are less at risk of VA loss when focal or grid treatment to reduce the macular oedema precedes scatter laser photocoagulation where this is possible. If this is not possible, focal or grid laser treatment should be applied at the first scatter laser treatment session.

This is discussed in Chapter 10 on maculopathy with proliferative DR.

Pregnancy

See Chapter 13 on pregnancy and diabetic retinopathy.

Renal failure

Treatment must be timed to fit in with renal dialysis or transplantation. It is also important to control hypertension.

Past history

The past history of retinopathy both in the eye for which scatter laser photocoagulation is being considered and in the fellow eye needs to be considered.

Follow-up after panretinal photocoagulation

In 1991, Blankenship[9] reported the 15-year argon laser and xenon photocoagulation results of Bascom Palmer Eye Institute's patients participating in the diabetic retinopathy study. Fifteen years after panretinal photocoagulation in the Diabetic Retinopathy Study, 86 (57%) patients had died, 14 (9%) could not be located, and 51 (34%) of 151 patients were examined to determine the long-term treatment effects. Eleven (58%) of the initially argon-treated and 13 (41%) of the initially xenon-treated eyes had 20/40 or better acuity, and 18 (95%) of the initially argon-treated and 26 (82%) of the initially xenon-treated eyes had 20/200 or better acuity. Of the control eyes 17 (33%) had 20/40 or better, and 30 (58%) had 20/200 or better acuity. Hence it was concluded that argon and xenon panretinal photocoagulation for diabetic retinopathy provide good results for at least 15 years.

Quantification of retinal ablation, use of one treatment session and lessons learnt from the UK National Diabetic Laser Treatment Audit

The DRS protocol for panretinal photocoagulation recommended 800–1600 argon laser burns of 500-micron spot size extending to or beyond the vortex ampullae for eyes with high risk characteristics. The ETDRS protocol for full scatter laser treatment was developed from this and recommended 1200–1600 argon laser burns of 500-micron spot size. The ETDRS recommended that the treatment should be performed in two or more episodes no more than 2 weeks apart, and that no more than 900 burns should be applied in one session. An estimate of the area of retina ablated can be described using the standard formula of πr^2 multiplied by the number of burns.

According to the DRS protocol the recommended amount of retina treated is equivalent to an area of 157–314 mm^2, whilst the lower limit for the full panretinal photocoagulation treatment as recommended by the ETDRS is equivalent to an area of 236 mm^2, with the same upper recommended area of 314 mm^2.

In 1998 Bailey[10,11] reported the results of the UK National Diabetic Retinopathy Laser Treatment Audit, which was a prospective survey of laser treatment for diabetic retinopathy throughout the United Kingdom. A total of 284 patients who were undergoing their first panretinal photocoagulation for proliferative retinopathy during a 2-month period in 1995 were followed up for a period of 9 months. For eyes with proliferative retinopathy, the retinal neovascularization had regressed fully in 50.8% of cases, whilst there had been no change or a deterioration in 10.3%. A VA of less than 6/60 at follow-up was present in 8.6% of eyes. There was a poor morphological outcome at follow-up (as defined by rubeosis, new tractional detachment or having had a vitrectomy) in 7.2%. Risk factors for poor morphological outcome were the presence of 'high risk characteristics', female sex and the presence of concurrent maculopathy at baseline. Regression of neovascularization was associated with greater areas of retinal ablation at the initial treatment session. It was considered that the ophthalmologist intended to give the initial panretinal photocoagulation in one sitting in 41.2% of cases and in 55.6% of cases it was intended to divide the initial treatment into more than one session, whilst in 3.2% of cases this information was not recorded. For the subgroup with the equivalent of high risk characteristics who were given their initial treatment in one session (n = 65), the median retinal area treated was 104.6 mm^2 (range 10.4–682.5 mm^2) or 377.6 mm^2 (range 37.6–2464 mm^2) if the quadraspheric lens had been used for all cases.

Unfortunately, UK ophthalmologists had been influenced by a publication by Hulbert and Vernon[12] in 1992 of 21 people with proliferative diabetic retinopathy who had received bilateral panretinal photocoagulation. They recommended burns of no larger than 200-micron real spot size and claimed that between 3000 and 3500 burns induced regression in all but severe cases. The reason given for the recommendations was that patients were more likely to pass the standards set for driving in the UK if the smaller spot size was used. This recommendation is considerably less than the recommendation of the DRS and ETDRS: 4997 burns of 200-micron spot size would be required to meet the equivalent area of retinal ablation to 800 burns of 500-micron spot size recommended in the DRS; and 7500 burns of 200-micron spot size would be required to meet the equivalent area of retinal ablation to 1200 burns of 500-micron spot size recommended in the ETDRS.

There is also concern from the UK audit about the percentage that intended to give their panretinal treatment in one session because of the risks of vision loss from macular oedema if large areas of retina were treated in one session and the apparent undertreatment of the subgroup of patients with high risk characteristics.

In fact some eyes do require more treatment than that recommended by the DRS. Reddy[13] studied 294 eyes of 182 patients treated with argon scatter laser treatment and followed up for a minimum of 1 year to quantitate the amount of retinal ablation required for regression of proliferative diabetic retinopathy. Regression was observed in 275 eyes (93%); 19 eyes (7%) failed to regress and eventually required vitrectomy. Panretinal photocoagulation alone successfully led to regression in 229 eyes (77%), whereas 46 eyes (15.6%) required both photocoagulation and peripheral anterior retinal cryotherapy. Low-treatment eyes received an average of 510 mm^2 of retinal ablation (2600 500-micron burns), and high-treatment eyes, 1280 mm^2 (6500 500-micron burns). More extensive treatment was required with more retinopathy risk factors. The authors concluded that the amount of initial treatment required for regression may be considerably more than that recommended by the DRS.

Recommended laser treatment settings using conventional non-pattern argon laser treatment

Following the DRS and ETDRS studies, refinement of scatter laser treatment for proliferative diabetic retinopathy has provided the following recommendations.

1 Argon laser photocoagulation using 1200–2000 burns of 500-micron spot size for an exposure time of 0.1 s.
2 Power is adjusted to obtain mild bleaching that does not spread to be appreciably larger than 500 microns.
3 This number of burns to be applied in two or more episodes at least 4 days apart but no less than 2 weeks apart.
4 No more than 900 burns are to be applied in a single setting.
5 The posterior extent of the initial scatter laser treatment is an oval area defined by a line passing 2 DDs above, temporal to and below the centre of the macula, and 500 microns from the nasal half of the disc margin. From this line scatter laser treatment extends peripherally to or beyond the equator avoiding direct treatment of major vessels (and chorioretinal scars if present).
6 When it is feared that vitreous haemorrhage may occur it is recommended that the inferior quadrants are treated first.
7 The treatment period should be completed within 6 weeks.

Other factors

Retinal dimensions

Davies[14] used a mathematical model of the emmetropic eye to calculate retinal dimensions corresponding to different angles of visual field. He suggested that it is theoretically possible to alter the pattern of PRP to avoid treatment in retinal areas concerned with the driving visual field whilst leaving the total number of burns constant. This has led many ophthalmologists to extend the area untreated to 1 DD or 1500 microns from the nasal edge of the disc margin.

Laser spot magnification factor and field of view of lens used

The laser spot magnification factor has a significant influence on the settings on the laser machine used. Many of the modern indirect laser lenses have a magnification factor of 1.9–2.0 and ophthalmologists are commonly using laser spot sizes of 200 microns with these lenses and hence the effective diameter of the beam is 380–400 microns once it has passed through one of these lenses. If an effective beam diameter lower than 500 microns is used, the number of burns needs to be increased as discussed in the section on quantification of retinal ablation.

The field of view of a retinal laser lens does alter the area of retina that is available to the operator to treat with that particular lens.

Examples of the manufacturer's advertised laser spot magnification factors and fields of view (taken from their respective websites) are given below.

- Volk's SuperQuad 160: 2.0× laser spot magnification factor; 160°–165° field of view.
- Volk's 130° QuadrAspheric lens: 1.92× laser spot magnification factor; 120°–144° field of view.
- Volk TransEquator: 1.44 laser spot magnification factor; 70°–84° field of view.
- Ocular Mainster PRP 165: 1.96× laser spot magnification factor; 165°–180° field of view.
- Ocular Mainster Wide Field: 1.5× laser spot magnification factor, 118°–127° field of view.

Duration of the burn

There has been an increasing tendency in 2008 for some operators to reduce the duration of the burn and increase the power to produce an apparently similar mild bleaching because of the clinical impression that this is more comfortable for the patient. The validity of this approach needs to be tested in a clinical trial setting as there is a theoretical risk that the width of the burn may be reduced by this approach and that more burns may therefore be required.

Number of treatment sessions

One of the ways in which the ETDRS[5] attempted to reduce harmful effects was the division of scatter treatment between two or more sittings. This was because in the DRS study 14.3% more argon-treated and 29.7% of xenon-treated eyes than controls had an early persistent loss of one or more lines. The likely cause of the loss of VA in the xenon-treated group was a persistent increase in macular oedema as a consequence of the increased intensity of treatment[15] in one session in the xenon-treated group. The alternative view suggested in a study by Doft and Blankenship[16] is that there is no major difference between groups in whom treatment was administered in a single session as compared with multiple sessions spaced over time in the effect of treatment on VA. The article stated that exudative retinal detachment, choroidal detachment and angle closure occurred more commonly in single-session treatment group eyes, but these effects were transient, and no long-term difference between treatment groups was found. The view of the current author is that treatment should be spaced over a minimum of two sessions unless there is a strong suspicion that the individual being treated might not attend for subsequent treatment sessions.

The pattern argon laser and the evidence behind the recommendations for this laser

Scatter laser photocoagulation involves the controlled destruction of the peripheral retina using targeted laser pulses. A full course of treatment typically requires two or more sessions, each lasting approximately 15 min (or longer with less experienced operators). With conventional methods of retinal laser photocoagulation, the ophthalmologist uses a mechanical joystick and foot pedal to deliver single 100-millisecond laser pulses to the peripheral retina.

Optimedia Corporation introduced the PASCAL (Pattern Scan Laser) Photocoagulator in June 2006, which is a frequency-doubled Nd : YAG diode-pumped solid state laser producing a wavelength of 532 nm. With the patterned scanning laser photocoagulation, the laser pulse time is reduced from 100 milliseconds to just 10–20 milliseconds, and automated multiple spots are produced with each depression of the foot pedal. Higher power is required for the shorter burns. From the main control panel, an LCD display with a touch-screen control is used to select from predetermined pattern types and administer up to 25 spots at a time for scatter laser treatment. The operator can select different arcs, circular grid patterns or sectors of grids for treatment, or use a rectangular array. Once the pattern is selected, a separate red beam is used for aiming and visualization of the placement before delivery. The touch screen interface is also used for selecting various parameters such as aim beam intensity, treatment laser power, exposure time, system status and shut down.

Blumenkranz et al.[17] conducted preclinical experiments with reduced pulse duration (10–100 ms) to determine retinal burn characteristics associated with these rapidly delivered light pulses. The histological appearance of light burns at 10–100 ms demonstrated that the damage is confined to the outer retina and retinal pigment epithelium. However at pulse durations >20 ms, significant diffusion of heat occurred with less localized homogenous lesions, histopathologically. The reduced pulse duration burns appear to produce less inner retinal (e.g. choroidal) injury and this may be the reason for the observation of less patient discomfort.

The potential advantages over conventional single spot laser are:

1 increased uniformity and precision of spot placement with less chance of overlap (a potential safety benefit)
2 reduced discomfort felt by the patient, which has been widely reported
3 reduced overall treatment duration/procedure time (thereby reducing costs).

What remains to be seen is whether these short-term observations translate into long-term benefits and improved outcomes overall. The above potential advantages might make it easier for ophthalmologists to follow the ETDRS guidelines once the studies have been done that translate this type of treatment to ETDRS guidelines. One aspect of concern in the article by Blumenkranz et al.[17] was the suggestion in the discussion section that the availability of a retinal photocoagulator capable of the rapid sequential application of a large number of spots makes single-session panretinal photocoagulation practically feasible. As stated in the section on number of treatment sessions above, the view of the current author is that treatment should be spaced over a minimum of two sessions unless there is a strong suspicion that the individual being treated might not attend for subsequent treatment sessions.

CASE HISTORY 3
Severe NVD in both eyes

This 28-year-old man (BMI 24) with type 1 diabetes since the age of 6 years had been referred after a visit to his optometrist with a diagnosis of proliferative diabetic retinopathy but failed to attend four clinic appointments that were sent to him. His most recent HbA1c result had been 9.4% and his blood pressure 115/84.

At the age of 29 years he presented with a sudden onset of a blurred patch in the vision of his right eye due to a vitreous haemorrhage from NVD and he showed signs of proliferative diabetic retinopathy in both eyes.

Laser treatment was commenced to each eye:
- right eye 1531 burns in two sessions, 710 burns of 350-micron size, 170 mW, 0.1 s, transequatorial lens (magnification factor 1.44), and 821 burns 200-micron size, 180 mW, 0.1 s, SuperQuad lens (magnification factor 2), argon laser;
- left eye 1442 burns in two sessions, 700 burns of 350-micron size, 190 mW, 0.1 s, transequatorial lens (magnification factor 1.44), and 742 burns 200-micron size, 190 mW, 0.1 s, SuperQuad lens (magnification factor 2), argon laser.

He then failed to attend five follow-up appointments. When he attended again 18 months later, photographs of his eyes showed the following (Fig. 9.12a–d).

He was then given further treatment to both eyes:
- right eye 850 burns, 200-micron size, 250 mW, 0.03 s, transequatorial lens (magnification factor 1.44), Pascale laser;
- left eye 875 burns, 200-micron size, 190 mW, 0.1 s, transequatorial lens (magnification factor 1.44), Pascal laser (Fig. 9.12e).

Further treatment is likely to be required.

CASE HISTORY 4
NVE in superotemporal retina with some macular ischaemia

This 44-year-old woman (BMI 41) with type 1 diabetes for 26 years was being followed up for moderate non-proliferative diabetic retinopathy. She developed an increasing right cataract, reducing her preoperative VA to 6/18 (20/60), but postoperatively her vision was noted to be worse at a level of 6/36 (20/180). A fluorescein angiogram demonstrated the presence of large NVE in her right superotemporal retina and a degree of macular ischaemia (Fig. 9.13).

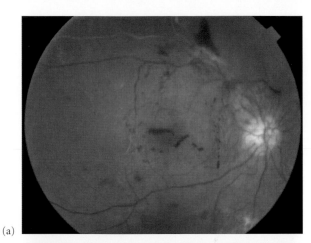

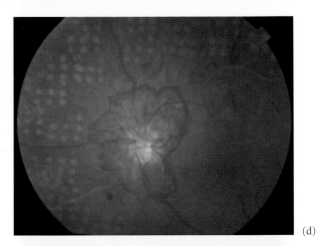

(a)

(d)

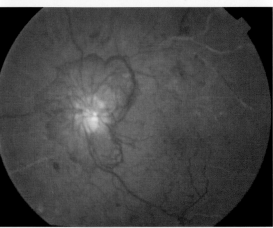

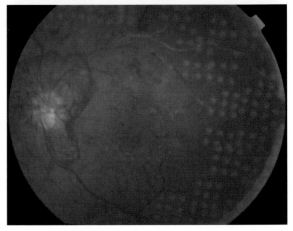

(b)

(e)

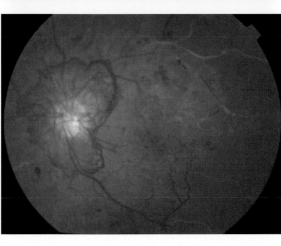

(c)

Fig. 9.12 Case history 3. (a) Right macula colour before treatment. (b) Left disc colour before treatment. (c) Left macula colour before treatment. (d) Left disc colour immediately after treatment. (e) Left macula colour immediately after treatment.

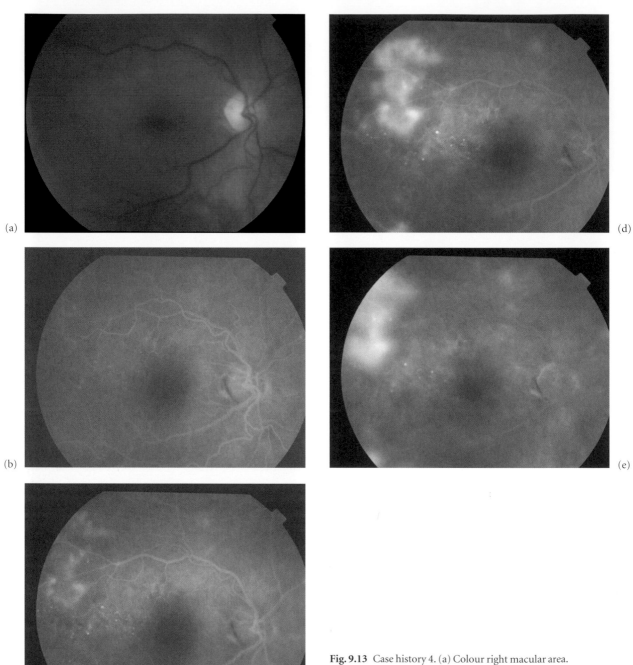

(a)

(b)

(c)

(d)

(e)

Fig. 9.13 Case history 4. (a) Colour right macular area. Fluorescein right macular area: (b) 35 s after injection; (c) 52 s after injection; (d) 1 min 45 s after injection; (e) 3 min 43 s after injection.

Her blood pressure readings had averaged 132/70 and her HbA1c results had improved from 12.3% to 10.6% over the previous 6 years. Her right retina was treated with panretinal photocoagulation using 1933 burns of 200-micron spot size using the SuperQuad 160 lens (magnification factor 2.0). The NVE gradually fibrosed over the subsequent 5 months and the vision has fortunately gradually improved to a level of 6/9 (20/30) over a 6-month period and has remained at this level.

CASE HISTORY 5
NVD treated with panretinal photocoagulation – attendance intermittent

This 42-year-old man with diabetes controlled by insulin (diagnosed at the age of 30 years), was referred by the retinal screening service with proliferative diabetic retinopathy in both eyes as can be seen in the colour and red-free photographs (Fig. 9.14). His attendance record

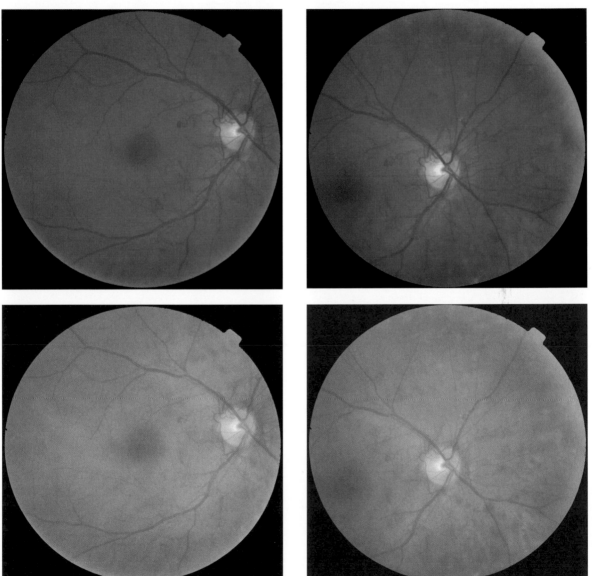

(a)

(b)

(c)

(d)

Fig. 9.14 Case history 5. (a) Colour photograph right macula. (b) Red-free photograph right macula. (c) Colour photograph right disc. (d) Red-free photograph right disc. (*Continued on p. 126*)

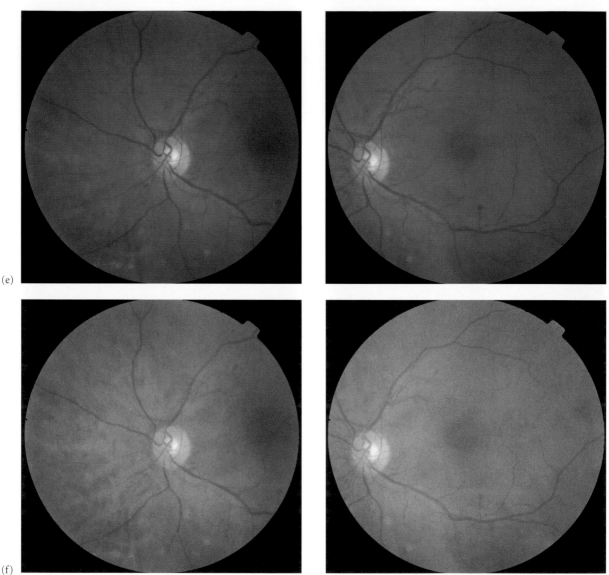

(e)

(f)

(g)

(h)

Fig. 9.14 (*Cont'd*) (e) Colour photograph left disc. (f) Red-free photograph left disc. (g) Colour photograph left macula. (h) Red-free photograph left macula.

over the last 2 years, since these photographs were taken, has made it very difficult to control the neovascularization with laser treatment.

CASE HISTORY 6
Posterior vitreous detachment with horseshoe-shaped tear at the site of NVE

A 62-year-old woman (BMI 20) with type 1 diabetes of 11 years' duration had been treated with panretinal photo-

coagulation to her left eye for proliferative diabetic retinopathy (NVE) 4 years before her current presentation. Her HBA1c had improved from 9.4% to 7.0% and her blood pressure from 153/77 to 136/68 over the previous 8 years. On this occasion she presented with a sudden onset of a 'blob' in the centre of the vision of her left eye and a greyish haze. The VA was 6/6 (20/20) and on examination a small haemorrhagic PVD was noted. One month later, an increase in blurriness was accompanied by occasional yellow flashes noted in half-light conditions. At that time

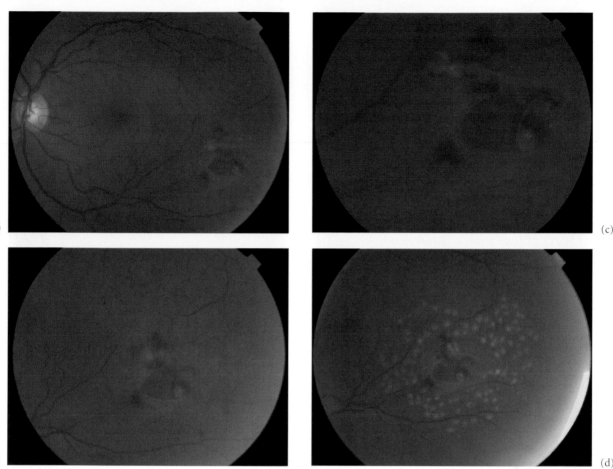

Fig. 9.15 Case history 6. (a) Avulsion of NVE leaving horseshoe tear: colour photograph. (b,c) Avulsion of NVE leaving horseshoe tear magnified: colour photographs. (d) Colour photograph taken immediately after laser treatment to encircle horseshoe tear.

the VA was 6/9 (20/30) and the source of the bleeding was noted to be a small patch of NVE in the left temporal retina. Some scatter laser treatment was given to some gaps in the previous panretinal laser treatment in the left temporal retina. At a subsequent follow-up visit 6 weeks later an operculated tear was noted (see Fig. 9.15a–c).

Argon laser treatment to encircle the retinal tear was undertaken:
• 126 burns, 210 mW, 100-micron size, argon laser, area centralis lens (Fig. 9.15d).

Patient experiences of laser

Many patients are very anxious about the possibility of having to receive laser treatment. Their experience can often be much improved by adequate explanations of the reasons for the laser treatment and what it involves.

If the patient remains very anxious following adequate explanation this can make laser treatment more difficult for both the patient and the ophthalmologist.

Anaesthesia for retinal laser

The vast majority of macular and panretinal laser treatments are performed without difficulty using a contact lens under topical anaesthesia. Macular laser usually causes little or no discomfort but panretinal laser can cause pain, particularly during prolonged treatment sessions or when using high-power settings in lightly pigmented eyes. Pain is often worse during retreatment sessions using a 'fill-in' pattern or when using long-wavelength diode lasers. Most patients characterize the pain associated with laser as brief, intermittent, sharp or piercing.

Randomized trials have found no benefit from oral[18] or

intramuscular analgesics[19] before panretinal photocoagulation compared with placebo, but peribulbar anaesthesia was very effective[19] at reducing pain. Sub-tenon injection of local anaesthetic is also effective[20] at reducing discomfort and eliminates the risk of globe perforation or damage to the orbital structures that can sometimes occur with sharp-needle techniques.

General anaesthesia is only very rarely required but can be useful when thorough bilateral treatment is urgently required or when treating patients with learning difficulties or those who, for whatever reason, cannot cope with laser under local anaesthesia.

The author's views on the treatment of NVD of less than a quarter of disc area

If signs of severe ischaemia are present, I would recommend panretinal photocoagulation. Venous beading in more than one quadrant, extensive retinal haemorrhages and opaque small arteriolar branches are signs suggesting severe retinal ischaemia, which suggest that these eyes are at greater risk of neovascularization.

If signs of severe ischaemia were not present I would perform a fluorescein angiogram to check that the NVD were definitely leaking and I would ask for peripheral retinal views to identify the extent of peripheral retinal ischaemia.

In the past I have watched some of these small NVD and in time they have got bigger or bled and become high risk. I, personally, have never seen one that has spontaneously resolved. I therefore have a low threshold for performing panretinal photocoagulation, especially as the complication rate that I have for performing a panretinal photocoagulation is considerably less than that reported in the DRS. I believe that this is because the extent of whitening (heaviness of the burn) that one currently uses with the recommended panretinal laser treatment is less than in the DRS.

The author's views on the treatment of NVE that have not haemorrhaged

There is no clearcut answer to this because each patient presents a different picture.

However, if signs of severe ischaemia are present, I would recommend panretinal photocoagulation. Venous beading in more than one quadrant, extensive retinal haemorrhages and opaque small arteriolar branches are signs suggesting severe retinal ischaemia, which suggest that these eyes are at greater risk of neovascularization.

If there are no signs of severe retinal ischaemia, I would perform a fluorescein angiogram asking for peripheral retinal views to identify the extent of peripheral retinal ischaemia. There are usually ischaemic signs peripheral to the NVE in the quadrant that the NVE have occurred. If the ischaemia was localized to this quadrant I would perform segmental laser treatment to the area of ischaemia peripheral to the NVE in this quadrant (this was recommended by Hamilton[21]). If the ischaemia was more extensive, I would consider which segments of ischaemic retina might require laser treatment.

ANTI-VEGF TREATMENTS

Ocular neovascularization (angiogenesis) and increased vascular permeability have been associated with vascular endothelial growth factor (VEGF). Neovascularization is dependent on the presence of VEGF; expression of VEGF in animal models is sufficient to induce neovascularization whereas inhibition reduces this effect. In humans ocular VEGF levels have been shown to rise with the growth and leakage of new vessels. This provides a therapeutic rationale for the targeting of VEGF in diabetic retinopathy.

However, there is a concern that VEGF does have a neuroprotective effect and that there might be neurological adverse effects if there is significant systemic absorption of these substances.

There are three potential VEGF inhibitors:
- pegaptanib (Macugen)
- ranibizumab (Lucentis)
- bevacizumab (Avastin).

Ranibizumab (Lucentis) is an antibody fragment derived from bevacizumab (Avastin), which is a full-length humanized monoclonal antibody against human VEGF currently used for treatment of several solid organ tumours (colorectal etc). These drugs have not been extensively studied in diabetic eye disease and there are only early reports of their use in diabetic retinopathy without any randomized controlled trials.

Favourable results have been reported with some regression of neovascularization and reduction in fluorescein leakage in studies by Arevalo,[22] Jorge,[23] Avery,[24] Mason[25] and Spaide[26] using bevacizumab and Adamis[27] using pegaptanib. The effect is only transient. Avery[24] reported that recurrent leakage was seen as early as 2 weeks after intravitreal injection in one case, whereas in other cases, no recurrent leakage was noted at last follow-up of 11 weeks. Arevalo[22] reported total regression of retinal neovascularization on fundus examination with absence of fluorescein leakage in 61.4% (27 eyes) after a mean of 28.4

weeks (range from 24 to 40 weeks). Adamis[27] reported that in 3 of 8 with regression, neovascularization progressed at week 52 after cessation of pegaptanib at week 30.

In view of the potential complications from intravitreal injections, extreme caution is advised in the use of this technique. Randomized controlled trials utilizing varying doses of the VEGF inhibitors are now required to assess the long-term efficacy, safety and to define optimum treatment regimens.

VITREOUS HAEMORRHAGE OBSCURING THE RETINAL VIEW

Two recent reports of vitrectomy case series, one from the USA[28] of 223 consecutive patients and the other from Austria[29] of 93 eyes with retinal disorders resulting from diabetic retinopathy have demonstrated that the commonest reason for vitrectomy, 68% in the first series and 86.1% in the second, is vitreous haemorrhage from active and significant proliferative diabetic retinopathy that makes it impossible to undertake the required scatter laser treatment without operative intervention. This is discussed in detail in Chapter 12 on the surgical approach to the diabetic eye.

CASE HISTORY 7
NVE with vitreous haemorrhage

This 43-year-old man with type 1 diabetes for 31 years had treatment for right clinically significant macular oedema at the age of 31 years.

At the age of 35 years he subsequently received panretinal photocoagulation to his right eye when small NVE were found in his right temporal retina, right inferonasal retina and right superior and superonasal retina. The treatment given was:

- 2022 burns, power 170–200 mW, size 350 microns, transequatorial lens (magnification factor 1.44), argon laser, spread over three sessions 1 week apart.

At the age of 39 years, he noticed a spot in the inferior vision of his right eye and clinical examination demonstrated the presence of a preretinal haemorrhage as shown in Fig. 9.16(a).

This preretinal haemorrhage then broke through into the vitreous 6 weeks later, reducing the right VA to 6/24 (20/80). Clinically, the vitreous haemorrhage interfered with the retinal view on slit-lamp biomicroscopy and an ultrasound B-scan was therefore undertaken (Fig. 9.16b).

A right pars plana vitrectomy was performed with a good postoperative visual result of 6/6 (20/20).

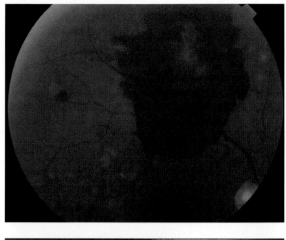
(a)

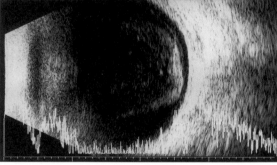
(b)

Fig. 9.16 Case history 7. (a) Preretinal haemorrhage later breaking into the vitreous to become a vitreous haemorrhage. (b) Vitreous haemorrhage: B-scan.

It is important to perform a B-scan on patients in whom one cannot view the retina due to a vitreous haemorrhage to exclude an underlying retinal detachment as shown in Fig. 9.17.

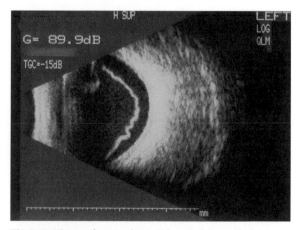

Fig. 9.17 Vitreous haemorrhage with underlying retinal detachment: B-scan.

CASE HISTORY 8
NVE in superotemporal retina and inferotemporal retina (not high risk proliferative)

A 45-year-old man (BMI 25) with type 2 diabetes controlled with oral hypoglycaemic medication was referred from the retinal screening service and was found to have small NVE in his right superotemporal and right inferotemporal retina. His VA was good at 6/6 (20/20). The fluorescein angiogram demonstrates ischaemia in the areas of retina peripheral to the NVE but the remaining retina did not show any significant signs of ischaemia (Fig. 9.18).

A decision was therefore made to treat the ischaemic peripheral areas superotemporal to the NVE and inferotemporal to the other patch of NVE in order to try and get these NVE to regress or fibrose.

Treatment was given to the peripheral retinal areas:
- right 690 burns, 200-micron size, 200 mW, 0.1 s, SuperQuad 160 lens, argon laser.

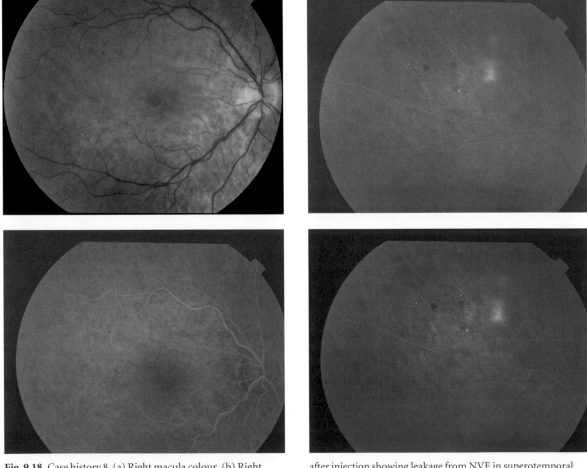

(a)

(b)

(c)

(d)

Fig. 9.18 Case history 8. (a) Right macula colour. (b) Right macula fluorescein 17 s after injection. (c) Right superior retina fluorescein 43 s after injection showing leakage from NVE in superotemporal retina. (d) Right superior retina fluorescein 55 s after injection showing leakage from NVE in superotemporal retina and some ischaemia peripheral to NVE. (*Continued on facing page*)

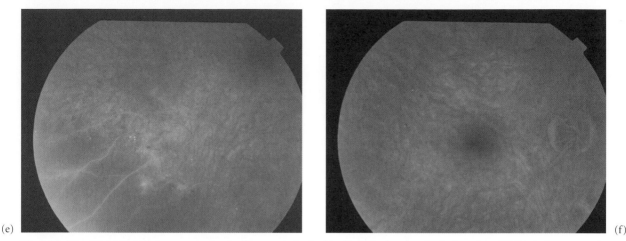

(e)   (f)

Fig. 9.18 (*Cont'd*) (e) Right inferotemporal retina fluorescein 3 min 34 s after injection showing leakage from NVE in inferotemporal retina and ischaemia peripheral to NVE. (f) Right macula fluorescein 4 min 17 s after injection.

PRACTICE POINTS

- In the treatment of neovascularization, involution of neovascularization is dependent upon a sufficient area of retinal ablation.[3,10]
- Panretinal laser treatment should be spaced over a minimum of two sessions unless there is a strong suspicion that the individual being treated might not attend for subsequent treatment sessions.

REFERENCES

1 Early worsening of diabetic retinopathy in the Diabetes Control and Complications Trial. *Arch Ophthalmol* 1998; **116**(7): 874–86.

2 The Diabetic Retinopathy Study Research Group. Preliminary report on effects of photocoagulation therapy. *Am J Ophthalmol* 1976; **81**(4): 383–96.

3 The Diabetic Retinopathy Study Research Group. Photocoagulation treatment of proliferative diabetic retinopathy. Clinical application of Diabetic Retinopathy Study (DRS) findings, DRS Report Number 8. *Ophthalmology* 1981; **88**(7):583–600.

4 The Diabetic Retinopathy Study Research Group. Indications for photocoagulation treatment of diabetic retinopathy: Diabetic Retinopathy Study Report no. 14. *Int Ophthalmol Clin* 1987; **27**(4): 239–53.

5 Early Treatment Diabetic Retinopathy Study Research Group. Early photocoagulation for diabetic retinopathy. ETDRS report number 9. *Ophthalmology* 1991; **98**(5 Suppl): 766–85.

6 McDonald HR, Schatz H. Macular edema following panretinal photocoagulation. *Retina* 1985; **5**(1): 5–10.

7 Mackie SW, Webb LA, Hutchinson BM, Hammer HM, Barrie T, Walsh G. Assessing the risk of failure to attain driving standards following laser photocoagulation. *Eur J Ophthalmol* 1994; **4**: 241.

8 Barsam A, Laidlaw A. Visual fields in patients who have undergone vitrectomy for complications of diabetic retinopathy. A prospective study. *BMC Ophthalmol* 2006; **6**: 5.

9 Blankenship GW. Fifteen-year argon laser and xenon photocoagulation results of Bascom Palmer Eye Institute's patients participating in the diabetic retinopathy study. *Ophthalmology* 1991; **98**(2): 125–8.

10 Bailey CC, Sparrow JM, Grey RH, Cheng H. The National Diabetic Retinopathy Laser Treatment Audit. III. Clinical outcomes. *Eye* 1999; **13**(Pt 2): 151–9.

11 Bailey CC, Sparrow JM, Grey RH, Cheng H. The National Diabetic Retinopathy Laser Treatment Audit. II. Proliferative retinopathy. *Eye* 1998; **12**(Pt 1): 77–84.

12 Hulbert MF, Vernon SA. Passing the DVLC field regulations following bilateral pan-retinal photocoagulation in diabetics. *Eye* 1992; **6**(Pt 5): 456–60.

13 Reddy VM, Zamora RL, Olk RJ. Quantitation of retinal ablation in proliferative diabetic retinopathy. *Am J Ophthalmol* 1995; **119**(6): 760–6.

14 Davies N. Altering the pattern of panretinal photocoagulation: could the visual field for driving be preserved? *Eye* 1999; **13**(Pt 4): 531–6.

15 Ferris FL 3rd, Podgor MJ, Davis MD. Macular edema in Diabetic Retinopathy Study patients. Diabetic Retinopathy Study Report Number 12. *Ophthalmology* 1987; **94**(7): 754–60.

16 Doft BH, Blankenship GW. Single versus multiple treatment sessions of argon laser panretinal photocoagulation for proliferative diabetic retinopathy. *Ophthalmology* 1982; **89**(7): 772–9.

17 Blumenkranz MS, Yellachich D, Andersen DE, Wiltberger MW, Mordaunt D, Marcellino GR *et al.* Semiautomated patterned scanning laser for retinal photocoagulation. *Retina* 2006; **26**(3): 370–6.

18 Vaideanu D, Taylor P, McAndrew P, Hildreth A, Deady JP, Steel DH. Double masked randomised controlled trial to assess the effectiveness of paracetamol in reducing pain in panretinal photocoagulation. *Br J Ophthalmol* 2006; **90**(6): 713–17.

19 Wu WC, Hsu KH, Chen TL, Hwang YS, Lin KK, Li LM *et al.* Interventions for relieving pain associated with panretinal photocoagulation: a prospective randomized trial. *Eye* 2006; **20**(6): 712–19.

20 Stevens JD, Foss AJ, Hamilton AM. No-needle one-quadrant sub-tenon anaesthesia for panretinal photocoagulation. *Eye* 1993; **7**(Pt 6): 768–71.

21 Hamilton A, Ulbig M, Polkinghorne P. *Management of Diabetic Retinopathy.* London: BMJ Publishing Group, 1996.

22 Arevalo JF, Wu L, Sanchez JG, Maia M, Saravia MJ, Fernandez CF *et al.* Intravitreal bevacizumab (avastin) for proliferative diabetic retinopathy: 6-months follow-up. *Eye* 2007; Sept 21. [Epub ahead of print]

23 Jorge R, Costa RA, Calucci D, Cintra LP, Scott IU. Intravitreal bevacizumab (Avastin) for persistent new vessels in diabetic retinopathy (IBEPE study). *Retina* 2006; **26**(9): 1006–13.

24 Avery RL, Pearlman J, Pieramici DJ, Rabena MD, Castellarin AA, Nasir MA *et al.* Intravitreal bevacizumab (Avastin) in the treatment of proliferative diabetic retinopathy. *Ophthalmology* 2006; **113**(10): 1695 e1–15.

25 Mason JO 3rd, Nixon PA, White MF. Intravitreal injection of bevacizumab (Avastin) as adjunctive treatment of proliferative diabetic retinopathy. *Am J Ophthalmol* 2006; **142**(4): 685–8.

26 Spaide RF, Fisher YL. Intravitreal bevacizumab (Avastin) treatment of proliferative diabetic retinopathy complicated by vitreous hemorrhage. *Retina* 2006; **26**(3): 275–8.

27 Adamis AP, Altaweel M, Bressler NM, Cunningham ET, Jr., Davis MD, Goldbaum M *et al.* Changes in retinal neovascularisation after pegaptanib (Macugen) therapy in diabetic individuals. *Ophthalmology* 2006; **113**(1): 23–8.

28 Lahey JM, Francis RR, Kearney JJ. Combining phacoemulsification with pars plana vitrectomy in patients with proliferative diabetic retinopathy: a series of 223 cases. *Ophthalmology* 2003; **110**(7): 1335–9.

29 Schrey S, Krepler K, Wedrich A. Incidence of rhegmatogenous retinal detachment after vitrectomy in eyes of diabetic patients. *Retina* 2006; **26**(2): 149–52.

10 Stage R3 with M1: proliferative diabetic retinopathy with maculopathy

Peter H. Scanlon

MANAGEMENT ISSUES – LASER FOR PROLIFERATIVE DR AND CONCURRENT MACULOPATHY

Results from the Diabetic Retinopathy Study[1] (DRS) demonstrated that scatter photocoagulation is associated with some loss of visual acuity (VA) soon after treatment and this was more common in eyes with pre-existing macular oedema. However, for eyes with high risk characteristics the DRS found that the benefits of treatment outweighed the possible side-effects of treatment as shown by the following results.

- In untreated eyes with high risk characteristics present at baseline and macular oedema present at baseline the 6-week risk of decrease in VA by two or more lines is 21.6%, 4-month 36.6%, 1-year 54.6% and 2-year 65.5%
- In argon-treated eyes with high risk characteristics present at baseline and macular oedema present at baseline the 6-week risk of decrease in VA by two or more lines is 14.6%, 4-month risk 26.1%, 1-year risk 32.6% and 2-year risk 46.3%. There was clearly a benefit from panretinal photocoagulation.

Increased macular oedema following panretinal photocoagulation was demonstrated by Meyers[2] and McDonald.[3]

A further report from the DRS[4] suggested that 'reducing macular oedema by focal photocoagulation before initiating scatter treatment and dividing scatter treatment into multiple sessions with less intense burns may decrease the risk of the visual loss associated with photocoagulation'.

Lee[5] combined treatment in two sessions consisting of an initial modified grid to the macula and panretinal photocoagulation to the inferior half of the peripheral retina, followed 2–4 weeks later by panretinal photocoagulation to the superior half. The study evaluated 52 patients and found that macular oedema resolved in 43 of 46 eyes (93%), and proliferative retinopathy was reduced in 25 of 29 eyes (86%) at the last examination.

The ETDRS[6] was designed to include a broad range of severity of retinopathy, from the mild non-proliferative to the mild proliferative stage but eyes with DRS high risk characteristics in either eye were ineligible. Eyes with mild non-proliferative retinopathy had to have macular oedema as well, which ranged from normal VA with hard exudates less than 1 DD from the foveal centre to eyes with a VA of 20/200 and extensive retinal thickening at the foveal centre, but this was not required for eyes with moderate or severe non-proliferative or mild proliferative. The ETDRS compared giving immediate panretinal photocoagulation with either simultaneous or delayed focal treatment. For eyes with macular oedema and more severe retinopathy the risk of severe visual loss in eyes assigned to deferral of photocoagulation was relatively high (6.5% at the 5-year visit). This risk was reduced to between 3.8% and 4.7% in the eyes assigned to early photocoagulation. The strategy associated with the least visual loss (both moderate and severe) was immediate mild scatter combined with immediate focal photocoagulation. The ETDRS did not include evaluation of a strategy that consisted of prompt focal photocoagulation with delayed scatter in eyes with clinically significant macular oedema and eyes that are approaching the high risk category.

It is therefore recommended that eyes needing scatter laser treatment and also having macular oedema are less at risk of VA loss when focal or grid treatment to reduce the macular oedema precedes scatter laser photocoagulation where this is possible. If this is not possible, focal or grid laser treatment should be applied at the first scatter laser treatment session.

A Practical Manual of Diabetic Retinopathy Management.
Peter H Scanlon, Charles P Wilkinson, Stephen J Aldington and David R Matthews. Published 2009 by Blackwell Publishing, ISBN 978-1-4051-7035-2.

Hamilton[7] recommended an exception to this approach for young patients with type 1 diabetes who have rapidly accelerating peripheral ischaemia associated with macular oedema that may resolve following panretinal photocoagulation.

Scatter laser treatment should not be delayed when the risk of vitreous haemorrhage or neovascular glaucoma seems high regardless of the status of the macula.

CASE HISTORY 1
NVD and NVE with maculopathy

A 41-year-old man (BMI 28) with type 1 diabetes of 30 years' duration was referred from the retinal screening programme when the photographs showed signs of proliferative diabetic retinopathy in both eyes and maculopathy in the left (Fig. 10.1).

(a)

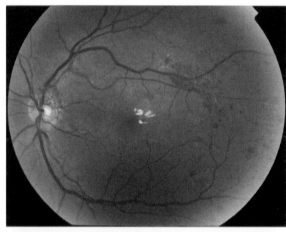

(b)

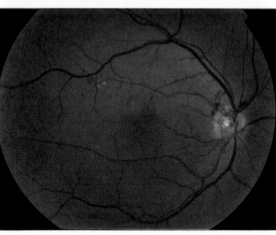

Fig. 10.1 Case history 1. Proliferative DR with maculopathy. (a) Left macula colour photograph. (b) Right macula colour photograph.

The left macular area was treated first:
• 23 burns of 100-micron size, 260 mW, 0.1 s, area centralis lens, argon laser.

Panretinal photocoagulation was commenced to both eyes at the first treatment session.
• In total 4010 burns, 2550 using the Transequator lens (magnification factor 1.44) and 350-micron spot size, and 1460 of 200-micron spot size using the SuperQuad 160 lens (magnification factor of 2.0) of average power 220 mW, have been required to control the neovascularization in his right eye.
• In total 4847 burns, 2303 using the Transequator lens (magnification factor 1.44) and 350-micron spot size and 2544 of 200-micron spot size using the SuperQuad 160 lens (magnification factor of 2.0) of average power 220 mW, have been required to control the neovascularization in the left eye.

His HbA1c has gradually improved from 10.1% to 8.1% over the last 5 years and his blood pressure was consistently satisfactory at 122/86 but has recently elevated to 153/92.

The exudates and CSMO in the left macular area cleared with the one course of focal laser treatment and his left corrected visual acuity has remained at 6/6 (20/20).

CASE HISTORY 2
NVD and NVE with maculopathy

This 59-year-old man with type 2 diabetes controlled on metformin 850 mg b.d. presented with a sudden onset of blurring of vision in his left eye (VA reduced to 6/24, 20/120). As the haemorrhage started to clear, a fluorescein angiogram (Fig. 10.2) showed NVD, NVE, severe ischaemia in the temporal retina and clinically significant macular oedema in the macular area.

Focal laser treatment was commenced to the area of retinal thickening on the temporal side of the left macula:
• 31 burns 100-micron size, 170 mW, 100 ms, area centralis lens, argon laser.

Panretinal photocoagulation was commenced at the same appointment following the macular laser treatment:
• three sessions giving a total of 2425 burns, which included 1620 burns of 350-micron spot size (average power 330 mW, spot size 200 microns) using the Transequator lens with a magnification factor of 1.44; and 805 burns of 200-micron spot size using the SuperQuad 160 lens with a magnification factor of 2.0.

With this treatment the VA improved over the next 5 months to a level of 6/9 (20/30) but there remained

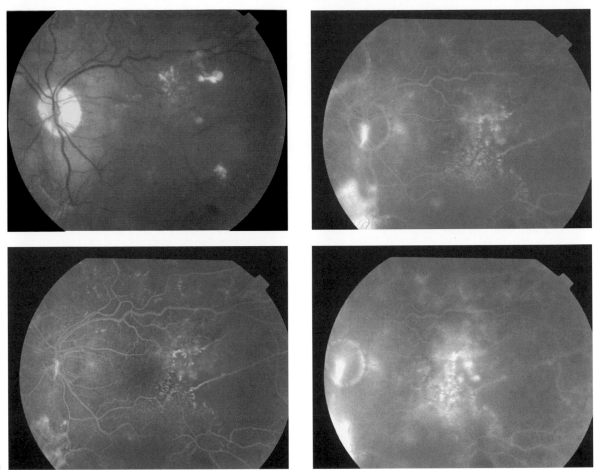

(a)

(c)

(b)

(d)

Fig. 10.2 Case history 2. Colour photograph left macular area (a). Fluorescein left macular area: (b) 29 s after injection; (c) 57 s after injection; (d) 4 min 15 s after injection.

some activity of the NVD and NVE, which required two further scatter laser treatments requiring a total of a further 1745 burns of 200-micron spot size using the SuperQuad 160 lens to control the neovascularization. His left VA subsequently stabilized at 6/12 (20/40). Over the 5 years, his HbA1c had varied between 8.4% and 8.1% and his blood pressure had varied between 195/78 and 138/83.

PRACTICE POINTS

• Where possible, treat clinically significant macular oedema by applying focal/grid photocoagulation before beginning scatter laser treatment.
• When the risk of vitreous haemorrhage or neovascular glaucoma seems high, combine treatment for clinically significant macular oedema by applying focal/grid photocoagulation for macular oedema with panretinal photocoagulation to the inferior half of the peripheral retina, followed 2 weeks later by panretinal photocoagulation to the superior half.
• In young patients with IDDM who have aggressive peripheral ischaemia associated with diffuse or cystoid macular oedema, commence panretinal photocoagulation before treating the macula to see if this resolves following panretinal photocoagulation. If the macular oedema does not undergo spontaneous resolution following panretinal photocoagulation, focal/grid laser treatment can then be considered depending on the extent of the remaining macular oedema.

REFERENCES

1 The Diabetic Retinopathy Study Research Group. Indications for photocoagulation treatment of diabetic retinopathy: Diabetic Retinopathy Study Report no. 14. *Int Ophthalmol Clin* 1987; **27**(4): 239–53.

2 Meyers SM. Macular edema after scatter laser photocoagulation for proliferative diabetic retinopathy. *Am J Ophthalmol* 1980; **90**(2): 210–16.

3 McDonald HR, Schatz H. Macular edema following panretinal photocoagulation. *Retina* 1985; **5**(1): 5–10.

4 Ferris FL 3rd, Podgor MJ, Davis MD. Macular edema in Diabetic Retinopathy Study patients. Diabetic Retinopathy Study Report Number 12. *Ophthalmology* 1987; **94**(7): 754–60.

5 Lee CM, Olk RJ, Akduman L. Combined modified grid and panretinal photocoagulation for diffuse diabetic macular edema and proliferative diabetic retinopathy. *Ophthalmic Surg Lasers* 2000; **31**(4): 292–300.

6 Early Treatment Diabetic Retinopathy Study Research Group. Early photocoagulation for diabetic retinopathy. ETDRS report number 9. *Ophthalmology* 1991; **98**(5 Suppl): 766–85.

7 Hamilton A, Ulbig M, Polkinghorne P. *Management of diabetic retinopathy*. London: BMJ Publishing Group, 1996.

11

The stable treated eye

Peter H. Scanlon

FOLLOWING TREATMENT OF MACULOPATHY

Following treatment of focal maculopathy

A good result following laser treatment[1] of focal exudative or focal/multifocal oedema is clearing of the areas of exudates and oedema. There are usually signs of clearing at the 3-month follow-up appointment, but clearing may continue for a further 3–6 months and hence, providing clearing has commenced by the first 3-month appointment, a decision does not need to be made at that appointment regarding further focal laser treatment until no further clearing is apparent.

Subsequent prognosis for the eye and vision will depend on control of systemic factors such as glucose,[2,3] hypertension[4] and lipids.[5]

It is not uncommon to successfully treat one area of leakage and subsequently find leakage appearing in a completely different area around the fovea of the same eye.

CASE HISTORY 1
Treated maculopathy

A 36-year-old man (BMI 27.4) with type 2 diabetes controlled with insulin from 6 months after diagnosis (at the age of 33 years), was referred from the retinal screening service with the following photographs of his left eye (Fig. 11.1a).

On examination he was found to have clinically significant macular oedema with retinal thickening <500 microns from the foveal centre. His HbA1c was 10.7% and his blood pressure 145/84, and the vision in this left

A Practical Manual of Diabetic Retinopathy Management.
Peter H Scanlon, Charles P Wilkinson, Stephen J Aldington and David R Matthews. Published 2009 by Blackwell Publishing, ISBN 978-1-4051-7035-2.

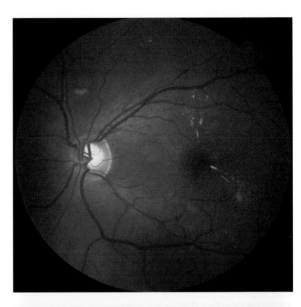

(a)

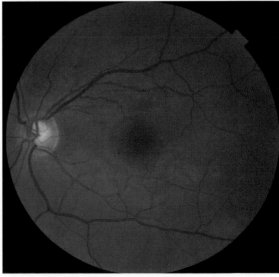

(b)

Fig. 11.1 Case history 1. (a) Focal maculopathy before treatment. (b) Treated focal maculopathy.

137

eye was good at 6/6 (20/20). He was given focal laser treatment to the left macular area:

- 15 burns, 500-micron size, 160 mW, 0.1 s, area centralis lens, argon laser were given to the areas of retinal thickening.

His visual acuity (VA) remained stable at 6/6 (20/20). The thickening and exudates cleared over the next 6 months. Eighteen months after the initial presentation, the HbA1c improved to 8.2% and a repeat photograph shows the improvement (Fig. 11.1b).

Following treatment of diffuse maculopathy

Treatment of diffuse diabetic macular oedema is generally much more difficult[6] and the results are not as good as treatment of focal maculopathy. Laser treatment is generally targeted at the areas of most leakage around the macular area. An individual treatment plan needs to be determined for each patient depending on the areas of leakage, the presence or absence of any cystoid changes, the level of peripheral ischaemia, the systemic blood pressure and the diabetic control. A successful result would be to see a gradual improvement in the leakage around the macular area because chronic oedema tends to cause pigment epithelial changes relating to damage to the photoreceptors in the central fovea and permanent loss of vision.

CASE HISTORY 2
Treated NVE proliferative DR with diffuse maculopathy

A 29-year-old man (BMI 27.7) diagnosed 1 month previously with type 2 diabetes and commenced on gliclazide 80 mg b.d. was seen by the retinal screening service and found to have VAs of right 6/6 (20,20), left 6/24 (20/80), and a diffuse macular oedema in his left eye. The colour photographs and fluorescein angiogram that were taken at presentation are shown in Fig. 11.2(a–i).

- Treatment was given to the left macular area with 23 burns 100-micron size, 170 mW, 0.1 s, area centralis lens, argon laser.

Six months later, the VAs were right 6/18 (20/60), left 6/36 (20/120), a diffuse macular oedema was present in both eyes and NVD were developing at both optic discs.

Further laser treatment was given to both macular areas:

- Right macular area: 18 burns, 100-micron size, 160 mW, 0.1 s, area centralis lens, argon laser.
- Left macular area: 24 burns, 100-micron size, 170–190 mW, 0.1 s, area centralis lens, argon laser.

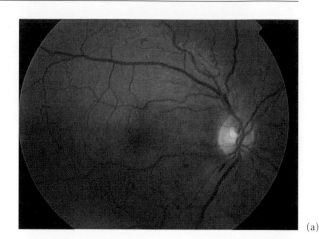

(a)

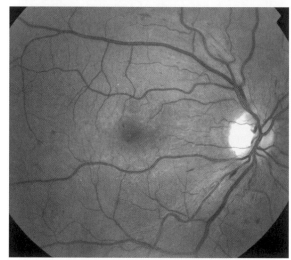

(b)

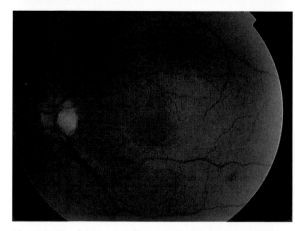

(c)

Fig. 11.2 Case history 2. Diffuse maculopathy at presentation: (a) right macular colour photograph; (b) right macular red-free photograph; (c) left macular colour photograph; (*Continued on facing page*)

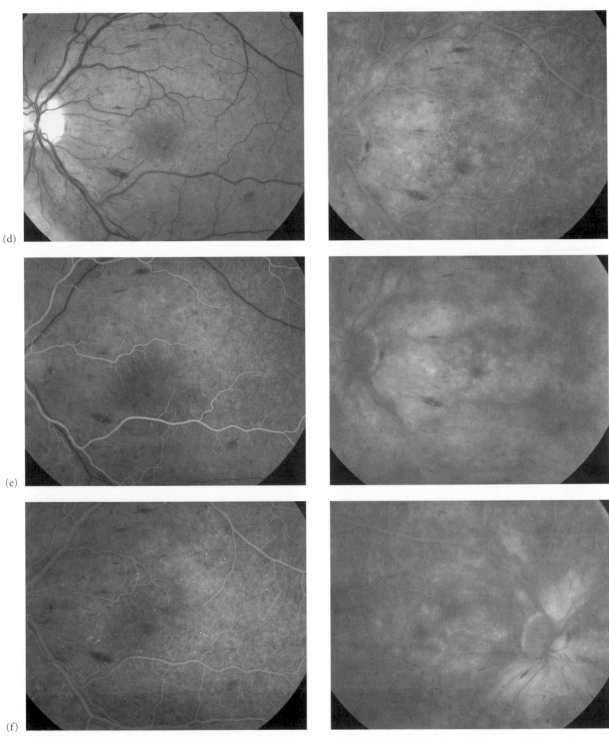

Fig. 11.2 (*Cont'd*) (d) left macular red-free photograph; (e) fluorescein left macular area 17 s after injection; (f) fluorescein left macular area 37 s after injection; (g) fluorescein left macular area 1 min 55 s after injection; (h) fluorescein left macular area 4 min 12 s after injection; (i) fluorescein right macular area 4 min 35 s after injection (*Continued on p. 140*)

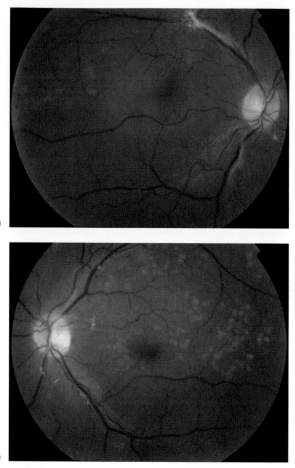

(j)

(k)

Fig. 11.2 (*Cont'd*) (j) stable treated right eye; (k) stable treated left eye.

Panretinal photocoagulation was commenced to each eye:

- Treatment given to the left eye was 3589 burns in four sessions, including 1625 burns, 350-micron size, trans-equatorial lens, 290 mW, and 1964 burns, 200-micron size, SuperQuad lens, 270 mW, argon laser.
- Treatment given to the right eye was 3586 burns in four sessions, including 1661 burns, 350-micron size, trans-equatorial lens, 240 mW, and 1925 burns, 200-micron size, SuperQuad lens, 210 mW, argon laser.

The neovascularization gradually settled, the macular areas improved over the next 12 months and the vision improved to a level of right 6/12, left 6/9. There is a small amount of preretinal fibrosis in the right macular area, which is the reason for the slightly reduced right vision.

Photographs of the retina were taken following the treatment, 4 years after the original presentation (Fig. 11.2j,k).

Ischaemic maculopathy

The modified ETDRS technique does recommend treating to all areas of diffuse leakage or non-perfusion (providing there is retinal thickening) within the area considered for grid treatment, but not within 500 microns of the foveal centre. However, if there is ischaemia that involves the central fovea, laser treatment in isolation is unlikely to improve the vision. Treatment of systemic hypertension does, in some patients, lead to an improvement or a stabilization of vision. It is therefore important that an ophthalmologist pays careful attention to the blood pressure in this group of patients. A good result in this group of patients is stabilization of the vision at a reasonable level.

An example of a patient with diabetes and hypertension whose maculopathy improved following treatment of his hypertension is described in the maculopathy section (Chapter 6, Case History 1).

FOLLOWING TREATMENT OF NVD OR NVE

NVD and NVE usually respond well to laser treatment. If involution of the vessels does not occur after a full panretinal photocoagulation, further scatter laser treatment is the recommended first approach. Involution of neovascularization is dependent upon a sufficient area of retinal ablation,[7,8] which depends on the extent of the retinal ischaemia. NVD are more likely to show signs of complete involution following laser treatment than NVE.

NVD or NVE may persist as thin fine vessels or 'ghost vessels' where no red blood corpuscles appear to pass through these vessels. If NVD or NVE persist, varying degrees of fibrosis surrounding the new vessel complex often occur. 'Ghost vessels' rarely progress or haemorrhage except when a posterior vitreous attachment occurs. This usually results in avulsion of the vessels from their stem and, once the haemorrhage clears, the vessels have been avulsed and recurrent haemorrhage does not therefore occur.

Vitreous haemorrhage may occur following scatter laser treatment and may be asymptomatic. The haemorrhage, if small and asymptomatic, often lies in the inferior vitreous cavity. A careful search needs to be made of the retina to determine the source of the haemorrhage to determine whether there is recurrent neovascularization, a partial or complete posterior vitreous detachment resulting in avulsion of new vessel complexes, or whether another source such as a retinal tear is the cause.

Following scatter laser treatment one is looking for the following signs.

1 Signs of adequate scatter laser photocoagulation scars
2 Signs of involution and finally disappearance of the new vessels where possible
3 Signs of lack of activity of the new vessel complex in the form of:
   • no further growth (and preferably involution as above)
   • no signs of red blood cells in the tips of the frond like ends of the new vessels
   • signs of fibrosis around the new vessel complex.
4 Looking at the overall venous calibre, signs of returning from a dilated and possibly beaded calibre back to a narrower width and absence of venous beading is an important sign of successful scatter laser treatment.
5 Absence of recurrent vitreous haemorrhages.
6 No new areas of neovascularization developing.
7 No signs of rubeosis iridis or neovascular glaucoma developing.

A good result following treatment of neovascularization is complete involution of the new vessels. It is more common to achieve this goal of complete involution in patients with NVD than NVE.

The second best result is incomplete involution of the new vessels with signs of lack of activity as described above, often associated with a degree of fibrosis.

CASE HISTORY 3
Treated NVD proliferative DR

A 25-year-old woman with type 1 diabetes of 18 years' duration was referred by her optometrist and she was found to have proliferative diabetic retinopathy in her left eye with small NVD (more than one-third disc area) and NVE (less than half disc area) in the superior and nasal retina.

• Treatment was given to the left eye with 1684 burns over two sessions, 500-micron size, 0.1 s, 230 m–280 mW, Karickhoff 4 mirror lens.

  The NVD regressed over the following 6 months and the NVE partially regressed and fibrosed.

  Six years after the initial presentation, proliferative diabetic retinopathy developed in the right eye with small NVD (more than one-third disc area) and NVE (less than half disc area) in the temporal retina.

• Treatment was given to the right eye with 2419 burns over 3 sessions, 200-micron size, 0.1 s, 170–190 mW, quadraspheric lens.

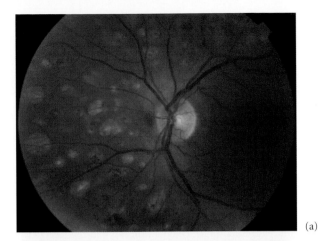
(a)

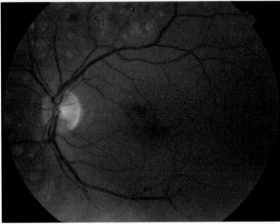
(b)

Fig. 11.3 Case history 3. Treated NVD proliferative DR: (a) left disc colour photograph; (b) left macula colour photograph.

The NVD regressed over the following 6 months and the NVE partially regressed and fibrosed.

Ten years after the initial presentation, this lady had a successful pregnancy with no deterioration in her stable treated retinae.

Her VAs have remained good at 6/6 (20/20) in each eye, her HbA1c results have been good at levels of between 6.7% and 7.3%, and her blood pressure has remained at an average of 125/81.

Photographs of her left retina are shown in Fig. 11.3.

CASE HISTORY 4
Treated NVE proliferative DR

A 23-year-old man (BMI 26) with type 1 diabetes of 22 years' duration was referred from retinal screening with possible new vessels in the superior retina of his left eye. Over the previous 2 years, his HbA1c result had varied between 9% and 10.5% and his blood pressure had averaged 139/80. A fluorescein angiogram confirmed that he had neovascularization in the superior retina and he also showed signs of extensive retinal ischaemia with severe IRMA in 2 other quadrants and venous beading in 2 quadrants. Panretinal photocoagulation was therefore commenced but despite extensive treatment, he required a vitrectomy for his left eye.

At the age of 26, photographs were taken of his right eye (Fig. 11.4a–c). The photographs show venous beading in an ischaemic area of right superior retina. New vessels had formed at the right disc and superotemporal retina, and panretinal photocoagulation was commenced to the right eye.

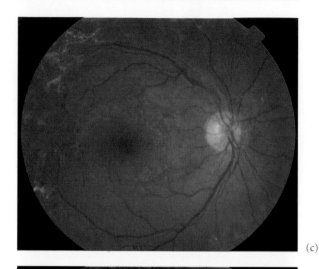

(c)

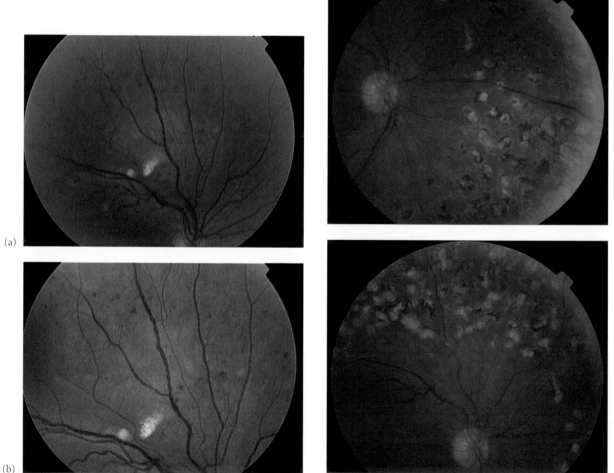

(a)

(b)

(d)

(e)

Fig. 11.4 Case history 4. Right superior colour photographs showing ischaemia before NVE developed (a,b). Treated NVE proliferative DR: (c) right macula colour; (d) right nasal colour; (e) right superior colour.

- Treatment was given to the right peripheral retina of right 3345 burns in four treatment sessions, 1895 using the transequatorial lens (magnification factor 1.44), 350-micron size, 250 mW, 0.1 s; and 1895 using the SuperQuad 160 lens (magnification factor 2), 200-micron size, 230 mW, 0.1 s, argon laser.
- Indirect laser was later given in theatre of right 1469 burns, 260–300 mW, 0.2 s.

This resulted in regression of the neovascularization and the following photographs (Fig. 11.4d–e).

The photograph of the superior retina after regression of the neovascularization (Fig. 11.4e) demonstrates that the venous calibre that was dilated and beaded has returned to a more normal calibre.

PRACTICE POINTS

- In the treatment of maculopathy, one aims to stabilize the vision using the treatment techniques recommended by the Early Treatment Diabetic Retinopathy Study and then paying careful control to systemic factors such as glucose,[2,3] hypertension[4] and lipids,[5] recognizing that the treatment of diffuse and ischaemic maculopathy is usually more difficult than treatment of focal maculopathy.[6]
- In the treatment of neovascularization, involution of neovascularization is dependent upon a sufficient area of retinal ablation.[7,8] When deciding how much laser to undertake in an individual patient the calibre of the venous circulation is an important determining factor as well as regression/fibrosis of any neovascularization.

REFERENCES

1 Early Treatment Diabetic Retinopathy Study Research Group. Treatment techniques and clinical guidelines for photocoagulation of diabetic macular edema. Early Treatment Diabetic Retinopathy Study Report Number 2. *Ophthalmology* 1987; **94**(7): 761–74.

2 Stratton IM, Kohner EM, Aldington SJ, Turner RC, Holman RR, Manley SE *et al.* UKPDS 50: risk factors for incidence and progression of retinopathy in Type II diabetes over 6 years from diagnosis. *Diabetologia* 2001; **44**(2): 156–63.

3 The Diabetes Control and Complications Trial Research Group. The effect of intensive treatment of diabetes on the development and progression of long-term complications in insulin-dependent diabetes mellitus. *N Engl J Med* 1993; **329**(14): 977–86.

4 Matthews DR, Stratton IM, Aldington SJ, Holman RR, Kohner EM. Risks of progression of retinopathy and vision loss related to tight blood pressure control in type 2 diabetes mellitus: UKPDS 69. *Arch Ophthalmol* 2004; **122**(11): 1631–40.

5 Lyons TJ, Jenkins AJ, Zheng D, Lackland DT, McGee D, Garvey WT *et al.* Diabetic retinopathy and serum lipoprotein subclasses in the DCCT/EDIC cohort. *Invest Ophthalmol Vis Sci* 2004; **45**(3): 910–18.

6 Kearns M, Hamilton AM, Kohner EM. Excessive permeability in diabetic maculopathy. *Br J Ophthalmol* 1979; **63**(7): 489–97.

7 Bailey CC, Sparrow JM, Grey RH, Cheng H. The National Diabetic Retinopathy Laser Treatment Audit. III. Clinical outcomes. *Eye* 1999; **13**(Pt 2): 151–9.

8 The Diabetic Retinopathy Study Research Group. Photocoagulation treatment of proliferative diabetic retinopathy. Clinical application of Diabetic Retinopathy Study (DRS) findings, DRS Report Number 8. *Ophthalmology* 1981; **88**(7): 583–600.

12 The surgical approach to the diabetic eye

Charles P. Wilkinson

INTRODUCTION

Although laser therapy for diabetic retinopathy is literally considered to be surgery, and although cataract surgery and other intraocular procedures are performed more frequently in diabetic eyes than in non-diabetic comparable cases, this chapter will be limited to vitrectomy, an intraocular procedure specifically aimed at the pathological features of diabetic retinopathy as well as their complications. Laser treatment for diabetic retinopathy is discussed in the chapters that describe specific stages of the disorder.

VITREOUS SURGERY (VITRECTOMY)[1-3]

The vitreous gel is a vital structural component in the pathogenesis of proliferative diabetic retinopathy (PDR) and selected cases of diabetic macular oedema (DME). The critical variable in these situations is the relationship between the posterior cortical surface (PCS) of the vitreous gel and the inner surface of the retina.

In PDR, extraretinal neovascular and fibrovascular tissue grow almost exclusively along the PCS (Fig. 12.1), and if the PCS has separated from the retina before the threat of neovascularization, literal PDR almost never occurs. In DME, most cases are probably not influenced significantly by the PCS, although there are a substantial percentage of cases in which it may be an important factor. In many of these, the PCS appears as a 'taut posterior hyaloid' and exerts more subtle traction upon the retinal surface than that typically associated with PDR. In addition, a relatively unusual syndrome occurs when a par-

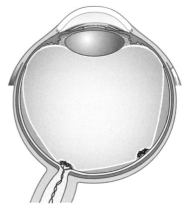

Fig. 12.1 Neovascularization on the optic nerve and elsewhere occurs at locations at which there are vitreoretinal interfaces.

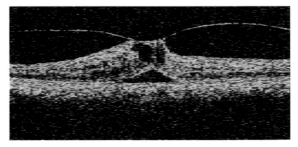

Fig. 12.2 OCT studies provide a means of more accurately identifying vitreoretinal traction forces that are occasionally responsible for DME. In this case a partial vitreous detachment and persistent traction upon the macula have caused marked macular thickening and a tiny retinal detachment.

tially detached PCS remains adherent to the macula and the resultant traction disturbs the permeability of central capillaries (Fig. 12.2). Finally, both an attached and a detached PCS may be associated with the formation of fibrocellular membranes that contract the inner surface of the macula and cause macular oedema and/or distortion.

A Practical Manual of Diabetic Retinopathy Management.
Peter H Scanlon, Charles P Wilkinson, Stephen J Aldington and David R Matthews. Published 2009 by Blackwell Publishing, ISBN 978-1-4051-7035-2.

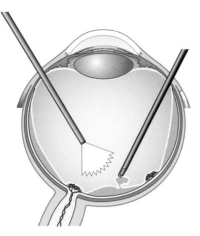

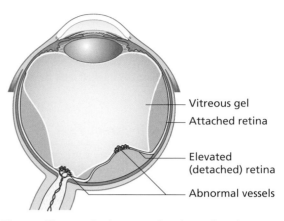

Vitreous gel
Attached retina
Elevated (detached) retina
Abnormal vessels

Fig. 12.3 Vitreous surgery usually includes three incisions for a cutting/aspiration device, an illumination system, and a continuous infusion site (not pictured). Vitreous haemorrhage in the gel is easily removed if the posterior vitreous cortical face is separated from the surface of the retina.

Fig. 12.4 Fibrovascular tissue growth and secondary changes in the vitreous gel cause traction at sites of vitreovascular attachments resulting in haemorrhage and traction retinal detachment. Retinal breaks and rhegmatogenous detachments can also occur.

TREATMENT TECHNIQUES FOR PDR

Contemporary vitrectomy techniques provide a means of removing vitreous haemorrhage and the PCS in a relatively safe and effective fashion. Most systems employ three small (20–25 gauge) entry 'ports' into the eye, and a cutting/suction device, an intraocular light source and an infusion cannula are inserted through these trans-scleral incisions (Fig. 12.3). In a right eye, these cutting instrument and light pipe are typically inserted 3–4 mm posterior to the limbus at approximately 10.30 and 2.15 respectively, with the infusion device inserted at approximately 8.30. Additional equipment, such as pics, scissors and forceps, are frequently substituted temporarily to replace the routine cutting device. Cataract surgery can be combined with vitrectomy if the lens opacity prevents an optimal view and in other selected cases.

The primary goals of vitreous surgery for PDR include removal of vitreous haemorrhage, wide excision of the PCS and associated neovascular tissue, and the elimination of epiretinal tissue and traction forces affecting macular function. In PDR, extraretinal neovascular and fibrovascular tissue grows almost exclusively along the posterior vitreous surface, as noted earlier. This proliferation often causes changes in the vitreous gel that result in separation of some of the cortical vitreous from the retina. The vitreous always remains attached to the anterior

retina at the vitreous base, and it frequently exhibits a funnel-shaped configuration that extends between the vitreous base anteriorly and posterior areas of neovascular proliferation. Variable portions of the posterior cortical vitreous remain near the plane of the retinal surface and bridge from one area of retinal neovascularization to another (Fig. 12.4). When little or no posterior vitreous detachment occurs, the proliferative tissue grows along the plane of the inner retinal surface, and widespread adhesions to the retina may develop. This fibrovascular tissue can contract, causing tangential traction on the retina and visual loss from swelling, distortion or displacement of the macula. Fibrovascular tissue growth and secondary changes in the vitreous gel cause traction resulting in further complications, including haemorrhage, traction retinal detachment, retinal breaks and rhegmatogenous retinal detachment.

If complete removal of vitreous haemorrhage and the posterior cortical vitreous with all attached fibrovascular tissue is accomplished without complications, further vasoproliferation on the posterior retina can usually be prevented, and reattachment of a detached retina can usually be accomplished. Removal of vitreous haemorrhage is relatively easily performed, and the most difficult surgical step in most vitrectomies for diabetic retinopathy is the removal of fibrovascular tissue from the surface of the underlying retina, a manoeuvre that is particularly difficult if the retina is also detached. These steps are usually performed with a variety of microsurgical vitrectomy instruments, including pics, forceps and scissors. Following successful vitreous surgery, extensive scatter laser photocoagulation is usually applied near the end of the procedure.

Removal of blood and vitreous gel

The posterior vitreous surface is frequently incised initially in an area of partial vitreous detachment and away from vitreoretinal attachments and/or areas of underlying retinal detachment. If non-clotted blood is present in the preretinal space behind the posterior vitreous surface, it is evacuated using an aspiration device. When there is little or no posterior vitreous detachment, portions of the posterior cortical vitreous can be elevated from the retina with a cutter, vitreoretinal pick, sharp bent-tipped needle or myringotomy knife (Fig. 12.5). Non-vascularized posterior hyaloid and immature proliferative membranes frequently can be bluntly dissected from the surface of the retina. Recently proliferating tissue is characterized by neovascularization with little or only translucent fibrous tissue. Older fibrovascular tissue becomes more white and opaque and more firmly adherent to the retina, and sharp dissection may be required.

Then the posterior vitreous surface is frequently excised around the circumference of its cone-like structure to relieve traction between the vitreous base and the posterior retina and zones of fibrovascular proliferation. Often, the edges of the posterior vitreous surface separate widely after it is cut, demonstrating that considerable traction was present preoperatively. At this stage, some surgeons prefer to remove as much of the cortical vitreous as possible, except for the anterior portion adjacent to the vitreous base and posterior remnants near areas of vitreoretinal attachment. Others remove the avascular gel at the same time that the fibrovascular tissue itself is excised.

Removal of fibrovascular tissue

'Delamination' and 'en bloc' are terms used to describe methods of dissecting epiretinal fibrovascular tissue from the surface of the retina. Using the delamination technique, surgeons initially remove all elevated cortical vitreous that is producing anteroposterior traction on posterior fibrovascular tissue. Vitreoretinal picks and scissors are then used to elevate and divide avascular portions of the more organized posterior vitreous cortex until only islands of tightly adherent fibrovascular tissue remain. Bimanual techniques are used to delaminate those focal membranes that appear to be excisable without major structural damage to the retina (Fig. 12.6). Other surgeons prefer the 'en bloc' technique, leaving portions of anterior vitreous gel intact, so that the residual anteroposterior traction will assist in the dissection of epiretinal tissue by elevating its edges (Fig. 12.7).

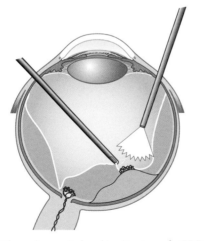

Fig. 12.5 The major surgical goal in vitrectomy for PDR is to separate and excise the posterior cortical vitreous surface and associated areas of fibrovascular proliferation from the retinal surface.

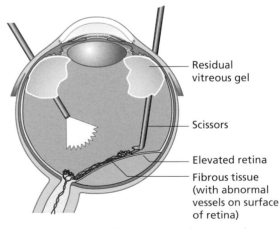

Residual vitreous gel

Scissors

Elevated retina

Fibrous tissue (with abnormal vessels on surface of retina)

Fig. 12.6 Segmentation 'delamination' techniques can be employed to remove fibrovascular proliferation from the surface of the retina.

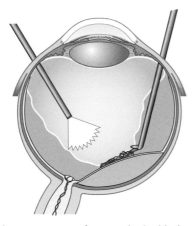

Fig. 12.7 Some surgeons prefer to employ 'en bloc' excision ('delamination') of fibrovascular tissue from the retinal surface. Vitreous traction can assist in elevating the abnormal vessels from portions of the retina.

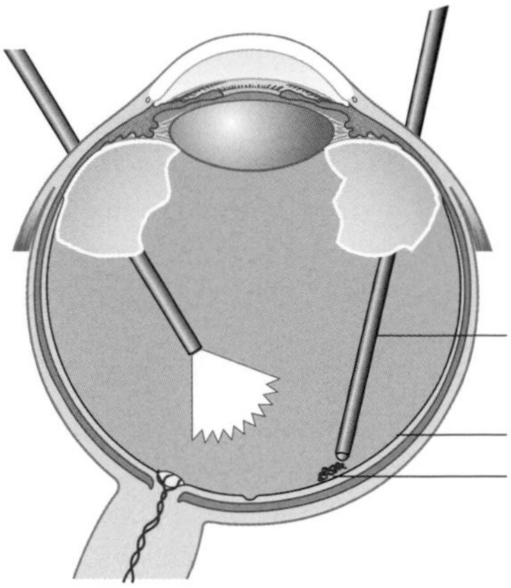

Fig. 12.8 Intraocular diathermy is employed to treat bleeding foci on the surface of the retina.

Removing all fibrovascular 'islands' is believed to reduce the frequency of postoperative bleeding, contraction of residual epiretinal membranes, recurrence of epiretinal proliferation and missed small retinal breaks. Therefore, 'segmentation' techniques, in which localized islands of epiretinal fibrovascular tissue are left following vitrectomy, have become less popular. Still, segmentation techniques are useful when the combination of relatively mature epiretinal tissue and atrophic retina results in a significant increase in risk of retinal breaks associated with complete epiretinal membrane dissection or when vascular membranes are located anteriorly and are difficult to remove safely. If no segmentation has been performed, the entire organized posterior cortical vitreous is usually removed in a single piece. Fibrovascular tissue attached to the optic nerve head is gently avulsed or excised from the nerve after all surrounding attachments to the retina have been eliminated. If retinal mobility associated with retinal detachment interferes with dissecting epiretinal tissue, a small amount of heavy perfluorocarbon liquid can be injected onto the posterior retina. This stabilizes the retina and makes delamination easier. Combinations of techniques are frequently employed, but the goal of removing the posterior cortical surface out to the vitreous base along with all fibrovascular membranes is always the same in these cases.

Intraoperative haemorrhage during segmentation and delamination is unfortunately not uncommon.

Unimanual or bimanual bipolar diathermy is routinely applied to sites of persistent bleeding other than the optic nerve (Fig. 12.8). The incidence of haemorrhage can be reduced by avoiding segmentation of highly vascularized membranes and ensuring that the patient's blood pressure is normal. Elevation of intraocular pressure is used to minimize bleeding during the dissection of vascularized tissue. Further elevation of intraocular pressure to a level above systolic blood pressure for 1–2 min will frequently stop persistent bleeding.

Treating retinal breaks and detachments

Retinal breaks with or without retinal detachment are treated before the operation is completed. Subretinal fluid is evacuated through suitable posterior breaks. This flattens the retina against the pigment epithelium, permitting transvitreal laser photocoagulation. Internal drainage of subretinal fluid also demonstrates whether all traction on the retina has been relieved. If the retina tends to redetach rapidly despite release of all fibrovascular tissue, the surgeon should search for thin avascular membranes peripheral to the sites of neovascularization and remove them. Drainage of subretinal fluid is frequently combined with fluid–gas exchange, and laser photocoagulation through the gas bubble is then applied around all retinal breaks. Most surgeons then add extensive scatter laser photocoagulation to the entire peripheral retina unless it has been heavily treated previously.

CASE HISTORY 1
Vitrectomy for severe vitreous haemorrhage and PDR

A 29-year-old Caucasian female with a long history of poorly controlled type 1 PDR and no prior laser therapy lost vision (reduced to 'hand movements') due to severe vitreous haemorrhage (Fig. 12.9). Although no retinal detachment was demonstrated on ultrasound studies, vitreous surgery was recommended because of visual loss and the presumed progression of PDR that would be expected without laser therapy. Vitreous surgery and intraoperative laser therapy eliminated the haemorrhage and responsible neovascularization, and vision has remained 20/30 for 3 years (Fig. 12.10).

CASE HISTORY 2
Vitrectomy for traction retinal detachment and vitreous haemorrhage due to PDR

A 57-year-old type 2 diabetic patient had received prior laser therapy for PDR, but progression had occurred, with traction retinal detachment and vitreous haemorrhage reducing vision to the level of less than 20/400 (Fig. 12.11). Vitreous surgery and intraoperative laser therapy eliminated the haemorrhage and fibrovascular neovascular tissue causing retinal detachment, and vision improved to 20/50, where it has remained for 18 months (Fig. 12.12).

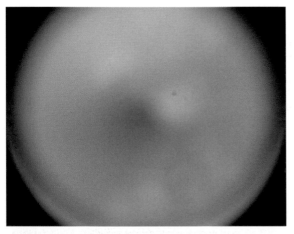

Fig. 12.9 Case history 1. Preoperative photograph of a massive vitreous haemorrhage associated with PDR.

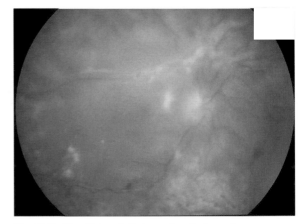

Fig. 12.11 Case history 2. Preoperative photograph demonstrating PDR with vitreous haemorrhage and traction retinal detachment.

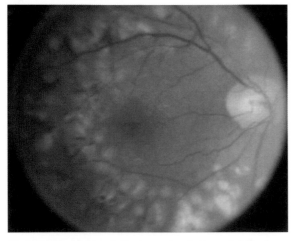

Fig. 12.10 Case history 1. Postoperative photograph following vitrectomy to remove a massive vitreous haemorrhage associated with PDR.

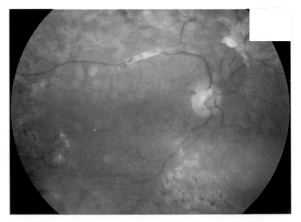

Fig. 12.12 Case history 2. Postoperative photograph of the retina seen in Fig. 12.11. Visual acuity has improved.

TREATMENT TECHNIQUES FOR DME[4,5]

Most cases of diabetic macular oedema are observed in eyes with NPDR and insignificant anterior–posterior vitreous traction upon the macula. However, in a subset of diabetic patients, macular oedema is associated with one or a combination of at least three syndromes in which vitreous traction upon the macula presumably causes permeability changes in the macular capillaries and subsequent macular thinkening. These include: (i) the so-called 'taut posterior hyaloid'; (ii) fibrocellular membranes that develop on the retina and then contract, distorting its surface; and (iii) the 'vitreomacular traction syndrome' (see Fig. 12.2 in which a partially detached cortical vitreous remains attached at the macula and exerts traction upon it).

In all of these situations, the surgical goals include removal of the posterior cortical vitreous surface and all epimacular membranes, and elimination of vitreomacular traction forces. This is usually accomplished with vitrectomy pics, forceps and scissors, as described earlier.

CASE HISTORY 3
Vitrectomy for DME associated with a taut posterior hyaloid and epiretinal membrane

A 59-year-old type 2 diabetic female developed progressive visual loss due to progressive DME in spite of two sessions of traditional laser photocoagulation and a single injection of intravitreal steroids. Vision was 20/200 (Fig. 12.13). There was no attachment of the posterior cortical vitreous to the macula, but vitreous surgery was performed to remove the modest epiretinal membrane and posterior cortical surface. The DME and visual acuity (VA) improved significantly to 20/60 over the following 2 months, and the latter has remained stable for 7 months (Fig. 12.14).

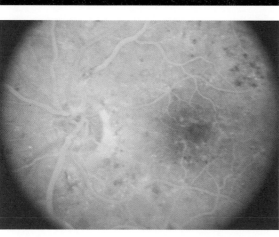

(a)

(b)

Fig. 12.13 Case history 3. (a) OCT image of the central retina (macula) in a patient with diabetic macular oedema (DME) associated with a taut posterior hyaloid and modest epiretinal membrane, neither of which is optimally visualized. The macula is approximately twice its normal thickness. No vitreomacular traction is apparent. (b) A fluorescein angiogram demonstrating leakage from many vessels.

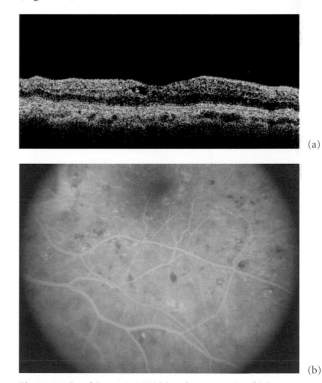

(a)

(b)

Fig. 12.14 Case history 3. OCT (a) and angiographic (b) images of the same case as demonstrated in Fig. 12.13 following vitreous surgery and removal of the preretinal tissue. Less oedema and leakage are present.

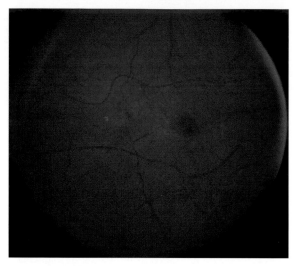

Fig. 12.15 Case history 4. Clinical photograph of the right eye of a patient with severe DME and vitreomacular traction syndrome whose OCT is depicted in Fig. 12.2.

CASE HISTORY 4
DME associated with a partially detached vitreous and vitreomacular traction

A 64-year-old female with type 2 diabetes developed a progressive loss of central vision due to macular oedema associated with severe vitreomacular traction (Figs 12.2 and 12.15). Vision was reduced to 20/100. Vitrectomy was performed to remove the vitreous gel and traction forces, and retinal oedema diminished as VA improved to 20/50 (Fig. 12.16). Subsequent laser treatment was applied to leaking vascular anomalies identified on the angiogram.

PRACTICE POINTS

- Both PDR and NPDR with macular oedema are indications for a variety of surgical options, and specific stages of retinopathy represent evidence-based indications for these procedures.
- Although PDR is usually managed initially with laser photocoagulation, vitrectomy procedures are invaluable in managing severe complications of PDR, including major vitreous haemorrhage and retinal detachment.
- Diabetic macular oedema is usually managed initially with laser photocoagulation, and vitrectomy is employed if vitreous or epimacular traction forces appear to be significant.

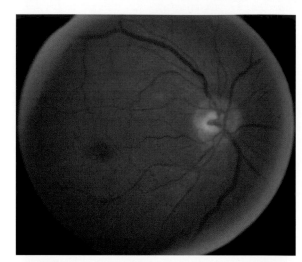

(a)

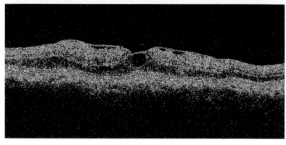

(b)

Fig. 12.16 Case history 4. (a) Clinical photograph and (b) OCT of the same patient as in Fig. 12.15 following vitreous surgery. The oedema has diminished and the traction forces have been eliminated.

REFERENCES

1 Eliot D, Lee M, Abrams G. Proliferative diabetic retinopathy: principles and techniques of surgical treatment. In: Ryan SJ, Wilkinson CP, eds. *Retina*, 4th edn. Philadelphia: Elsevier Mosby, 2006: 2413–50.

2 Smiddy W, Flynn H. Vitrectomy for diabetic retinopathy. In: Flynn HW Jr, Smiddy W, eds. *Diabetes and Ocular Disease. Past, Present, and Future Therapies*. San Francisco: American Academy of Ophthalmology, 2000: 155–80.

3 Cooper B, Shah GK, Grand MG, Bakal J, Sharma S. Visual outcomes and complications after multiple vitrectomies for diabetic vitreous hemorrhage. *Retina* 2004; **24**(1): 19–22.

4 daCruz L, Gregor Z. Surgery in the treatment of cystoid macular edema. In: *Retina*, 4th edn. Philadelphia: Elsevier Mosby, 2006: 2633–44.

5 Rosenblatt BJ, Shah GK, Sharma S, Bakal J. Pars plana vitrectomy with internal limiting membranectomy for refractory diabetic macular edema without a taut posterior hyaloid. *Graefes Arch Clin Exp Ophthalmol* 2005; **243**(1): 20–5.

13 Pregnancy and the diabetic eye

Peter H. Scanlon

RISK FACTORS FOR PROGRESSION OF DIABETIC RETINOPATHY DURING PREGNANCY

Progression of diabetic retinopathy may occur during pregnancy. The worsening of retinopathy during pregnancy can be quite significant and may require photocoagulation during pregnancy, more frequently in those patients with pre-existing diabetic retinopathy. The known risk factors for progression of diabetic retinopathy in pregnancy are summarized below.

Pregnancy is independently associated with progression of diabetic retinopathy

Two studies found pregnancy to be independently associated with progression of diabetic retinopathy.

A prospective study[1] was undertaken within the Wisconsin Epidemiological Study of Diabetic Retinopathy in 1990 to determine the effect of pregnancy on diabetic retinopathy. Insulin-taking diabetic women were enrolled; one group was comprised of 171 pregnant women, the other group was comprised of 298 women who were not pregnant. Women were evaluated on referral and again in the postpartum period. 133 pregnant women and 241 non-pregnant women attended and had gradable photographs at both visits. The severity of diabetic retinopathy was based on grading of fundus photographs of seven standard photographic fields. The glycosylated haemoglobin, duration of diabetes, current age, diastolic blood pressure, number of past pregnancies and current pregnancy status were evaluated as risk factors for progression of diabetic retinopathy. After adjusting for glycosylated haemoglobin, current pregnancy was significantly associated with progression ($p < 0.005$, adjusted odds ratio 2.3).

In the Diabetes Control and Complications Trial (DCCT) in 2000, a multicentre controlled clinical trial that compared intensive treatment with conventional diabetes therapy, 180 women who had 270 pregnancies and 500 women who did not become pregnant were studied during an average of 6.5 years of follow-up. Women assigned to the conventional treatment group were changed to intensive therapy if they were planning pregnancy or as soon as possible after conception. Fundus photography was performed every 6 months. Compared with non-pregnant women, pregnant women had a 1.63-fold greater risk of any worsening of retinopathy from before to during pregnancy ($p < 0.05$) in the intensive treatment group; the risk was 2.48-fold greater for pregnant vs. not pregnant women in the conventional group ($p < 0.001$). Although individual patients had transient worsening of retinopathy during pregnancy, which persisted for as long as 12 months post-pregnancy, at the end of the DCCT, mean levels of retinopathy in subjects who had become pregnant were similar to those in subjects who had not become pregnant within each treatment group. Hence it was concluded that because pregnancy in type 1 diabetes induces a transient increase in the risk of retinopathy, increased ophthalmological surveillance is needed during pregnancy and the first year postpartum. The long-term risk of progression of early retinopathy, however, does not appear in this study to be increased by pregnancy.

Baseline severity of retinopathy

The baseline severity of retinopathy is a risk factor for progression of retinopathy during pregnancy. In the Diabetes in Early Pregnancy Study,[2] 155 diabetic women were followed from the periconception period to 1 month postpartum. In the 140 patients who did not have proliferative retinopathy at baseline, progression of

A Practical Manual of Diabetic Retinopathy Management.
Peter H Scanlon, Charles P Wilkinson, Stephen J Aldington and David R Matthews. Published 2009 by Blackwell Publishing, ISBN 978-1-4051-7035-2.

retinopathy was seen in 10.3% of patients with no retinopathy, 21.1% with microaneurysms only, 18.8% with mild nonproliferative retinopathy, and 54.8% with moderate-to-severe nonproliferative retinopathy at baseline, respectively. Proliferative retinopathy developed in 6.3% with mild and 29% with moderate-to-severe baseline retinopathy. These findings are supported by two further studies.

Phelps[3] monitored 35 women with insulin-dependent diabetes mellitus for changes in diabetic retinopathy in 38 pregnancies. Of patients with no retinopathy at baseline, 3/13 developed retinopathy during pregnancy; 13/20 with background retinopathy at baseline showed progression of retinopathy during pregnancy; 2/20 developed proliferative retinopathy. All five patients with proliferative retinopathy at baseline deteriorated during pregnancy.

Rosenn[4] followed 154 women with type 1 diabetes through pregnancy and found progression of diabetic retinopathy in 18/78 (23%) with no retinopathy, 28/68 (41%) with background retinopathy and 5/8 (63%) with proliferative retinopathy at baseline.

Poor metabolic control at conception

Poor metabolic control at conception is a risk factor for progression of diabetic retinopathy in pregnancy. In the Diabetes in Early Pregnancy Study,[2] the risk for progression of diabetic retinopathy was increased by initial glycosylated haemoglobin elevations as low as 6 SD above the control mean. This increased risk may be due to suboptimal control itself or to the rapid improvement in metabolic control that occurred in early pregnancy.

Rapid improvement of glycaemic control

Rapid improvement of glycaemic control *may* be a contributing factor in worsening of retinopathy as shown in four studies.[2–5]

The effect of rapid improvement in glycaemic control is impossible to separate from the effect of elevated glycosylated haemoglobin levels at conception and the associated increased proportion of retinopathy (both mild and severe) that occurs in this group of patients. The progression of retinopathy following commencement of intensive treatment has also been observed in non-pregnant adults with diabetes.[6] The established benefits of excellent diabetic control during pregnancy clearly outweigh the relatively minor effects noted in the fundi of the majority of patients who do not have significant pre-existing retinopathy.

Poor metabolic control during pregnancy or the early postpartum period

This is a risk factor for progression as shown in four studies.[1,4,5,7] Tight glycaemic control is recommended to avoid progression of retinopathy. Attention should be given to the period after delivery where the tight regulation may be more difficult to achieve.

Duration of diabetes

Longer duration of diabetes is a risk factor for progression of retinopathy during pregnancy as shown in three studies.[4,8,9] The effect of duration of diabetes on progression of retinopathy during pregnancy is difficult to separate from the effect of the severity of retinopathy at conception as the two are correlated. For example, the Diabetes in Early Pregnancy Study[2] found that the baseline retinopathy level was a significant risk factor for progression (p = 0.025) but duration of diabetes was not (p = 0.10).

Chronic hypertension and pregnancy-induced hypertension

Chronic and pregnancy-induced hypertension are risk factors for progression of retinopathy during pregnancy.

Rosenn[4] followed 154 women with type 1 diabetes through pregnancy and found progression of diabetic retinopathy in 11/29 (25%) with no hypertensive disorder, 11/22 (50%) with pregnancy-induced hypertension and 11/18 (61%) with chronic hypertension with or without superimposed pregnancy-induced hypertension.

LASER TREATMENT BEFORE CONCEPTION AND DURING PREGNANCY

Dibble[8] studied 55 insulin-dependent diabetic patients throughout pregnancy with serial retinal examinations by ophthalmoscopy and photographs. During gestation 3/19 patients (16%) with minimal or background retinopathy and 6/7 patients (86%) with untreated proliferative retinopathy experienced deterioration of their eye disease. In four patients with proliferative retinopathy, progression of retinal disease was arrested with photocoagulation during pregnancy. Only 1/6 who had received laser treatment before pregnancy experienced progression of her retinopathy.

POSTPARTUM REGRESSION

Postpartum regression of diabetic retinopathy does occur in a proportion of patients.

In the study by Rosenn[4] of 154 women with type 1 diabetes followed through pregnancy, 51 women had progression of retinopathy during pregnancy of which seven developed PDR. Thirteen women experienced postpartum regression. None of the women who developed PDR during pregnancy experienced postpartum regression.

RECOMMENDATIONS FOR RETINAL ASSESSMENT BEFORE AND DURING PREGNANCY

1 Annual screening for diabetic retinopathy is recommended in the preconception period.
2 It is recommended that screening in the preconception period should include annual mydriatic digital photography to provide a hard copy for comparison purposes. In the UK two 45° fields are taken (one macula centred and one disc centred).
3 Women with type 1 and type 2 diabetes should be offered mydriatic retinal assessment at the first antenatal clinic visit and again at 28 weeks' gestation. Digital photography is recommended at these visits to provide a hard copy for comparison purposes.
4 If any diabetic retinopathy is present at booking an additional screen should be performed at 16–20 weeks.
5 If diabetic retinopathy is found to be present in early pregnancy, careful ophthalmological supervision is required depending on the level of retinopathy both during pregnancy and for at least 6 months postpartum.

CASE HISTORY 1
Proliferative diabetic retinopathy in pregnancy

A 32-year-old woman with type 1 diabetes (diagnosed aged 13 years) presented to the eye clinic with blurred vision in her left eye. Her HbA1c was 8.6% and her blood pressure was 139/89. Her visual acuities (VAs) were right 6/6 (20/20), left 6/9 (20/30). A fluorescein angiogram was undertaken (Fig. 13.1). This showed leakage in the both macular areas with extensive ischaemic changes.
- Left focal laser treatment was commenced in the first instance: left macular area, 23 burns, 100-micron size, 120 mW, 0.1 s, area centralis lens, argon laser.

Six weeks after initial presentation, neovascularization had started to develop at the left optic disc and the patient

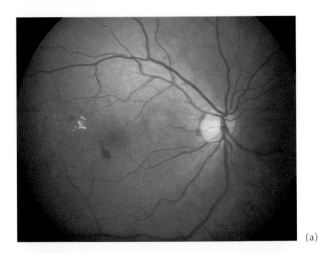

(a)

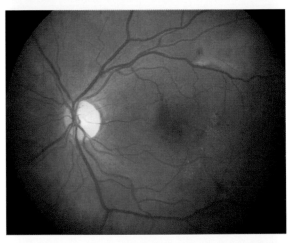

(b)

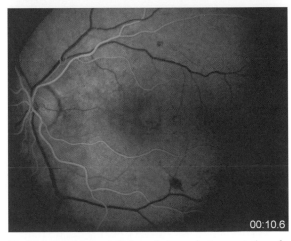

00:10.6 (c)

Fig. 13.1 Case history 1. Colour photograph at presentation of (a) right macula and (b) left macula. Fluorescein angiograms at presentation of: (c) left macula 10 s; (*Continued on p. 154*)

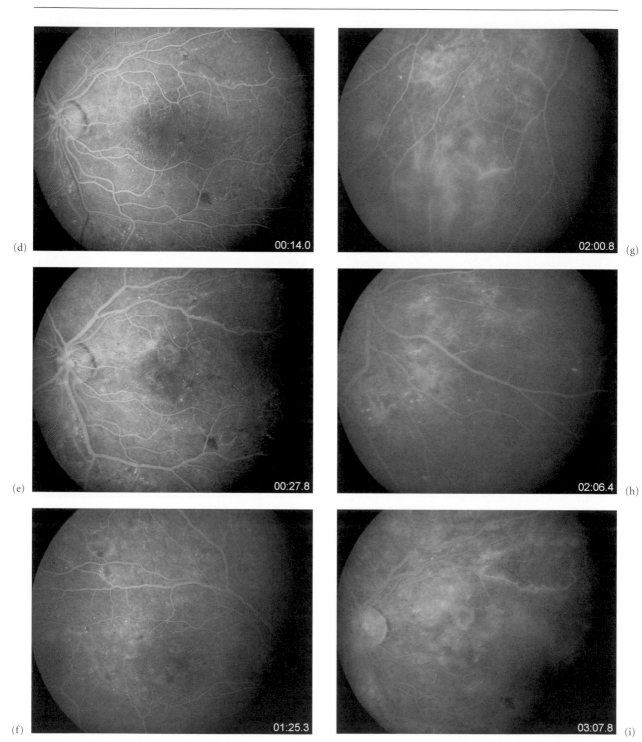

Fig. 13.1 (*Cont'd*) (d) left macula 14 s; (e) left macula 27 s; (f) right macula 1 min 25 s; (g) right inferior 2 min 00 s; (h) right inferonasal 2 min 06 s; (i) left macula 3 min 07 s; (*Continued on facing page*)

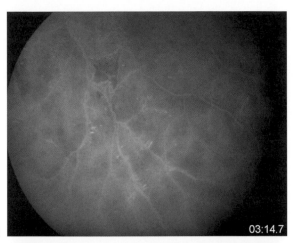

(j)

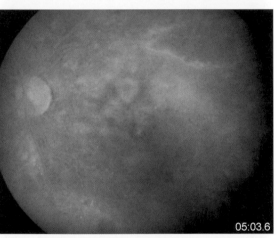

(k)

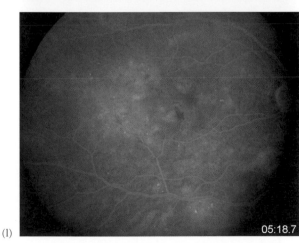

(l)

Fig. 13.1 (*Cont'd*) (j) left inferotemporal 3 min 14 s; (k) left macula 5 min 03 s; (l) right macula 5 min 18 s.

had a positive pregnancy test (5/40). Panretinal photocoagulation was given to the left eye.

- Left panretinal laser treatment: 1529 burns were given in two sessions 1 week apart, 200-micron size, 160–180 mW, SuperQuad lens (magnification factor 2), argon laser.

Clinically significant macular oedema was diagnosed in the right eye and 8 weeks after initial presentation (7/40):

- 14 burns, 100-micron size, 110 mW, 0.1 s, area centralis lens, argon laser were given as focal laser treatment to the right macular area.

Twenty weeks after initial presentation (19/40), NVD had started to develop at the right disc (more than one-third disc diameter). Panretinal photocoagulation was commenced to the right retina:

- right panretinal laser treatment, 1426 burns in two sessions 1 week apart, 320-micron size, 160–180 mW, trans-equatorial lens (magnification factor 1.44), argon laser.

At 38/40 weeks she delivered a healthy boy.

Her HbA1c results were mostly improved during pregnancy with results of 7.8%, 7.2%, 7.1%, 7.3%, 7.5%, 6.2%, 10.8%, 7.2%, 6.1% and 7.5%.

Ten days postpartum a vitreous haemorrhage developed in the right eye, requiring a right vitrectomy operation 4 months postpartum. At the time her blood pressure was 141/79 and HbA1c 5.2%. Indirect laser was given in theatre to the left eye.

Ten months postpartum she required a right phaco-emulsification of cataract with posterior chamber intra-ocular lens implant.

Twelve months postpartum her VA is 6/12 (20/40), left 6/6 (20/20).

CASE HISTORY 2
Diabetic retinopathy in pregnancy

A 29-year-old woman with type 1 diabetes for 21 years was seen in the eye clinic with mild nonproliferative diabetic retinopathy. Her blood pressure was 138/74 and HbA1c 8.8. The following photographs were taken (Fig. 13.2a–d).

The following year she was seen in the eye clinic when 11/40 weeks pregnant. The fundi did not appear to have changed and no photographs were taken. Images were taken at 25/40 weeks (Fig. 13.2e–h), 29/40 weeks (Fig. 13.2i–j) and 34/40 weeks (Fig. 13.2k–n).

The retinal appearance gradually settled during the postpartum period.

One year postpartum, no treatment having been given, further images were taken (Fig. 13.2o–r).

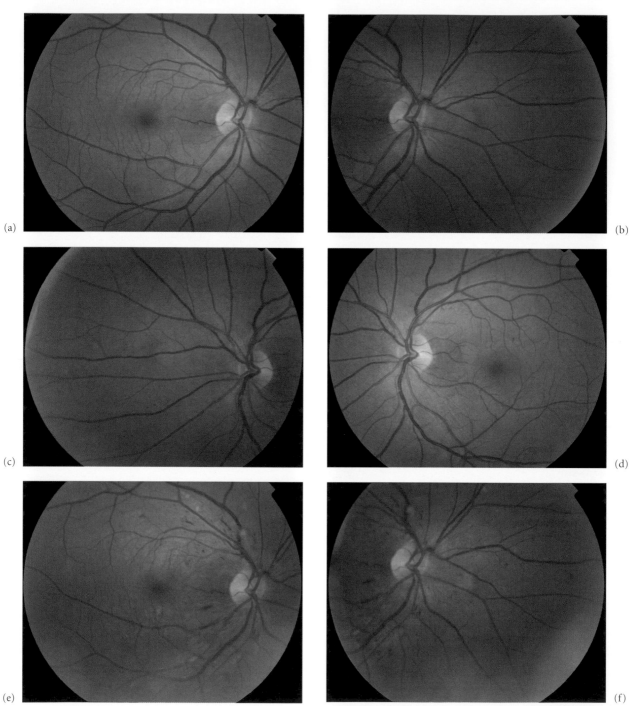

Fig. 13.2 Case history 2. (a) Right macula colour before pregnancy. (b) Right nasal colour before pregnancy. (c) Left nasal colour before pregnancy. (d) Left macula colour before pregnancy. (e) Right macula colour at 25/40 weeks. (f) Right nasal colour at 25/40 weeks. (*Continued on facing page*)

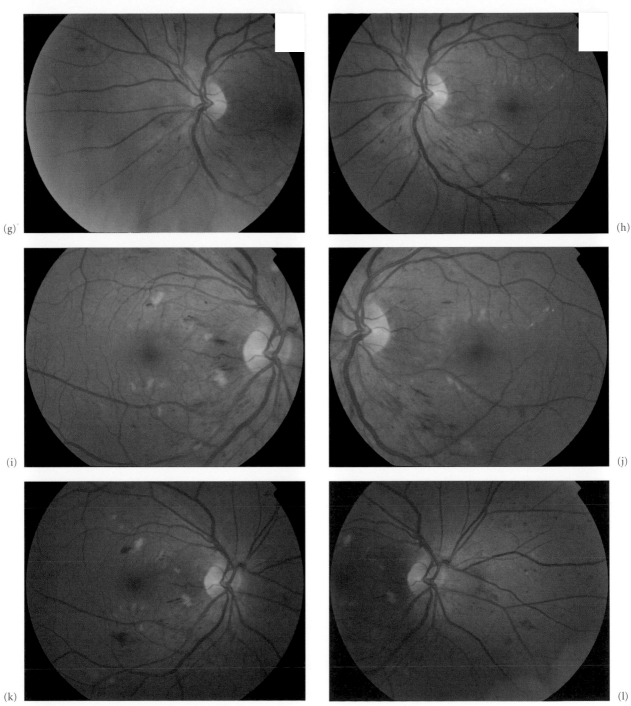

Fig. 13.2 (*Cont'd*) (g) Left nasal colour at 25/40 weeks. (h) Left macula colour at 25/40 weeks. (i) Right macula colour at 29/40 weeks. (j) Left macula colour at 29/40 weeks. (k) Right macula colour at 34/40 weeks. (l) Right nasal colour at 34/40 weeks. (*Continued on p. 158*)

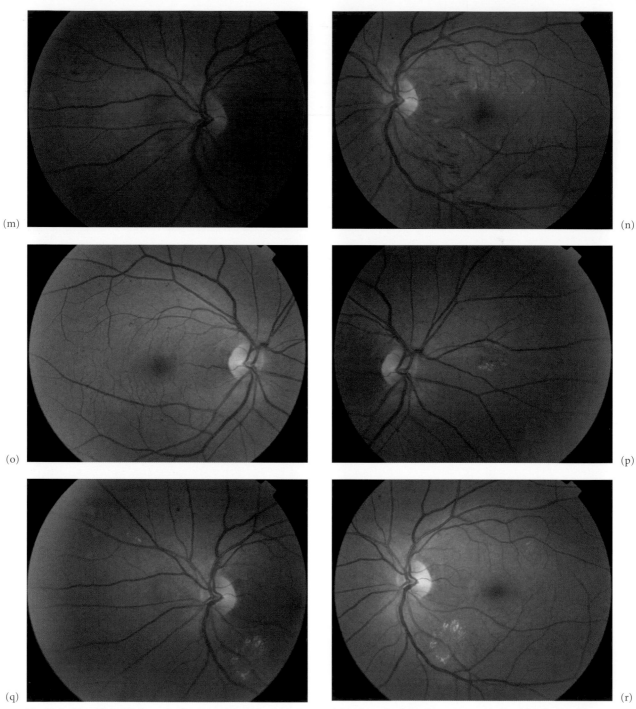

(m)

(n)

(o)

(p)

(q)

(r)

Fig. 13.2 (*Cont'd*) (m) Left nasal colour at 34/40 weeks. (n) Left macula colour at 34/40 weeks. (o) Right macula colour at 1 year post partum. (p) Right nasal colour at 1 year post partum.

(q) Left nasal colour at 1 year post partum. (r) Left macula colour at 1 year post partum.

Her VA remained good at 6/6 (20/20), right and left, throughout this time.

PRACTICE POINTS

- Women with type 1 diabetes should be encouraged to plan pregnancies early in life.
- Improving metabolic control before conception is recommended both for the mother and for the infant.
- Improving metabolic control during pregnancy is recommended both for the mother and for the infant.
- Control of hypertension both before conception and during pregnancy is recommended both for the mother and for the infant.
- It is recommended that, if a patient is found to have significant retinopathy before conception, pregnancy is delayed where possible until appropriate laser treatment has been applied and good metabolic control has been achieved for a 9-month period to overcome any effects of the early worsening phenomenon. Photocoagulation before pregnancy may protect against rapidly progressive proliferative retinopathy. Aggressive treatment of proliferative retinopathy developing in pregnancy may prevent further progression of the disease.

REFERENCES

1 Klein BE, Moss SE, Klein R. Effect of pregnancy on progression of diabetic retinopathy. *Diabetes Care* 1990; **13**(1): 34–40.
2 Chew EY, Mills JL, Metzger BE, Remaley NA, Jovanovic-Peterson L, Knopp RH *et al.* Metabolic control and progression of retinopathy. The Diabetes in Early Pregnancy Study. National Institute of Child Health and Human Development Diabetes in Early Pregnancy Study. *Diabetes Care* 1995; **18**(5): 631–7.
3 Phelps RL, Sakol P, Metzger BE, Jampol LM, Freinkel N. Changes in diabetic retinopathy during pregnancy. Correlations with regulation of hyperglycemia. *Arch Ophthalmol* 1986; **104**(12): 1806–10.
4 Rosenn B, Miodovnik M, Kranias G, Khoury J, Combs CA, Mimouni F *et al.* Progression of diabetic retinopathy in pregnancy: association with hypertension in pregnancy. *Am J Obstet Gynecol* 1992; **166**(4): 1214–18.
5 The Diabetes Control and Complications Trial Research Group. Effect of pregnancy on microvascular complications in the diabetes control and complications trial. *Diabetes Care* 2000; **23**(8): 1084–91.
6 Early worsening of diabetic retinopathy in the Diabetes Control and Complications Trial. *Arch Ophthalmol* 1998; **116**(7): 874–86.
7 Lauszus F, Klebe JG, Bek T. Diabetic retinopathy in pregnancy during tight metabolic control. *Acta Obstet Gynecol Scand* 2000; **79**(5): 367–70.
8 Dibble CM, Kochenour NK, Worley RJ, Tyler FH, Swartz M. Effect of pregnancy on diabetic retinopathy. *Obstet Gynecol* 1982; **59**(6): 699–704.
9 Temple RC, Aldridge VA, Sampson MJ, Greenwood RH, Heyburn PJ, Glenn A. Impact of pregnancy on the progression of diabetic retinopathy in type 1 diabetes. *Diabet Med* 2001; **18**(7): 573–7.

14 Low vision and blindness from diabetic retinopathy

Peter H. Scanlon

DEFINITIONS OF BLINDNESS

USA

'Legal blindness' is defined in the United States as best corrected visual acuity (VA) in the better eye worse than or equal to 20/200 or a visual field extent of less than 20° in diameter. Vision impairment is defined as having a best corrected VA of 20/40 or worse vision in the better-seeing eye.

World Health Organization

'Legal blindness' is defined in the same way as in the United States: i.e. a best corrected VA in the better eye worse than or equal to 20/200.

UK

Definitions of blindness and partial sight in the UK are as follows.

Blindness (severely sight impaired):
- acuity below 3/60
- acuity better than 3/60 but below 6/60 with a very restricted visual field.

Partial sight (sight impaired):
- from 3/60 to 6/60 with a full field
- up to 6/24 with moderate restriction of visual field (e.g. glaucoma)
- 6/18 or better with a gross field defect (e.g. hemianopia) or a marked constriction of the field (e.g. retinitis pigmentosa).

From 2005 the Certificate of Visual Impairment is the new form used in the UK (replacing the BD8) to register people as severely sight impaired (blind) or sight impaired (partially sighted). The definitions remain as above (Fig. 14.1).

A Practical Manual of Diabetic Retinopathy Management.
Peter H Scanlon, Charles P Wilkinson, Stephen J Aldington and David R Matthews. Published 2009 by Blackwell Publishing, ISBN 978-1-4051-7035-2.

USA

Vision Problems in the US is a publication produced jointly by 'Prevent Blindness America' (a volunteer eye health organization) and the National Eye Institute. The 2002 publication reported that legal blindness affects more than one million Americans aged 40 and older and affects black people more frequently than white. Hispanics have higher rates of visual impairment than other races but not blindness. The overall national rate of blindness in the total US population aged 40 and older is 2.85%, varying between 1.3% in Alaska and 3.74% in North Dakota. The 2002 report estimated the numbers of people in the US with mild or worse diabetic retinopathy as 5,353,233, of whom 74% were white, 10% black, 10% Hispanic and 6% of other ethnicity. This can be compared to the 2000 US Census figures: total US population aged 40 years of 119,386,252, of whom 78% were white, 10% black, 7% Hispanic and 5% of other ethnic backgrounds.

Diabetic retinopathy is a leading cause of adult blindness in the US, reported by Fong[1] *et al.* in 2004 to result in blindness for over 10,000 people with diabetes per year. Moss[2] reported the 10-year incidence of blindness in the Wisconsin Epidemiological study of Diabetic Retinopathy to be 1.8%, 4.0% and 4.8% in the younger-onset, older-onset taking insulin, and older-onset not taking insulin groups, respectively. Respective 10-year rates of visual impairment were 9.4%, 37.2% and 23.9%. The *Diabetes 2000* programme of the American Academy of Ophthalmology (AAO) was established to disseminate the recommendations of various nationwide controlled studies[3–6] that demonstrate that effective therapy exists for diabetic retinopathy, and also the preferred practice patterns (PPP) for diabetic retinopathy, in an effort to improve the overall quality of care for patients with diabetes and those specifically at risk of diabetic retinopathy. A review of clinicians'[7] practice patterns over time suggests that practitioners are becoming increasingly

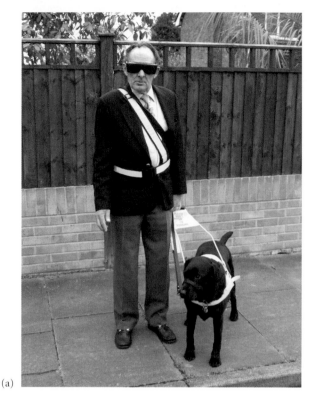
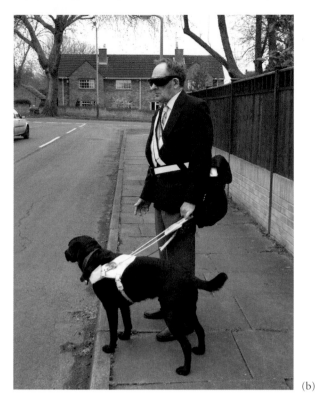

(a)   (b)

Fig. 14.1 (a,b) A blind patient using his guide dog.

aware of *Diabetes 2000* and are adopting the guidelines outlined within the PPP.

The report used data from the 1996–2002 Medical Expenditure Panel Survey of people aged 40 years and older. The majority (70,711) of the 77,511 participants over the 7 years reported no visual impairment; 6288 reported visual impairment; 512 reported being blind.
- Of the 70,711 reporting no visual impairment, 9% were diagnosed with diabetes.
- Of the 6288 reporting visual impairment, 18% were diagnosed with diabetes.
- Of the 512 reporting blindness, 22% were diagnosed with diabetes.

Europe

In 1990, the St Vincent Declaration[8] recognized diabetes and diabetic retinopathy to be a major and growing European health problem, a problem at all ages and in all countries. The first of the 5-year targets that were unanimously agreed by Government Health Departments and patient organizations from all European countries was to reduce new blindness due to diabetes by one-third or more.

In 2002, Kocur[9] reported that in people of working age in Europe, diabetic retinopathy is the most frequently reported cause of serious visual loss.

A conference took place in Liverpool, UK in November 2005 to review progress in the prevention of visual impairment due to diabetic retinopathy since the writing in 1989 and publication in 1990 of the St. Vincent Declaration. Formal invitations were sent to all known diabetes and ophthalmology organizations in 43 countries in Europe, and official national representatives of 29 European countries attended. Each country was asked to submit a poster that reviewed their current position.

In posters from the first group of countries, Denmark, England, Finland, Iceland, Northern Ireland, Norway, Scotland, Sweden and Wales, the reported prevalence of diabetes varied between 2.9% and 4.7%. However, in Turkey the reported prevalence of diabetes was 7.2% and in the Czech Republic 7%.

Over the past 15 years most countries appear to have made genuine progress in an effort to reduce blindness due to diabetic retinopathy. However there were certain key issues that affected some European countries more than others:

- lack of data
- inadequate resources
- lack of awareness and education
- lack of coordination and communication within the individual health system.

In 1995, Evans[10] reported on the causes of blindness and partial sight in England and Wales from an analysis of all registration forms for the year April 1990 to March 1991. Among people of working age (ages 16–64), diabetes was the most important cause of blindness (13.8%), with 11.9% due to diabetic retinopathy.

In 2006, Bunce[11] repeated this analysis of all registration forms for the year April 1999 to March 2000. Overall, the age-specific incidence of all three leading causes (age-related macular degeneration, glaucoma and diabetic retinopathy) had increased since 1990–1991, with changes in diabetic retinopathy being the most marked, particularly in the over-65s where figures had more than doubled. In the figures from 1999–2000, diabetic retinopathy was again reported as the commonest cause of severe visual impairment (combining blind and partial sight registrations) in the working age group.

In the year April 1999 to March 2000, a total of 813 people were registered blind and 1414 people registered partially sighted due to diabetic retinopathy, making a total registered with visual impairment as 2227. A publication[12] from a clinic in Birmingham, UK suggested that only 55% of eligible people are registered because of the voluntary nature of the registration and the individual variations in interpretation by ophthalmologists. Hence, one might assume that the actual number of people who should have been registered as blind or partially sighted in England in the year April 1999 to March 2000 should have been 4049 people. Of concern in the Bunce[11] paper was that the numbers in the age group 16–64 had increased from 1.26 in 1990–91 to 2.05 per 100,000 population in 1999–2000; in the age group 65–74 had increased from 7.28 to 15.06; in the age group 75–84 had increased from 8.27 to 17.08; and in the age group 85 and over had increased from 3.92 to 11.02. This may be partly explained by increased ascertainment and diabetic patients living longer.

One would hope that the screening programme that has been introduced and implemented across the UK in 2003–2007 will start to have an impact on these figures, as it is reported to have done in the Newcastle area since the introduction of their retinal screening programme in 1986.

The most progress in reduction of blindness has been made in Iceland where the prevalence of legal blindness from diabetic retinopathy dropped from 4.0% to 0.5% over 15 years, beginning in 1980. The prevalence of diabetes is relatively low in Iceland (2.9%), and the country has a very strong centralized medical system regarding all aspects of diabetes care and screening. However, the example that Iceland has shown is that optimal management is very effective in preventing and/or reducing severe complications of diabetes.

Other reports of successful reductions of blindness have come from Poland[13] and Sweden.[14]

World

As stated above, the World Health Organization definition of blindness is the same as that in the United States, i.e. a best corrected VA in the better eye worse than or equal to 20/200.

In 2001, Cunningham[15] reported that 45 million people worldwide fulfil the World Health Organization's criteria for blindness. More than 90% of all blind and visually disabled people live in the developing world, where common causes of bilateral vision loss include cataract, glaucoma, trachoma, vitamin A deficiency and onchocerciasis. Additional causes of bilateral vision loss, which together comprise nearly one-quarter of all blindness, and which affect people in both developed and developing nations, include diabetic retinopathy and macular degeneration.

COSTS OF BLINDNESS DUE TO DIABETIC RETINOPATHY

In 2003, Meads[16] reported the costs of blindness and equated the published estimates of the annual cost of blindness in diabetic retinopathy to December 2002 rates:

- Foulds' 1983 estimate[17] was inflated to £7433 in 2002 costs (converts to 14,654 US dollars)
- Dasbach's 1991 estimate[18] was inflated to £5391 in 2002 costs (converts to 10,628 US dollars)
- Wright's 2000 estimate[19] was inflated to £7452 (£4070–£11,250) in 2002 costs (converts to 14,690 US dollars with a range of 8023–22,183 US dollars).

He suggested that much of the uncertainty in any sensitivity analysis of the cost of blindness in older people was associated with the cost of residential care because the excess admission to care homes caused by poor vision was impossible to quantify at that time. In the publication *The Economic Impact of Vision Problems* produced by Prevent

Blindness America in 2007, it reported that visual impairment, compared to no visual impairment, is associated with over $1000 of excess annual medical expenses and a little more than a day of informal care days. Blindness, compared to no visual impairment, is associated with over $2000 of excess annual medical expenditures per year and to more than 5 extra days of informal care from someone outside the household. Excess medical expenses are tied mainly to home healthcare expenditures, particularly from private providers. The authors also published a paper[20] that reported the annual total financial burden of major adult visual disorders in the US as $35.4 billion and reported that the annual governmental budgetary impact is $13.7 billion.

COSTS OF TREATMENT FOR DIABETIC RETINOPATHY

Brown[21] reported results from a retrospective literature review that demonstrated that ophthalmic interventions for diabetic retinopathy and other eye diseases are cost-effective because of the substantial value that ophthalmic interventions confer to patients for the resources expended. In another publication[22] he reported that laser surgical procedures, such as for diabetic retinopathy, appear to be especially cost-effective as a group.

REDUCED VISION AND QUALITY OF LIFE

There is a substantial prevalence of vision-related quality of life impairment in both the UK[23] and USA. Major complications relating to diabetes are in general associated with worse health-related quality of life[24] and with lower utility scores, although Brown[25] found that visual loss seems to cause a similar diminution in self-assessed quality of life in those who do and do not have serious associated systemic comorbidities. A review of evidence[26] evaluating the effect of diabetic retinopathy and diabetic macular oedema on health-related quality of life found several articles that demonstrated both a qualitative and a quantitative reduction in health-related quality of life in persons with diabetic retinopathy.

A study of reported symptoms and quality-of-life impacts in patients having laser treatment for sight-threatening diabetic retinopathy showed that fewer of the multitreatment patients were free of symptoms at their post-treatment follow-up interviews (13% compared to 26% of first treatment patients), which cascaded into a variety of life impacts.[27] Concurrent progression of both

the underlying diabetes and the eye disease adds other progressive complications and life impacts into the picture. First-time-treatment patients reported both relief in visual disturbances and a general decrease in level of anxiety associated with the worry about what the treatment would be like. Multitreatment patients seemed to have considerably less pain and anxiety about the treatment, but their anxiety and worry appears to grow in relation to their increasing visual disturbances and daily life limitations. Their worry or fear tended to be more focused on the progression of their condition.

LOW VISION REHABILITATION

Despite major advances in treatment and early detection of diabetic eye disease, the ageing demographic and increased incidence of diabetes is resulting in greater numbers of diabetic visually impaired people in the population.[28]

Low vision aids (LVAs) have been shown[29,30] to be useful in aiding important near and distance daily living tasks, and in contributing to increased quality of life in those using them.

Low vision clinics in the UK have been traditionally hospital based with LVAs supplied on permanent loan to patients. This service has historically been patchy,[31] and following national consultation[32] in the UK and the formation of local low vision services committees, a number of clinics have evolved[32,33] to suit local need and are increasingly multidisciplinary with the involvement of rehabilitation, mobility and voluntary services amongst others.

Low vision assessments typically encompass detailed task and lifestyle analysis, measurement of functional vision, the selection of an appropriate LVA and development of modified approaches to attempt the task, and the providing of information to access additional support.

Identifying a need or task is often attempted on a problem-solving basis and correctly defining a suitable activity is known to affect the successful use of LVAs. Chosen or preferred tasks are patient specific and may be divided into spot or rapid tasks such as looking at a cooker dial or shop price, and prolonged tasks such as reading a book or newspaper. A greater level of magnification is normally required for the latter.[34] Tasks are significantly influenced by lifestyle. An elderly diabetic patient living alone may raise issues about viewing medication and reading their mail and correspondence, whilst a younger person of working age may be more concerned with work-related visual problems.

Information about a patient's visual function is used in conjunction with this to select an initial aid to attempt a given task. Useful measures of visual function for all low vision assessments include best corrected VA (preferably logMAR[35]), near acuity and basic visual field assessment. Peak contrast sensitivity function using an assessment tool such as the Peli-Robson chart, with all the letters of the same size and contrast decreasing from the top to the bottom, has been shown to be a useful tool for selecting a preferred eye for viewing.[36] An assessment of reading speed may be valuable.[37]

There are many hundreds of low vision aids commercially available,[38] in different designs and magnification availability. They can be divided into different categories. Hand magnifiers are relatively inexpensive, portable, easy to use and widely accepted. If the patient has a hand tremor or has difficulty in maintaining a good grip, then stand magnifiers (often with internal illumination) can be more useful. To obtain the largest field of view for a given magnification and to maintain a 'hands-free' approach, for example when reading a chapter of a book, an aid that involves reading close with a high spectacle reading aid or slightly further away with a spectacle microscope, might be tried initially. If the longest possible working distance is required, a near telescope (usually Galilean) would be the first LVA of choice; these are normally spectacle mounted. If a distance task is identified, then a distance telescope (either Galilean or astronomical with a righting device) can be tried. These are usually hand-held devices and magnification of up to 8× can be commonly utilized, if the user has a reasonably steady hand. More modern telescopic devices have been developed with an autofocus facility for distance and near, although the considerable cost has limited their supply from most clinics.

CCTV reading aids electronically magnify print onto a TV screen and have enabled many more people to be able to read print. Simpler devices that plug into the user's own TV have become available for a couple of hundred pounds (US $366), as opposed to several thousand for the most sophisticated models. Portable pocket video devices have become increasingly popular for spot tasks.

The development of enlargement software for computers (which can often be used in conjunction with speech synthesis) has enabled many visually impaired people to embrace modern technology and has revolutionized the way they can access information. There are a number of commercially available products.

Finally, there are many non-optical ways of tackling visual difficulties, including optimum task lighting and use of contrast to make cooking easier for a person with visual impairment, a template for signing a name or cheque, a device that buzzes when a cup is filled, talking scales and watches, bumper stickers for cooker dials and road signs (displaying the canes symbol) to aid crossing roads. Examples of this last group are available from social services as part of the community care provision, and many low vision clinics have direct access to these services.

Low vision clinics are often able to supply written information about sight loss, and the availability of local services such as clubs and support groups, for example newly registered groups as well as computer access and large print text. They can provide a gateway to additional support and information from other agencies such as the RNIB Directory of Low Vision Services in the UK,[39] the Disability Employment Advisers (DEAs) in most local job centres and the Access to Work programme which provides advice and equipment to visually impaired people in the work place.

Low vision aids have been shown to be beneficial in the rehabilitation of those who have lost acuity because of diabetic retinopathy changes, and those who have temporary reduction in sight. In a recent study[40], LVAs have been shown to be more successful for patients with visual difficulties related to diabetic retinopathy than those with age-related macular degeneration. This was thought to be related to a more useable central field and lack of a dense central scotoma in most cases.

Successful usage of correctly selected LVAs is relatively high and considered cost-effective[41], and many people are able to continue to live independently and carry out everyday tasks if the right help has been made available.[42,43]

CASE HISTORY 1
Blindness due to diabetic retinopathy

This 83-year-old woman (BMI 32) with type 2 diabetes diagnosed at the age of 62 years started initially on tablets and is now controlled on insulin.

She presented to the ophthalmology department at the age of 72 years with extensive haemorrhages and oedema in her right macular area and a reduced VA to a level of right 6/36 (20/180). The left VA was satisfactory at 6/9 (20/30). At the time her blood pressure was elevated at 180/110 and, although she had been treated with insulin since the age of 64 years, her blood sugars had been consistently high at her diabetic clinic appointments running between 10.9 and 20.7 mmol/L. Her blood pressure had also been poorly controlled, with readings recorded of 200/95, 200/85 and 180/110.

At 72 years, laser treatment was given to the extensive thickening in the right macular area:

- right 95 burns, 100-micron size, 170–240 mW, area centralis lens, argon laser.

The right vision improved a little to 6/24 (20/80) and the retinal thickening reduced but no further visual improvement occurred.

At 73 years, blurring then started to develop in the left eye and photographs were taken (Fig. 14.2a–d). Extensive oedema was present in both macular areas and the VAs were right 6/60 (20/200), left 6/18 (20/60).

Treatment was given to the right macular area:

- right 160 burns, 100-micron size, 150 mW, area centralis lens, argon laser.

Treatment was given to the left macular area:

- left 70 burns, 100-micron size, 130–150 mW, area centralis lens, argon laser.

Unfortunately the vision did not improve and the vision in her left eye subsequently deteriorated over the next 18 months to a level of 3/60 despite one further laser treatment to her left eye of left 85 burns, 100-micron size, 180 mW, area centralis lens, argon laser.

She was registered on the partial register of visual impairment.

At 73 years, panretinal photocoagulation was commenced to the right eye because of the increasing signs of peripheral retinal ischaemia. Treatment was given:

- right 2022 burns, 500-micron size, 260–300 mW, Karickhoff 4-mirror lens, argon laser over three sessions separated by 1 week.

Subsequent photographs were taken at the age of 76 years (Fig. 14.2e–h).

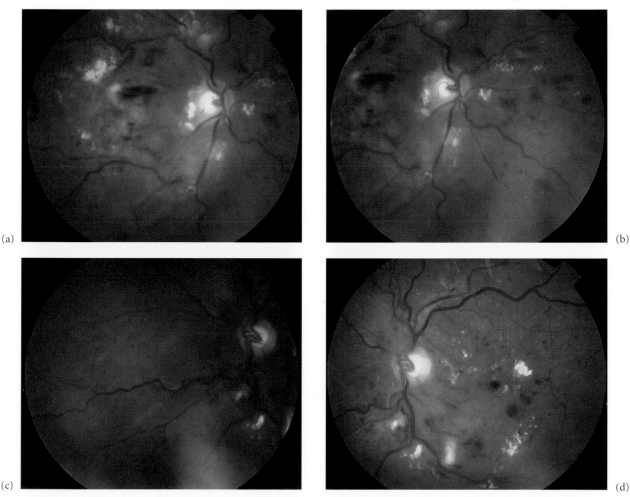

(a) (b) (c) (d)

Fig. 14.2 Case history 1. (a) Right macula, (b) right nasal, (c) left nasal, (d) left macula, at age 72 years. (*Continued on p. 166*)

At 77 years, her VA had fallen to right 'counting fingers' and left 1/60 (3/200) due to severe ischaemic maculopathy. There were also signs of increasing ischaemia in her left retina. Panretinal photocoagulation was therefore commenced to the left eye:

- right 2275 burns, 200-micron size, 250–300 mW, Quadraspheric lens, argon laser over two sessions separated by 1 week.

She was registered on the full register of visual impairment.

Subsequent photographs were taken at the age of 81 years (Fig. 14.2i–l).

HbA1c results that have been recorded in the last 10 years have been 9.9, 9.5, 11.4, 11.4, 10.6, 11.0, 8.5, 10.0, 10.6, 12.9, 8.6 and 10.8%.

Blood pressure results that have been recorded in the last 10 years have been 170/90, 150/82, 176/60, 181/88, 164/100, 155/85, 140/70, 165/95, 130/70, 118/68, 150/82, 138/70, 153/71, and 212/93.

In this woman, the combination of difficulties with glycaemic control, blood pressure control and the development of ischaemic maculopathy that has been difficult to treat with conventional argon laser treatment have led to this loss of vision.

CASE HISTORY 2
Blindness associated with renal failure

A 64-year-old woman with type 2 diabetes (diagnosed aged 50 years) had had her condition controlled by diet until the age of 59 years, had been on glibenclamide until the age of 63 years and had started on insulin 8 months before presentation at the eye clinic with blurred vision

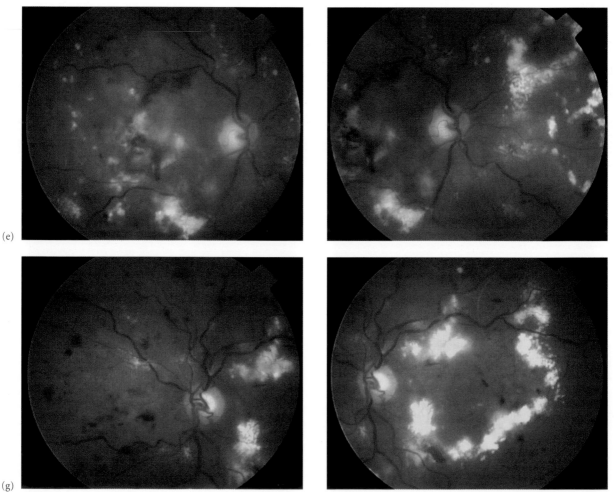

(e)

(f)

(g)

(h)

Fig. 14.2 (*Cont'd*) (e) Right macula, (f) right nasal, (g) left nasal, (h) left macula, at age 73 years. (*Continued on facing page*)

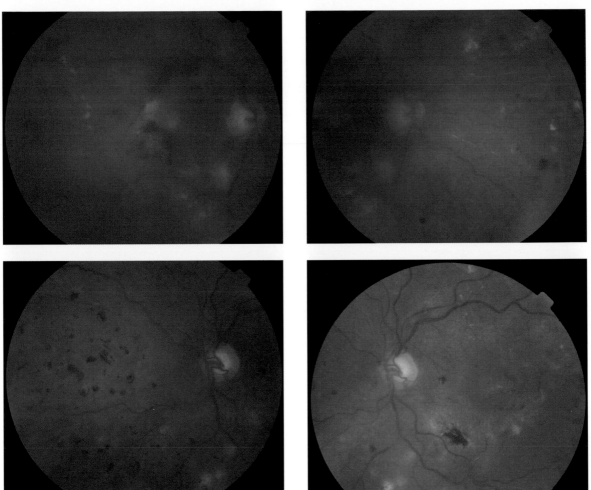

(i)

(j)

(k)

(l)

Fig. 14.2 (*Cont'd*) (i) Right macula, (j) right nasal, (k) left nasal, (l) left macula, at age 81 years.

that had become progressively worse over the previous 4 months. The VA was found to be right 4/60 (14/200), left 5/60 (17/200).

Colour photographs and a fluorescein angiogram were taken (Fig. 14.3).

Extensive leakage is present in both macular areas with generalized breakdown of the blood–retina barrier and profuse early leakage from the entire capillary bed of the posterior pole. Her blood pressure was found to be 190/82. She was known to have had poor glycaemic control for a number of years. Attempts were made to control her blood pressure and her treatment regime consisted of insulatard, amlodipine 5 mg, furosemide 40 mg, rosuvastatin 10 mg and olmesartan 40 mg, all once daily.

Laser treatment was given to both macular areas:
• right eye, 79 burns, 100-micron size, 310 mW, 0.1 s, area centralis lens, argon laser;

• left eye, 59 burns, 100-micron size, 260 mW, 0.1 s, area centralis lens, argon laser.

Four months later further laser treatment was given to the left eye:
• left eye, 66 burns, 100-micron size, 360 mW, 0.1 s, area centralis lens, argon laser

and an intravitreal injection of triamcinolone was given to the right eye followed 4 weeks later by:
• right eye, 50 burns, 100-micron size, 460 mW, 0.1 s, area centralis lens, argon laser.

However, the VAs did not improve, remaining at a level of right 1/60 (3/200), left 2/60 (7/200), and the patient was placed on the full register for visual impairment, 6 months after her initial presentation. She was seen in the low vision clinic to assist her with visual aids.

Eighteen months after her presentation to the eye clinic and 6 months after her registration, she was referred to

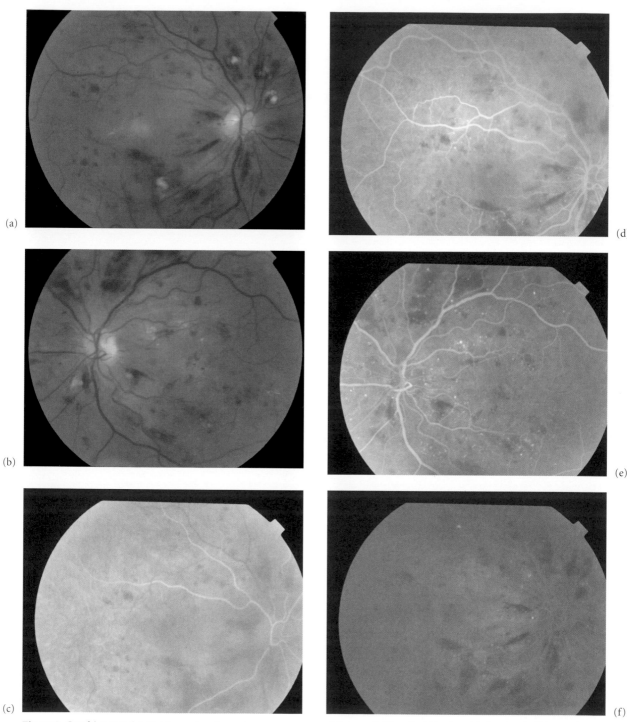

Fig. 14.3 Case history 2. (a) Right macula colour at presentation. (b) Left macula colour at presentation. (c) Fluorescein right macula 21 s after injection. (d) Fluorescein right macula 28 s after injection. (e) Fluorescein left macula 35 s after injection. (f) Fluorescein right macula 2 min 38 s after injection. (*Continued on facing page*)

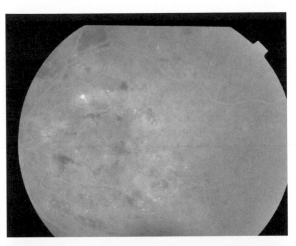

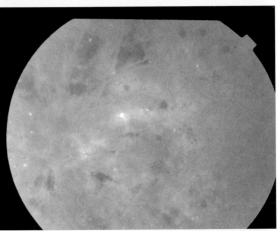

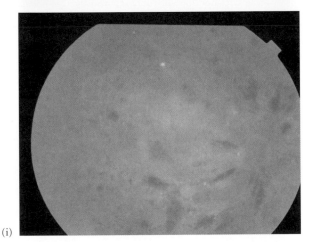

Fig. 14.3 (*Cont'd*) (g) Fluorescein left macula 2 min 59 s after injection. (h) Fluorescein left macula 3 min 57 s after injection. (i) Fluorescein right macula 4 min 29 s after injection.

the renal physician with an Hb of 8.6 g/dL and an eGFR of 22 mL/min.

Two months later, when she was admitted for a blood transfusion and a renal biopsy, her creatinine was 453 μmol/L, her eGFR was 9 mL/min and her blood pressure was 160/70. The renal biopsy showed severe diabetic renal disease with little surviving kidney. One month later she began renal dialysis, which she is currently having three times per week.

She remains one of my most cheerful patients.

PRACTICE POINTS

- In the Wisconsin study,[44] proliferative retinopathy occurred in 67% of people with type 1 diabetes for 35 or more years. One would therefore expect that two-thirds of people with type 1 diabetes would need laser treatment for proliferative diabetic retinopathy during their lifetime. In the same study, the 4-year incidence of panretinal photocoagulation was 2.5 times higher than the rate of macular laser.
- In patients with type 2 diabetes, the rate of proliferative diabetic retinopathy is not as high but it is estimated that 1 in 3 patients with type 2 diabetes will develop sight-threatening diabetic retinopathy requiring laser during their lifetime.
- The prevalence of blindness is influenced by duration of diabetes, blood glucose and pressure control, and by the presence or absence of screening and preventive laser treatment.
- Achieving a high compliance as has been done in Iceland can lower the risk of blindness to very low levels.

REFERENCES

1 Fong DS, Aiello LP, Ferris FL 3rd, Klein R. Diabetic retinopathy. *Diabetes Care* 2004; **27**(10): 2540–53.
2 Moss SE, Klein R, Klein BE. Ten-year incidence of visual loss in a diabetic population. *Ophthalmology* 1994; **101**(6): 1061–70.
3 The Diabetic Retinopathy Study Research Group. Indications for photocoagulation treatment of diabetic retinopathy: Diabetic Retinopathy Study Report no. 14. *Int Ophthalmol Clin* 1987; **27**(4): 239–53.
4 Early Treatment Diabetic Retinopathy Study research group. Photocoagulation for diabetic macular edema. Early Treatment Diabetic Retinopathy Study report number 1. *Arch Ophthalmol* 1985; **103**(12): 1796–806.
5 The Diabetes Control and Complications Trial Research Group. The effect of intensive treatment of diabetes on the development and progression of long-term complications in

insulin-dependent diabetes mellitus. *N Engl J Med* 1993; **329**(14): 977–86.

6 The Diabetic Retinopathy Vitrectomy Study Research Group. Early vitrectomy for severe vitreous hemorrhage in diabetic retinopathy. Two-year results of a randomized trial. Diabetic Retinopathy Vitrectomy Study report 2. *Arch Ophthalmol* 1985; **103**(11): 1644–52.

7 Khadem JJ, Buzney SM, Alich KS. Practice patterns in diabetic retinopathy: part 1: analysis of retinopathy follow-up. *Arch Ophthalmol* 1999; **117**(6): 815–20.

8 Diabetes care and research in Europe: the Saint Vincent declaration. *Diabet Med* 1990;**7**(4):360.

9 Kocur I, Resnikoff S. Visual impairment and blindness in Europe and their prevention. *Br J Ophthalmol* 2002;**86**(7): 716–22.

10 Evans J. Causes of blindness and partial sight in England and Wales 1990–1991. London: OPCS, 1995:1–29.

11 Bunce C, Wormald R. Leading causes of certification for blindness and partial sight in England and Wales. *BMC Public Health* 2006; **6**: 58.

12 Barry RJ, Murray PI. Unregistered visual impairment: is registration a failing system? *Br J Ophthalmol* 2005; **89**(8): 995–8.

13 Bandurska-Stankiewicz E, Wiatr D. Diabetic blindness significantly reduced in the Warmia and Mazury Region of Poland: Saint Vincent Declaration targets achieved. *Eur J Ophthalmol* 2006; **16**(5): 722–7.

14 Backlund LB, Algvere PV, Rosenqvist U. New blindness in diabetes reduced by more than one-third in Stockholm County. *Diabet Med* 1997; **14**(9): 732–40.

15 Cunningham ET, Jr. World blindness–no end in sight. *Br J Ophthalmol* 2001;**85**(3):253.

16 Meads C, Hyde C. What is the cost of blindness? *Br J Ophthalmol* 2003; **87**(10): 1201–4.

17 Foulds WS, MacCuish ATB. Diabetic retinopathy in the west of Scotland: its detection and prevalence, and the cost-effectiveness of a proposed screening programme. *Health Bulletin* 1983; **41**(6): 318–26.

18 Dasbach EJ, Fryback DG, Newcomb PA, Klein R, Klein BE. Cost-effectiveness of strategies for detecting diabetic retinopathy. *Med Care* 1991; **29**(1): 20–39.

19 Wright SE, Keeffe JE, Thies LS. Direct costs of blindness in Australia. *Clin Experiment Ophthalmol* 2000; **28**(3): 140–2.

20 Rein DB, Zhang P, Wirth KE, Lee PP, Hoerger TJ, McCall N *et al.* The economic burden of major adult visual disorders in the United States. *Arch Ophthalmol* 2006; **124**(12): 1754–60.

21 Brown GC, Brown MM, Sharma S, Brown H, Smithen L, Leeser DB *et al.* Value-based medicine and ophthalmology: an appraisal of cost–utility analyses. *Trans Am Ophthalmol Soc* 2004; **102**: 177–85; discussion 185–8.

22 Brown MM, Brown GC, Sharma S. Value-based medicine and vitreoretinal diseases. *Curr Opin Ophthalmol* 2004; **15**(3): 167–72.

23 Frost A, Eachus J, Sparrow J, Peters TJ, Hopper C, Davey-Smith G *et al.* Vision-related quality of life impairment in an elderly UK population: associations with age, sex, social class and material deprivation. *Eye* 2001; **15**: 739–44.

24 Coffey JT, Brandle M, Zhou H, Marriott D, Burke R, Tabaei BP *et al.* Valuing health-related quality of life in diabetes. *Diabetes Care* 2002; **25**(12): 2238–43.

25 Brown MM, Brown GC, Sharma S, Hollands H, Landy J. Quality of life and systemic comorbidities in patients with ophthalmic disease. *Br J Ophthalmol* 2002; **86**(1): 8–11.

26 Sharma S, Oliver-Fernandez A, Liu W, Buchholz P, Walt J. The impact of diabetic retinopathy on health-related quality of life. *Curr Opin Ophthalmol* 2005; **16**(3): 155–9.

27 Scanlon PH, Martin ML, Bailey C, Johnson E, Hykin P, Keightley S. Reported symptoms and quality-of-life impacts in patients having laser treatment for sight-threatening diabetic retinopathy. *Diabet Med* 2006; **23**(1): 60–6.

28 Bunce C, Wormald R. Leading causes of certification for blindness and partial sight in England & Wales. *BMC Public Health* 2006; **6**: 58.

29 Wolffsohn JS, Cochrane AL. Design of the low vision quality-of-life questionnaire (LVQOL) and measuring the outcome of low-vision rehabilitation. *Am J Ophthalmol* 2000; **130**(6): 793–802.

30 Wolffsohn JS, Cochrane AL, Watt NA. Implementation methods for vision-related quality of life questionnaires. *Br J Ophthalmol* 2000; **84**(9): 1035–40.

31 Ryan B, McCoughan L. *Our Better Vision: What People Need From Low Vision Services in the UK.* London: RNIB, 1999.

32 Low Vision Services Consensus Group. *Low Vision Services: Recommendations for Future Service Delivery in the UK.* London: RNIB, 1999: 1–32.

33 *Framework for a Multidisciplinary Approach to Low Vision.* London: The College of Optometrists, 2001.

34 Rumney NJ. Using visual thresholds to establish low vision performance. *Ophthalmic Physiol Opt* 1995; **15**(Suppl 1): S18–24.

35 Bailey IL, Lovie JE. New design principles for visual acuity letter charts. *Am J Optom Physiol Opt* 1976; **53**(11): 740–5.

36 Leat SJ, Woodhouse JM. Reading performance with low vision aids: relationship with contrast sensitivity. *Ophthalmic Physiol Opt* 1993; **13**(1): 9–16.

37 Whittaker SG, Lovie-Kitchin J. Visual requirements for reading. *Optom Vis Sci* 1993; **70**(1): 54–65.

38 Gill JM, Muthiah N, Silver JH, Gould ES. *Equipment For Blind and Partially Sighted Persons: an International Guide.* London: Royal National Institute for the Blind and Moorfields Eye Hospital, 1997.

39 *Low Vision Services in the UK.* http://info.rnib.org.uk/EyeHealth/LowVision.htm. RNIB, 2008.

40 Fröhlich SJ. Age-related macula degeneration and diabetic retinopathy: differences in optical rehabilitation. *Klinische Monatsblätter für Augenheilkunde* 2005; **222/4**: 337–41.

41 Shuttleworth GW, Dunlop A, Collins JK, James CRH. How effective is an integrated approach to vision rehabilitation? *B J Ophthalmol* 1995; **79**: 719–23.

42 Leat SJ, Fryer A, Rumney NJ. Outcome of low vision aid provision: the effectiveness of a low vision clinic. *Optom Vis Sci* 1994; **73**(3): 199–206.

43 Del'Aune W, Welsh R, Williams M. A national outcomes assessment of the rehabilitation of adults with visual impairments. *J Vis Impair Blind* 2000; **94**: 281–91.

44 Klein R, Klein BE, Moss SE, Davis MD, DeMets DL. The Wisconsin epidemiologic study of diabetic retinopathy. II. Prevalence and risk of diabetic retinopathy when age at diagnosis is less than 30 years. *Arch Ophthalmol* 1984; **102**(4): 520–6.

15 Future advances in the management of diabetic retinopathy

Peter H. Scanlon

MODERN AND FUTURE MEDICAL THERAPIES

Current attempts to manage patients with diabetic retinopathy are aimed at preserving vision and reducing progression of the disease by appropriate management of glucose, blood pressure, weight and lipids, and laser treatment at the appropriate stage in the disease process. There are a number of ongoing studies including further studies of angiotensin-converting enzyme (ACE) inhibitors and angiotensin receptor blockers that may give more information on possible reductions of retinopathy progression and the effect of lipid control on the progression of diabetic retinopathy.

A recent study has suggested that use of fenofibrate in type 2 diabetes might reduce the need for laser treatment of diabetic retinopathy over a 5-year period. However, one needs to be cautious with the interpretation of the results because this was a tertiary outcome of a trial that failed its primary outcome of coronary heart disease death or non-fatal myocardial infarction, and the numbers of events, particularly in the substudy, were small. The results would, however, support a study specifically designed for the purpose.

There has been hope in recent years that emerging treatments will provide additional treatment options for control of the progression of diabetic retinopathy.

Protein kinase C (PKC) inhibitors

In 2003 Ciulla[1] wrote a review article on novel therapies for diabetic retinopathy and diabetic macular oedema (DR/DME). He described several biochemical mechanisms, including protein kinase C-beta activation, increased vascular endothelial growth factor production, oxidative stress and accumulation of intracellular sorbitol and advanced glycosylation end-products, that may contribute to the vascular disruptions that characterize DR/DME. He suggested that inhibition of these pathways holds the promise of intervention for DR at earlier non-sight-threatening stages.

In 2005, Joy[2] described the use of ruboxistaurin mesylate which, by inhibiting excessive activation of certain PKC isoforms, has the potential to reduce the burden of microvascular complications for patients with diabetes.

In 2005 the PKC-DRS Study Group[3] reported on a multicentre double-masked randomized placebo-controlled study of 252 subjects with moderately severe to very severe non-proliferative diabetic retinopathy (NPDR) given placebo or orally administered PKC-beta isoform-selective inhibitor ruboxistaurin (RBX 8, 16, or 32 mg/day) for 36–46 months. In this clinical trial, 32 mg/day RBX was well tolerated and significantly ($p = 0.012$) reduced the risk of moderate visual loss (doubling of the visual angle) but did not prevent DR progression.

In 2006, the PKC-DRS Study Group[4] reported results from 685 patients randomized at 70 clinical sites. Sustained moderate visual loss occurred in 9.1% of placebo-treated patients versus 5.5% of ruboxistaurin-treated (32 mg/day) patients (40% risk reduction, $p = 0.034$) with moderately severe to very severe non-proliferative diabetic retinopathy. Mean visual acuity (VA) was better in the ruboxistaurin-treated patients after 12 months.

In summary, although the study did not lead to a statistically significant effect on the primary endpoint of DR progression or application of focal photocoagulation, it displayed a trend towards a positive effect on moderate visual loss. Thus, initial clinical trial data suggest that PKC

A Practical Manual of Diabetic Retinopathy Management.
Peter H Scanlon, Charles P Wilkinson, Stephen J Aldington and David R Matthews. Published 2009 by Blackwell Publishing, ISBN 978-1-4051-7035-2.

inhibitors are safe and can be well tolerated in humans and may have beneficial effects in preventing visual loss from diabetic retinopathy. However, the actual efficacy of the PKC inhibitor and the patient populations responsive to the treatment must be clarified in ongoing clinical trials. The US Food and Drug Administration granted an approval letter for this treatment following the above studies; however, another trial is required before final approval.

The use of intravitreal vascular endothelial growth factor (VEGF) inhibitors

The currently available VEGF inhibitors are:
- pegaptanib (Macugen)
- ranibizumab (Lucentis)
- bevacizumab (Avastin).

The use of these agents is described in Chapter 9 on proliferative DR and Chapter 6 on maculopathy.

TECHNOLOGICAL ADVANCES IN IMAGING

Three-dimensional OCT

Optical coherence tomography (OCT) is an imaging technique that interprets the 'time of flight' and intensity of reflected optical waves using interferometry. OCT uses wavelengths between 600 nm and 2000 nm, and the modern light sources vary between superluminescent diodes, mode-locked lasers and photonic crystal fibres.[5]

The light beam is split into a reference beam and a signal beam. The reference beam is reflected from a mirror and the signal beam is back-scattered from the sample under investigation. By analysis of the reflected interference signal, it is possible to perform imaging at different depths within the sample. Early descriptions of the use of OCT in normal retinae and in diabetic maculopathy were by Hee *et al.*[6–8]

Because of its high level of resolution, OCT is particularly suitable for retinal thickness measurements, offering penetration to approximately 2–3 mm with micrometer-scale axial and lateral resolution. OCT images can be presented as either cross-sectional images or topographic maps. A cross-sectional or B-mode image is constructed from many A-scans, which are a combination of reflectivity profiles and depth. To facilitate interpretation a false colour scheme is added in which bright colours such as red and green correspond to highly reflective areas and darker colours such as blue and black correspond to areas of lower reflectivity. With the early OCT machines that use the above principles of A- and B-mode imaging, tomographic maps are produced by obtaining six consecutive cross-sectional scans at 30° angular orientations in a radial spoke pattern centred on the fovea. A similar false colour scheme to aid interpretation, as described above for the B-mode images, is used for the tomographical maps.

The ability to capture similar images to OCT depth information in slices of the tissue at orientations perpendicular to the optic axis (*en-face* images, or C-scans) was described by Podoleanu,[9] and later T-scanning (transverse priority) images have been described by Cucu.[10] This method and other methods have provided three-dimensional OCT images, which have provided the ability to construct 3D volumes at different depths. The application of these techniques has been described by Wojkowski[11] and Podoleanu.[9] See Fig. 15.1.

OCT has provided ophthalmologists with depth resolution in imaging the diabetic retina only previously possible in post-mortem histological slides. This technique is likely to develop further to provide even greater image resolution, interpretation and analysis, and enable ophthalmologists to understand and treat microscopic pathology in a way that would previously have been impossible.

Combining these techniques with other imaging techniques, such as the advances in oximetry described below, may further develop our understanding of and ability to treat sight-threatening diabetic retinopathy.

Retinal oximetry

There has been widespread application of spectral and hyperspectral imaging systems in biomedicine, including cytogenetics,[12] pathology[13] and oncology.[14] Hyperspectral imaging has also been used in studies in medicine because of an appreciation of dissimilar spectral signatures in oxygenated and deoxygenated haemoglobin. Hyperspectral oximetric studies have encompassed a variety of subspecialties, from its application to assessing haemorrhagic shock[15] and tissue perfusion[16] to the assessment of microvascular disease in the diabetic foot[17] and in sickle cell anaemia.[18] The application of hyperspectral technology in the functional analysis of living tissues has extended into ophthalmology,[19,20] with qualitative and quantitative oxygen saturation assessments being extracted from distinctive haemoglobin spectral signatures within retinal blood vessels, which may provide further information relating to the physiological mechanisms underlying the progression and treatment of diabetic retinopathy.

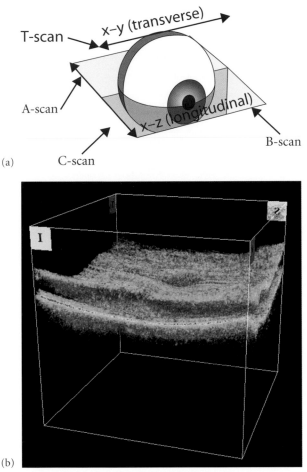

(a)

(b)

Fig. 15.1 Three-dimensional optical coherence tomography. (a) Diagram to demonstrate A-scan, B-scan, T-scan and C-scan axes, (b) 3-D OCT of a patient with diffuse macular oedema

The causal linkage between retinal ischaemia and ocular neovascularization has been recognized and widely accepted by the ophthalmic community since the early pioneering work of Ashton[21] and many others. Histopathological studies were followed by the development of fluorescein angiography of the retinal vessels, Doppler flowometry, digital retinal photography, scanning laser ophthalmoscopy and biochemical analyses. However, the mechanism by which laser treatment improves the prognosis of sight-threatening diabetic retinopathy is ill-understood. The Early Treatment Diabetic Retinopathy Study (ETDRS) demonstrated that focal (direct/grid) laser photocoagulation reduces moderate vision loss caused by diabetic macular oedema (DME) by 50% or more. The hypotheses that have developed to explain the mechanism of action of focal laser treatment have included the closure of leaky microaneurysms and, with the reduced retinal tissue following photocoagulation, autoregulation results in decreased retinal blood flow with lower fluid flow, resulting in decreased oedema.[22] Others have suggested that the reduced retinal blood flow is due to improved oxygenation following photocoagulation.[23] Biochemical and physiological studies suggest that the resolution of the oedema may also result from changes in the biochemical processes within the retinal pigment epithelium.[24]

Oximetry maps represent a semiquantitative spectral analysis technique using a linear unmixing algorithm to classify areas of the retina where there is high blood oxygen saturation. In a normal retina this spectral classification technique identifies major retinal arterioles that have high blood oxygen saturation in red. In the venules of a normal retina there is lower blood oxygen saturation and the classification technique identifies these areas in black.

An early example of the type of images that can be recorded from a patient with proliferative diabetic retinopathy is shown in Fig. 15.2.

CASE HISTORY 1
Proliferative diabetic retinopathy

This 42-year-old man with type 2 diabetes controlled on tablets was referred from retinal screening. On examination, he was found to have a VA of right 6/12 (20/40), left 6/9 (20/30), right clinically significant macular oedema and neovascularization in his right eye.

Colour photographs of each eye, fluorescein angiography photographs and oximetry images are shown in Fig. 15.2(a–i).

The oximetry maps of a diabetic patient are shown with respective colour fundus and fluorescein angiography photographs. This patient has new vessels in the nasal and inferotemporal retina of the right eye. The oximetry map shows that some nasal veins have been classified in red indicating abnormally high venular blood oxygenation in areas of the retina where new vessels have grown. This suggests focal alterations in the consumption of oxygen in retinal tissues associated with proliferative diabetic retinopathy. This technique is in the early stages of development and further refinements to the analysis techniques are being developed to allow one to make accurate assessments of the quantitative oxygen saturation in the vasculature.

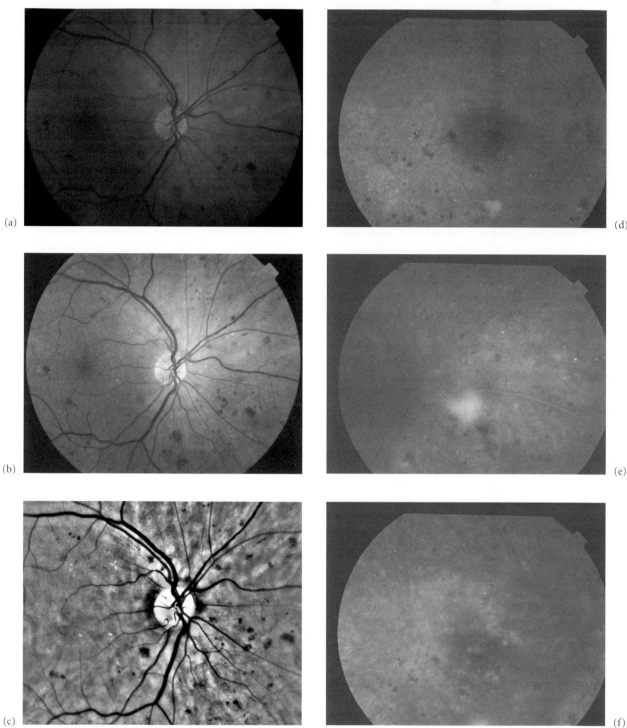

Fig. 15.2 (a) Colour photograph right disc and macula.
(b) Red-free photograph right disc and macula. (c) Oximetry
images right disc area (including macula). (d) Fluorescein right
macula 54 s after injection. (e) Fluorescein right disc 2 min 26 s
after injection. (f) Fluorescein right macula 3 min 40 s after
injection. (*Continued on facing page*)

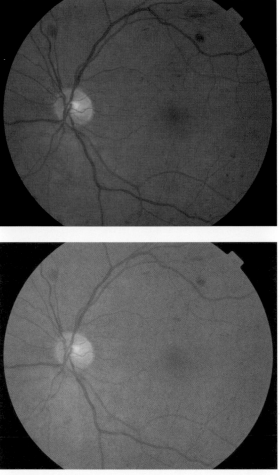

(g)

(h)

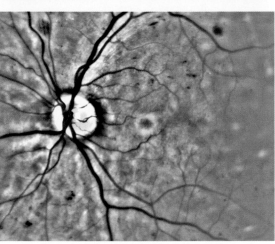

(i)

Fig. 15.2 (*Cont'd*) (g) Colour photograph left macula. (h) Red-free photograph left macula. (i) Oximetry images left disc area (including macula).

For eyes with a combination of proliferative diabetic retinopathy and maculopathy, the ETDRS compared giving immediate panretinal photocoagulation with either simultaneous or delayed focal treatment and found that the former strategy was associated with the least visual loss.[25] The Diabetic Retinopathy Study[26] (DRS) suggested that 'perhaps eliminating or reducing retinal thickening by applying focal photocoagulation for macular oedema before beginning scatter laser treatment might reduce the risk of visual loss'. Some ophthalmologists make an exception to this approach, especially for young patients with insulin-dependent diabetes mellitus who have aggressive peripheral ischaemia associated with macular oedema that may resolve following panretinal photocoagulation.[27] This approach has been supported by a study by Okano[28] who measured disc-to-macula transit time (DMTT) to evaluate the retinal circulation by means of rapid serial fluorescein angiography, employing a scanning laser ophthalmoscope. He found that retinal circulation is retarded in diabetic retinopathy and that this retardation improves after panretinal photocoagulation. Einar Stefansson presented his theory[29] that the clinical effect of retinal photocoagulation is based on the effect the treatment modality has on retinal oxygenation.

Retinal oximetry measurements may help us to better understand the mechanisms by which laser treatment benefits patients with both proliferative diabetic retinopathy and maculopathy, and may become more widely used in ophthalmology in the future.

THE INFLUENCE OF ELECTRONIC MEDICAL RECORDS

Paper-based medical records with unstructured free text data entry are still the norm in hospitals throughout the world. Data in such records are inconsistently recorded and frequently duplicated, and cannot easily be shared or collated to improve the quality and consistency of patient care or deliver a local or national audit of the standard of care.

The success of the UK National Screening Programme[30] for sight-threatening diabetic retinopathy in terms of reducing blindness and visual impairment depends both on the efficient management of screening programmes and the delivery of optimal care in hospital eye services. In the UK minimum datasets to support excellent care of diabetic retinopathy have been agreed on a national basis and implemented in electronic medical records (EMR) systems. Previous national audits[31–33] in the UK have shown that the standards of laser treatment do vary but, without EMR, ongoing audits that have the potential to improve standards of care and outcomes are very difficult.

Well-designed EMR[34,35] are able to improve the quality of care by being available anywhere, any time, and can improve consistency by encouraging or forcing structured data entry of all mandatory data items. In the context of the hospital eye clinic, ophthalmologists can be made to consistently record the severity of each clinical sign of diabetic retinopathy and maculopathy and the EMR will then grade the findings according to ETDRS, international or NSC classifications at every visit. Decision support functions can help guide the clinician regarding appropriate follow-up intervals or the need to register the patient as visually impaired.

Once clinical, laser and laboratory data have been recorded at multiple visits and shared between screening programmes, primary care and hospital settings, timeline charts can display multiple parameters such as VA, blood pressure and current medication to give the clinician an immediate graphical display of the clinical progress of each patient.[36] With EMR, detailed audit of clinical outcomes can be delivered on a local or national[37] level.

The transition to EMR is a major cultural change for doctors that has universally occurred in primary care and is beginning to happen in hospitals.

PRACTICE POINT

• The advances in technology discussed in this chapter offer exciting new prospects for future diagnosis and treatment of patients with sight-threatening DR.

REFERENCES

1 Ciulla TA, Amador AG, Zinman B. Diabetic retinopathy and diabetic macular edema: pathophysiology, screening, and novel therapies. *Diabetes Care* 2003; **26**(9): 2653–64.

2 Joy S, Scates A, Bearelly S, Dar M, Taulien C, Goebel J *et al.* Ruboxistaurin, a protein kinase C beta inhibitor, as an emerging treatment for diabetes microvascular complications. *Ann Pharmacother* 2005; **39**(10): 1693–9.

3 PKC-DRS. The effect of ruboxistaurin on visual loss in patients with moderately severe to very severe non-proliferative diabetic retinopathy: initial results of the Protein Kinase C beta inhibitor Diabetic Retinopathy Study (PKC-DRS) multicenter randomized clinical trial. *Diabetes* 2005; **54**(7): 2188–97.

4 Aiello LP, Davis MD, Girach A, Kles KA, Milton RC, Sheetz MJ *et al.* Effect of ruboxistaurin on visual loss in patients with diabetic retinopathy. *Ophthalmology* 2006; **113**(12): 2221–30.

5 Podoleanu AG. Optical coherence tomography. *Br J Radiol* 2005; **78**(935): 976–88.

6 Hee MR, Izatt JA, Swanson EA, Huang D, Schuman JS, Lin CP *et al.* Optical coherence tomography of the human retina. *Arch Ophthalmol* 1995; **113**(3): 325–32.

7 Puliafito CA, Hee MR, Lin CP, Reichel E, Schuman JS, Duker JS *et al.* Imaging of macular diseases with optical coherence tomography. *Ophthalmology* 1995; **102**(2): 217–29.

8 Hee MR, Puliafito CA, Duker JS, Reichel E, Coker JG, Wilkins JR *et al.* Topography of diabetic macular edema with optical coherence tomography. *Ophthalmology* 1998; **105**(2): 360–70.

9 Podoleanu AG, Dobre GM, Cucu RG, Rosen R, Garcia P, Nieto J *et al.* Combined multiplanar optical coherence tomography and confocal scanning ophthalmoscopy. *J Biomed Opt* 2004; **9**(1): 86–93.

10 Cucu R, Podoleanu A, Rogers J, Pedro J, Rosen R. Combined confocal/en face T-scan-based ultra high-resolution optical coherence tomography in vivo retinal imaging. *Optics Letters* 2006; **31**(11): 1684–6.

11 Wojkowski M, Srinivasan V, Fujimoto J, Ko T, Schuman J, Kowalczyk A *et al.* Three dimensional retinal imaging with high speed ultra high resolution optical coherence tomography. *Ophthalmology* 2005; **112**(10): 1734–46.

12 Nuffer LL, Medvick PA, Foote HP, Solinsky JC. Multispectral/hyperspectral image enhancement for biological cell analysis. *Cytometry A* 2006; **69**(8): 897–903.

13 Schultz RA, Nielsen T, Zavaleta JR, Ruch R, Wyatt R, Garner HR. Hyperspectral imaging: a novel approach for microscopic analysis. *Cytometry A* 2001; **43**(4): 239–47.

14 Martin ME, Wabuyele MB, Chen K, Kasili P, Panjehpour M, Phan M *et al.* Development of an advanced hyperspectral imaging (HSI) system with applications for cancer detection. *Ann Biomed Eng* 2006; **34**(6): 1061–8.

15 Cancio LC, Batchinsky AI, Mansfield JR, Panasyuk S, Hetz K, Martini D *et al.* Hyperspectral imaging: a new approach to the diagnosis of hemorrhagic shock. *J Trauma* 2006; **60**(5): 1087–95.

16 Zuzak KJ, Schaeberle MD, Lewis EN, Levin IW. Visible reflectance hyperspectral imaging: characterization of a non-invasive, in vivo system for determining tissue perfusion. *Anal Chem* 2002; **74**(9): 2021–8.

17 Greenman RL, Panasyuk S, Wang X, Lyons TE, Dinh T, Longoria L *et al.* Early changes in the skin microcirculation and muscle metabolism of the diabetic foot. *Lancet* 2005; **366**(9498): 1711–17.

18 Zuzak KJ, Gladwin MT, Cannon ROr, Levin IW. Imaging hemoglobin oxygen saturation in sickle cell disease patients using noninvasive visible reflectance hyperspectral techniques: effects of nitric oxide. *Am J Physiol Heart Circ Physiol* 2003; **285**(3): 1183–9.

19 Mordant DJ, Al Abboud I, Harvey AR, McNaught AI. Hyperspectral Imaging of the Human Retina – Oximetric Studies. *Invest Ophthalmol Vis Sci* 2007; **48**: E-abstract 148.

20 Mordant DJ, Al Abboud I, Harvey AR, McNaught AI.

Quantitative Spectral Imaging of the Retina. *Invest Ophthalmol Vis Sci* 2007; **48**: E-abstract 148.

21 Ashton N. Arteriolar involvement in diabetic retinopathy. *Br J Ophthalmol* 1953; **37**: 282–92.

22 Wilson DJ, Finkelstein D, Quigley HA, Green WR. Macular grid photocoagulation: an experimental study on the primate retina. *Arch Ophthalmol* 1988; **106**: 100–5.

23 Arnarsson A, Stefansson E. Laser treatment and the mechanism of oedema reduction in branch retinal vein occlusion. *Invest Ophthalmol Vis Sci* 2000; **41**: 877–9.

24 Ogata N, Tombran-Tink J, Jo N, Mrazek D, Matsumura M. Upregulation of pigment epithelium-derived factor after laser photocoagulation. *Am J Ophthalmol* 2001; **132**: 427–9.

25 Early Treatment Diabetic Retinopathy Study Research Group. Early photocoagulation for diabetic retinopathy. ETDRS report number 9. *Ophthalmology* 1991; **98**(5 Suppl): 766–85.

26 DRSRG. Macular oedema in Diabetic Retinopathy Study patients. *Ophthalmology* 1987; **94**: 754–60.

27 Hamilton AMP, Ulbig MW, Polkinghorne P. *Management of Diabetic Retinopathy*. London: BMJ Publishing Group, 1996.

28 Okano T. The evaluation of retinal circulation in advanced diabetic retinopathy before and after panretinal laser photocoagulation by scanning laser ophthalmoscope. *Proc SPIE Intern Soc Opt Eng* 2005; **5967**: 5967C 1–5.

29 Stefansson E. Ocular oxygenation and the treatment of diabetic retinopathy. *Surv Ophthalmol* 2006; **51**(4): 364–80.

30 Gillow JT, Gray JA. The National Screening Committee review of diabetic retinopathy screening. *Eye* 2001; **15**(Pt 1): 1–2.

31 Bailey CC, Sparrow JM, Grey RH, Cheng H. The National Diabetic Retinopathy Laser Treatment Audit. III. Clinical outcomes. *Eye* 1999; **13**(Pt 2): 151–9.

32 Bailey CC, Sparrow JM, Grey RH, Cheng H. The National Diabetic Retinopathy Laser Treatment Audit. I. Maculopathy. *Eye* 1998; **12**(Pt 1): 69–76.

33 Bailey CC, Sparrow JM, Grey RH, Cheng H. The National Diabetic Retinopathy Laser Treatment Audit. II. Proliferative retinopathy. *Eye* 1998; **12**(Pt 1): 77–84.

34 Davidescu L, Ignat F, Popescu GL. Computer program for medical records of patients with diabetic retinopathy. *Oftalmologia* 2005; **49**(4): 74–9.

35 DeBry PW. Considerations for choosing an electronic medical record for an ophthalmology practice. *Arch Ophthalmol* 2001; **119**(April): 590–6.

36 Young RJ, Khong CK, Vaughan NJ, New J, Roxburgh M. The evolution of diabetes information systems. *Diabet Med* 2002; **19**(Suppl 4): 6–12.

37 Jaycock P, Johnston RL, Taylor H, Adams M, Tole DM, Galloway P *et al*. The Cataract National Dataset electronic multi-centre audit of 55,567 operations: updating benchmark standards of care in the United Kingdom and internationally. *Eye* 2007; Nov 23. [Epub ahead of print].

16 Other retinal conditions that are more frequent in diabetes

Stephen J. Aldington & Peter H. Scanlon

HYPERTENSION

Systemic hypertension is all too frequently coexistent with diabetes mellitus so it is often difficult or impossible to clearly differentiate which is the cause of a particular retinal lesion. To further complicate the matter, many of the observable early retinal changes caused by systemic hypertension such as arterial sclerosis and changes to arteriovenous crossing points are very similar to those found in the common ageing processes.

Hence in younger patients it can usually be assumed that visible arteriolar narrowing and attenuation are likely to be hypertensive in origin, whereas in older patients this may not be so clear cut.

Hypertensive retinopathy shares several common lesions with diabetic retinopathy, principally retinal haemorrhage, cotton wool spots, hard exudates and apparent vascular occlusions. Microaneurysms, intra-retinal microvascular abnormalities (IRMA) and venous beading are not, however, features commonly associated with hypertension. In the absence of widespread 'dot and blot' diabetic retinopathy, hypertensive retinopathy can usually be differentiated as nerve-fibre layer 'streak' or 'flame-shaped' haemorrhages frequently surrounding and pointing towards the optic disc, and associated (nerve-fibre layer) cotton wool spots, also surrounding the optic disc. The presence of these features when observed with coexistent widespread arteriolar constriction is usually associated with prolonged chronic exposure to systemic hypertension.

In acute systemic hypertension, however, whilst the major retinal arterioles are usually relatively unaffected, there is almost always a far more aggressive microvascular manifestation with severe flame- and even deep retinal haemorrhage, widespread peripapillary cotton wool spots and the presence of middle layer hard exudates. It is not uncommon to also observe quite marked swelling of the optic nerve head in these cases and, in its most severe manifestation, hard exudate development and coalescence in the form of a partial or full hypertensive macular exudate star (Fig. 16.1).

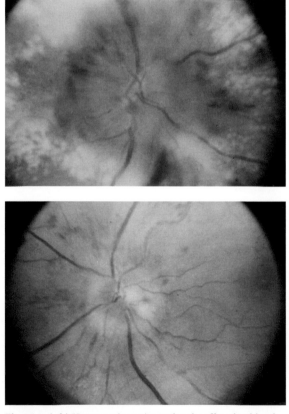

(a)

(b)

Fig. 16.1 (a,b) Hypertensive retinopathy: the effect that blood pressure alone can have on the eyes.

A Practical Manual of Diabetic Retinopathy Management.
Peter H Scanlon, Charles P Wilkinson, Stephen J Aldington and David R Matthews. Published 2009 by Blackwell Publishing, ISBN 978-1-4051-7035-2.

RETINAL ARTERIAL OCCLUSIONS

Occlusion of a retinal artery can have acute, profound and long-lasting effects on visual function. When the occlusion is limited to a relatively small artery or arteriole, the damage and effect will be localized and indeed may not be sufficient to be symptomatic, at least not initially. Occlusion of larger arteries delivering blood to quadrants or entire superior or inferior hemifields of the eye, or worse still, occlusion of the central retinal artery itself, however, is always symptomatic and visual loss of some degree is usually inevitable.

Patients presenting with retinal arterial occlusions almost always do so complaining of just one affected eye (at that time). However, recurrence or subsequent occlusion of vessels in the fellow eye is common.

Clinical examination of the fundi and colour imaging are the common investigative techniques. Fluorescein angiography can be used, although this is of little additional diagnostic value, particularly in cases of central retinal artery occlusion (CRAO). Fluorescein transit times would be very significantly greater, if they can be assessed at all. Major arteries usually do become perfused to some degree eventually, although the majority of this is likely to come about through retrograde flow from the venous and capillary networks with little from direct arterial flow.

In all cases of vascular occlusion, a careful assessment of associated underlying systemic clinical conditions such as diabetes, temporal arteritis, hypertension or atherogenic diseases is necessary and investigations such as full blood count, erythrocyte sedimentation rate, blood glucose and carotid ultrasonography are often indicated.

CASE HISTORY 1
Arteriolar occlusion in diabetes associated with hypertension

This 65-year-old woman with type 2 diabetes (diagnosed at age 59 years) controlled with tablets and a history of hypertension controlled with perindopril 8 mg o.d. and bendrofluazide 2.5 mg o.d. presented with a sudden onset of a blob in front of the central vision of her right eye and a visual acuity (VA) reduced to 6/24 (20/80). Figure 16.2 shows colour and fluorescein angiogram photographs taken of her right eye.

The cause of these changes is a small arteriolar occlusion leading to a small area of ischaemia giving rise to the cotton wool spot demonstrated on the colour photograph. The cotton wool spot gradually cleared over the

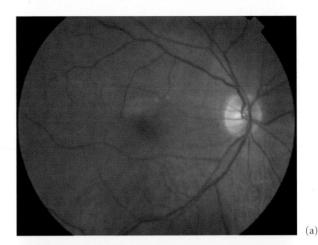
(a)

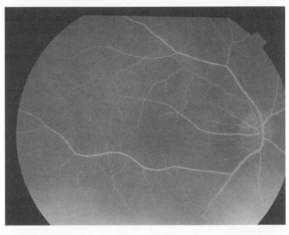
(b)

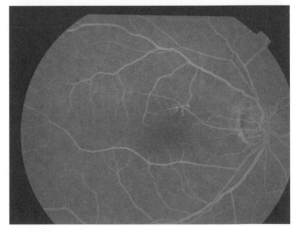
(c)

Fig. 16.2 Case history 1. (a) Colour photograph of right macular area showing cotton wool spot just above right central fovea due to small arteriolar occlusion. Fluorescein right macular area: (b) 21 s after injection of dye; (c) 29 s after injection of dye; (*Continued on p. 180*)

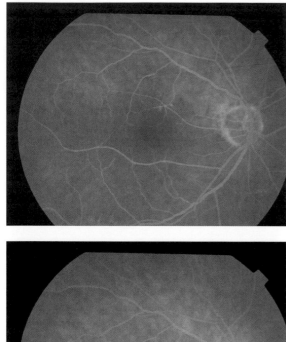

(d)

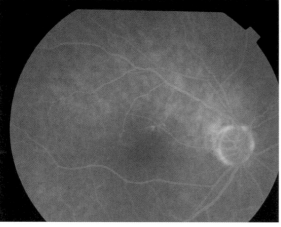

(e)

Fig. 16.2 (*Cont'd*) (d) 57 s after injection of dye; (e) 2 min 41 s after injection of dye.

next 2 months but unfortunately the vision remained at the reduced level of 6/24 (20/80).

Central retinal artery occlusion (CRAO)

Occlusion of the central retinal artery (CRAO) is most frequently caused by blockage of the artery by either local thrombosis or emboli originating from either the heart or carotid artery. Occlusion in younger adult patients, though less frequent, is more likely to be associated with cardiovascular instability whilst that occurring in the elderly population is more commonly associated with arteriosclerosis.

Occlusion of the central artery requires the blockage to have occurred in the retrobulbar region of the eye, before bifurcation of the central artery as it enters the visible

globe. As such, the occlusion is in itself not visible to the examining observer. Much less frequently, CRAO is caused by vascular spasm of the artery itself, although this diagnosis is often controversial as rarely is a patient seen clinically whilst the spasm is occurring and indeed spontaneous return to normality is quite common. However relatively rare such cases of arterial spasms may be, recurrence is not uncommon and potential permanent occlusion is often the outcome, with resultant very severe visual loss in the affected eye.

Clinically, the appearance is one of a very pale yellowish retina, cloudy and with increased general opacity and gross swelling of and around the optic disc (Fig. 16.3a).

A classic characteristic of CRAO, however, is the often marked 'cherry-red spot', delineating the fovea. This is caused by the contrast between the redness of the still-patent choroidal capillary circulation serving the fovea against the whiteness of the totally occluded retinal arterial circulation in the surrounding region and the associated oedema. Retinal arteries frequently appear thin and attenuated (Fig. 16.3b).

Whilst total visual loss in an eye compromised by CRAO is not always inevitable, the final outcome may be reduction of visual function to a level of simple perception of light in that eye at best. Indeed, such a reduction in visual function occurs very quickly, within minutes or certainly hours, of the actual arterial occlusion. Patients complain of visual loss in the affected eye which frequently takes the appearance of a total dimming and contraction of visual perception from the periphery towards the visual axis, usually over the course of just a few minutes. The longer a CRAO remains undiagnosed but potentially treatable, the greater the risk of permanent severe visual loss.

In some cases of CRAO, a significant amount of central vision may actually be retained due to the fortunate coexistence of one or more cilioretinal arteries. These are found in upwards of 15% of otherwise normal eyes. They are arterial vessels arising from the posterior ciliary circulation, i.e. before the origination of the central retinal artery, and as such are independent of that retinal vascular supply route. If a pre-existing cilioretinal artery happens to supply the macular region, the patient may be fortunate enough to retain posterior pole blood supply and hence some macular function (Fig. 16.3c).

Whilst acute CRAO can be diagnosed through sudden visual changes and by retinal examination of the affected eye, previously 'resolved' CRAO is often more difficult to diagnose on examination. Key visible features may include asymmetrical vascular appearance between the

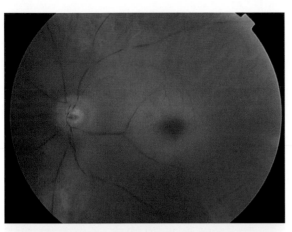

(a)

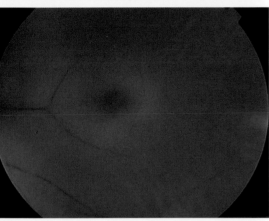

(b)

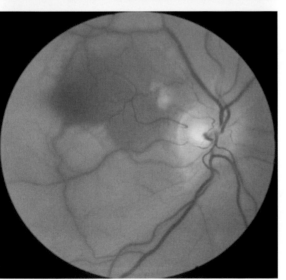

(c)

Fig. 16.3 (a) Central retinal artery occlusion (CRAO). (b) Cherry-red spot. (c) CRAO with a pre-existing cilioretinal artery supplying the macular region.

affected and fellow eye, marked persistent attenuation of vessels in the affected eye and often a residual pale optic disc. Detection of lipid-like deposits along arterial walls is another not uncommon finding.

Branch retinal artery occlusion (BRAO)

As for the central retinal artery, there can be occlusion of a branch retinal artery (BRAO). As these occur in vessels within the visible retinal circulation, however, their point of actual occlusion can usually be determined and observed directly.

Small arteriolar branches, major branches, quadrants or indeed entire hemifields of the eye may be affected dependent on the exact point of occlusion. In cases where the occlusion is caused by an embolus, the relative size will usually determine how far along the retinal arteriolar circulation the blockage will occur. Local thrombosis or vessel wall spasm-induced occlusions, however, can occur largely anywhere along the arterial tree.

On examination, the retinal appearance is dependent on the size of the arterial vessel compromised by the occlusion. Occlusions following the first or second bifurcations of the central retinal artery within the margins of the optic disc would affect an entire hemifield or one quadrant respectively (Fig. 16.4a).

More distal occlusions would usually affect progressively smaller regions of the retinal circulation (Fig. 16.4b).

The classical appearance would be marked whitening of the affected retinal region, although some smaller arterioles within affected areas may still appear to be patent, but this is due to retrograde filling of the end arterioles from the uncompromised venous circulation. The actual point of occlusion can often be clearly determined.

Arterial emboli

Circulating microemboli are relatively common. Should one of these find its way to the ocular circulation, it will inevitably become trapped, frequently causing damage and often it can be detected and imaged.

Emboli are formed from a variety of sources although cholesterol/fibrin or platelet emboli are by far the most common. Small emboli frequently travel considerable distances through the retinal arterial tree before lodging and causing a localized occlusion (Fig. 16.5a–e).

Most are asymptomatic and cause no noticeable visual defect, although uniocular transient or short-term visual loss is most likely to be embolitic in cause, even if the culprit is no longer detectable on examination.

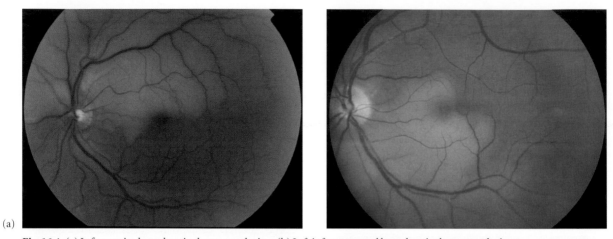

(a)

(b)

Fig. 16.4 (a) Left superior branch retinal artery occlusion. (b) Left inferotemporal branch retinal artery occlusion.

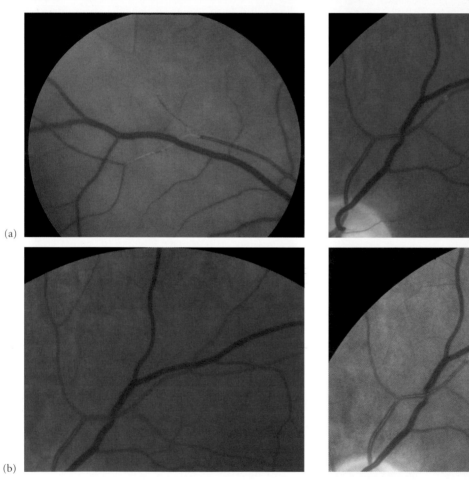

(a)

(c)

(b)

(d)

Fig. 16.5 (a) Fibrinoplatelet arterial embolus. (b) Left superotemporal artery appearance before asymptomatic cholesterol emboli. (c) Left superotemporal artery appearance after asymptomatic cholesterol emboli. (d) Red-free photograph of left superotemporal artery appearance after asymptomatic cholesterol emboli. (*Continued on facing page*)

(e)

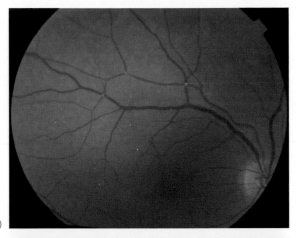

(f)

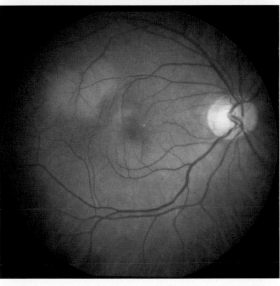

Fig. 16.5 (*Cont'd*) (e) Multiple emboli lodging at junctions in arterial tree. (f) Multiple emboli causing pale areas of oedema in areas of retinal ischaemia.

Larger emboli can, and do of course, cause occlusion of major arterioles and arteries, with the effects on vision noted in the preceding sections (Fig. 16.5f).

RETINAL VENOUS OCCLUSIONS

As diabetic retinopathy is classically associated with disease and early damage to the venous blood supply, the incidence of retinal venous occlusions is higher in patients with diabetes than in age-matched non-diabetic persons. Retinal vein occlusion, however, even in the non-diabetic population, is a common cause of retinal pathology and subsequent visual loss.

As for retinal arterial occlusions, the extent and severity of retinal damage in venous occlusions is largely dependent on the size of the vein occluded and on whether partial or total occlusion has occurred.

Retinal vein occlusions are most commonly seen affecting one or more quadrants of the eye, most commonly the superior or inferior temporal quadrant, but almost always affect only one eye at a single presentation.

The usual uniocular presentation of a patient with vein occlusion is a key criterion on which to base a differential diagnosis. Retinal lesions and damage caused by systemic conditions such as diabetes, hypertension or age-related macular degeneration are generally bilateral and affect both eyes with relatively equal vigour at any particular point in time. Not only the type and severity of lesions but also the location and indeed absence of some abnormal retinal features must be taken into account.

In many cases of coexistent diabetic retinopathy and vein occlusion (particularly of a branch vein), it proves to be impossible to differentiate whether any particular retinal lesion or feature is likely to be caused by the effect of systemic diabetes or by localized venous occlusion. This is usually of little relevance in a clinical context, however.

Venous occlusions are not caused by emboli because to do so, the embolus would have had to traverse the entire branching and reducing arterial system and cross through the capillary bed before affecting the venous side of the circulatory system.

Central retinal vein occlusion

Central retinal vein occlusion (CRVO) is a severe or total outflow obstruction to the main vein leaving the eye. This occurs out of sight of the observer and happens within the confines of the retrobulbar region of the optic disc. The acute and chronic damage done by a CRVO is, however, clearly visible.

In older patients, CRVO is commonly associated with diabetes, hypertension and arteriosclerosis. In some cases the entering central retinal artery, lying in close association to the leaving central retinal vein, can create sufficient pressure on the vein to cause a near- or total occlusion. In younger patients, occlusion is sometimes associated with systemic conditions such as sarcoidosis, Behçet's disease or a general phlebitis causing an inflammatory response. In many cases, particularly in the young, the exact cause remains unclear.

Severe or total occlusions affecting the central retinal vein have a marked appearance on clinical examination of the retina. Most common findings include large quantities of very dark red retinal haemorrhage surrounding the optic disc. These peripapillary haemorrhages are usually flame-shaped, with their principal axis pointing to the centre of the optic disc as they are haemorrhages involving the superficial, nerve-fibre layer. Moving outwards towards the retinal periphery, the appearance is of large numbers and clusters of deep dark blot haemorrhages, indicating substantial damage also to the deeper retinal layers. Multiple retinal infarcts and ischaemic retina can usually also be seen and gross venous engorgement is commonplace. Should the macular region actually be visible (through retinal haemorrhaging), oedematous swelling is a common feature. The optic disc may well be swollen. Visual loss is common (Fig. 16.6a–d).

CASE HISTORY 2
Central retinal vein occlusion in diabetes

This 58-year-old man with type 2 diabetes diagnosed 8 years ago, was controlled on metformin 1000 mg t.d.s., with gliclazide 40 mg b.d. added more recently. Over the previous 5 years his diabetes had been poorly controlled with HbA1c values of 11.2%, 12.1% and 10.5%, but the most recent value following the introduction of gliclazide had been 6.3.

He had a left phacoemulsification of cataract at the age of 57 years and 1 week postoperatively his vision was good at 6/9 (20/30) unaided. However, 1 month postoperatively he developed a left central retinal vein occlusion with a reduced VA of 6/24 (6/80). The photographs show the signs of central retinal vein occlusion in his left eye (Fig. 16.6e–f).

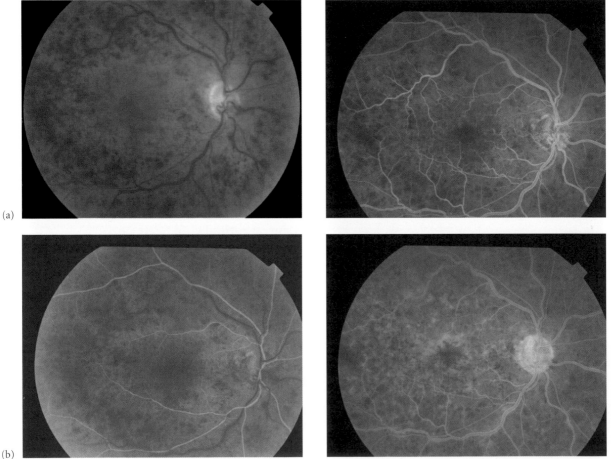

(a)

(b)

(c)

(d)

Fig. 16.6 Case history 2. Right central retinal vein occlusion: (a) colour photograph; (b) fluorescein 29 s after injection; (c) fluorescein 45 s after injection; (d) fluorescein 4 min 5 s after injection. (*Continued on facing page*)

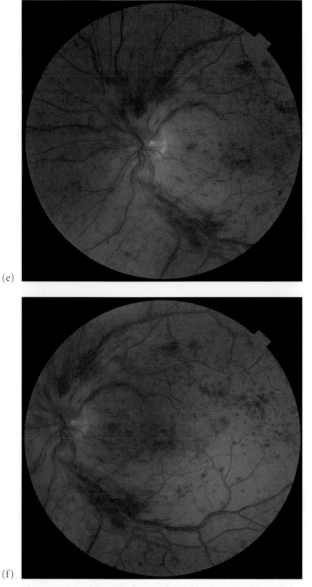

(e)

(f)

Fig. 16.6 (*Cont'd*) (e) Left central retinal vein occlusion: colour photograph left nasal view. (f) Left central retinal vein occlusion: colour photograph left macular view.

The timing of the central retinal vein occlusion 1 month after the cataract operation was felt to be coincidental.

In situations where the central retinal vein is not totally occluded, the retinal appearance is usually rather quieter. Some venous engorgement is still usually present but fewer peripheral deep blot and considerably fewer nerve-

fibre layer haemorrhages are visible. Infarcts as cotton wool spots are not particularly common and areas of apparent retinal ischemia are fewer. In the early stages and in relatively mild CRVO, noticeable visual loss may not have occurred.

In some cases, whilst the central retinal vein actually is mostly or totally occluded, some outflow from the affected eye is maintained through new collateral or existing cilioretinal vessels on the optic disc, linking the retinal circulation to that of the choroid and providing some outflow from the eye via the vortex veins. Development of true collateral vessels, however, is usually a feature of long-standing vein occlusion and these tortuous remnants on the optic disc are often the sole remaining visible feature of a long-resolved CRVO. That and reduced VA in the eye.

Visual loss from CRVO is generally caused by either extensive retinal capillary closure and ischaemia, with or without subsequent neovascularization, or by subsequent macular oedema. Some improvement of visual function over time is common, particularly in cases of macular oedema, although the individual outcome varies considerably. What is essential, however, is continued monitoring of the patient and assessment of both the affected and fellow eye; both the posterior and crucially the anterior segments. Central retinal vein occlusion, through widespread retinal ischaemia, is frequently associated with subsequent development of iris neovascularization and ultimately rubeotic glaucoma. With the coexisting insult of diabetes-induced retinal ischaemia, such patients must receive long-term follow-up and monitoring.

Clinical examination and colour retinal imaging for recording purposes are always appropriate. Fluorescein angiography is an added advantage, although in profound cases little retinal detail may be visible due to overlying haemorrhage. In cases of suspected macular oedema, OCT investigations are particularly beneficial as they are not affected by other retinal lesions.

No direct or effective treatment is currently available for CRVO although attention to an underlying systemic condition is essential. Anticoagulants such as heparin and aspirin have been tried but with little general effect. Treatment may, however, be required for complications that may develop such as retinal or iris neovascularization.

Branch retinal vein occlusion (BRVO)

Occlusion of a retinal branch vein (BRVO) is a relatively common finding, particularly in patients with diabetes; it most frequently affects the superior or inferior temporal arcades to create a quadrant occlusion. An occlusion involving the major vein immediately before the last bifurcation (rejoining, actually) on the optic disc causes a defect which affects either the upper or lower hemifield of the eye. The unaffected portion or portions of the eye are most usually relatively, if not totally, normal. Occlusion of smaller retinal venules causes damage to a correspondingly narrower and more restricted region with much more localized lesions.

Branch vein occlusions affecting an entire quadrant most commonly occur at an arteriovenous crossing point close to the optic disc. Arterial compression, with the artery usually crossing over the related vein, causes relative or total venous occlusion. Another cause of venous occlusion, particularly in the nasal retina, is when the vein becomes severely constricted due to it passing over the steep edge of the optic rim in cases of deeply cupped glaucomatous discs. Occlusion of smaller and more peripheral veins is thought to be linked to phlebitis and other inflammatory insults, although the susceptible arteriovenous crossing cannot be ruled out even in these cases.

Clinical examination of a branch vein occlusion in an otherwise normal eye (i.e. in the absence of any other confounding features) reveals lesions and retinal features which are very localized and are restricted to the retinal area drained by the affected vein (Fig. 16.7).

Laser treatment is indicated if neovascularization develops in the distribution of an occluded vein. Focal laser treatment may be indicated for persistent localized macular oedema.

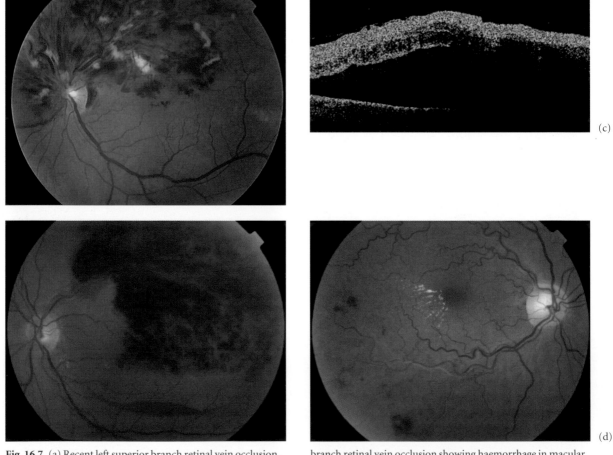

(a)

(b)

(c)

(d)

Fig. 16.7 (a) Recent left superior branch retinal vein occlusion. (b) Left superior branch retinal vein occlusion with haemorrhage in macular area. (c) OCT line scan–left superior branch retinal vein occlusion showing haemorrhage in macular area. (d) Older right inferotemporal branch retinal vein occlusion. (*Continued on facing page*)

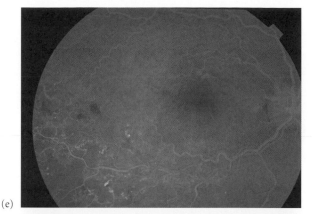

(e)

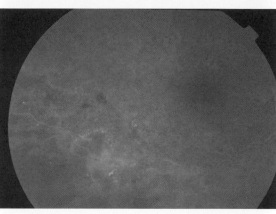

(f)

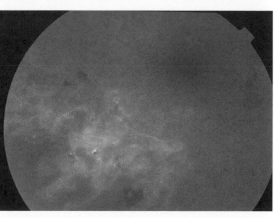

(g)

Fig. 16.7 (*Cont'd*) (e) Older right inferotemporal branch retinal vein occlusion: fluorescein angiogram 37 s after injection showing ischaemia in distribution of occluded vein. (f) Older right inferotemporal branch retinal vein occlusion: fluorescein angiogram 1 min 58 s after injection showing ischaemia and leakage in the distribution of occluded vein. (g) Older right inferotemporal branch retinal vein occlusion: fluorescein angiogram 3 min 31 s after injection showing ischaemia and leakage in the distribution of occluded vein.

ANTERIOR ISCHAEMIC OPTIC NEUROPATHY

Anterior ischaemic optic neuropathy (AION) usually causes a sudden loss of vision because of ischaemia of the anterior part of the optic nerve. It is more common in people with diabetes and/or high blood pressure. It needs to be differentiated from temporal arteritis, which is an arteritic cause requiring urgent treatment to prevent involvement of the other eye.

Patients should be advised to pay careful attention to their blood pressure control and to avoid smoking.

CASE HISTORY 3
Anterior ischaemic optic neuropathy in diabetes

A 64-year-old man with type 2 diabetes controlled with metformin 1 g twice a day, and a history of hypertension controlled with atenolol 100 mg once daily, noticed a sudden loss of vision in his left eye when he started to shave one morning. On examination his VA was found to be 6/12, and the optic disc showed oedema, more marked inferiorly with splinter haemorrhages at the disc margin (Fig. 16.8a).

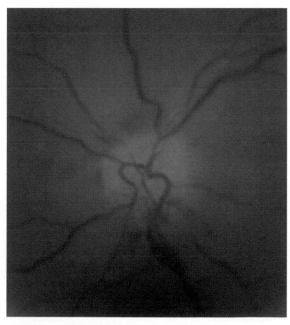

(a)

Fig. 16.8 Case history 3. Anterior ischaemic optic neuropathy. (a) Colour photograph of disc showing blurring and haemorrhage of inferior disc margin. (*Continued on p. 188*)

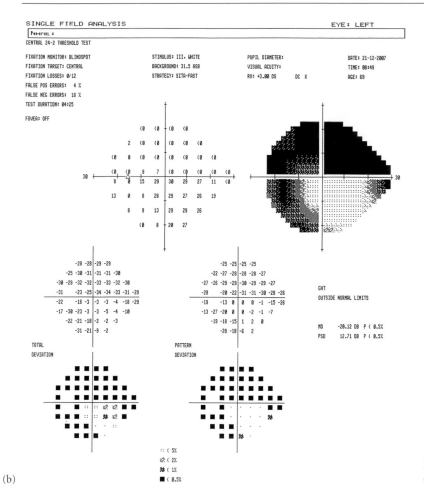

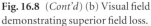

Fig. 16.8 (*Cont'd*) (b) Visual field demonstrating superior field loss.

(b)

Within 2–3 months the optic disc swelling resolved spontaneously and the disc became pale. The left visual field shows loss of the superior field and some nasal loss inferiorly (Fig. 16.8b).

ASTEROID HYALOSIS

Asteroid hyalosis is a primarily unilateral disorder (bilateral in only 9%), occurring more frequently in men (almost twice the frequency), and in older patients. The condition is usually asymptomatic and only mildly affects VA even when it is difficult for the ophthalmologist to get a good view of the retina.

On examination, refractile yellow-white particles (asteroid bodies) are seen in the vitreous; they are composed of a mixture of calcium, phosphorus and oxygen showing a composition similar to those found for hydroxyapatite with the presence of chondroitin-6-sulfate at the periphery of asteroid bodies.[1]

An association between diabetes mellitus was suggested by Cockburn,[2] and in a large study of 12,205 patients Bergren[3] found diabetes mellitus in 29 of the patients with asteroid hyalosis (29%), as compared to 10 of 101 (10%) control subjects (p = 0.0007). However, this association has been disputed by Moss[4] in the Beaver Dam Eye study where an association was found with greater body mass (p = 0.02) and higher alcohol consumption (p = 0.03), but not with diabetes.

Asteroid hyalosis is a benign condition in itself and never leads to severe vision loss. Hence the presence of asteroid hyalosis usually only needs to be documented. Any significant visual loss in a person with asteroid hyalosis requires further investigation and treatment of any associated condition.

Interestingly, although the retinal view may be limited using slit-lamp biomicroscopy and colour photography, one often finds that a surprisingly good view is obtained on fluorescein angiography as shown in Case History 4.

CASE HISTORY 4
Macular oedema in a patient with asteroid hyalosis in diabetes

This 75-year-old man with type 2 diabetes for 11 years, controlled with insulin, noticed a gradual loss of vision in his right eye, which was known to have asteroid hyalosis. On examination, the VA was reduced to 6/60 and scattered haemorrhages and microaneurysms were noted in his right fundus, but the macular area was difficult to view adequately because of the asteroid hyalosis. His blood pressure was 181/64 and his HbA1c was 8.5%.

The colour photographs (Fig. 16.9a,b) show the asteroid bodies on the anterior view and the difficulty in obtaining a clear colour photograph of the macular area. A fluorescein angiogram demonstrates that good fluorescein pictures can often be obtained in patients with asteroid hyalosis and that in this particular case marked cystoid macular oedema is present (Fig. 16.9c–f).

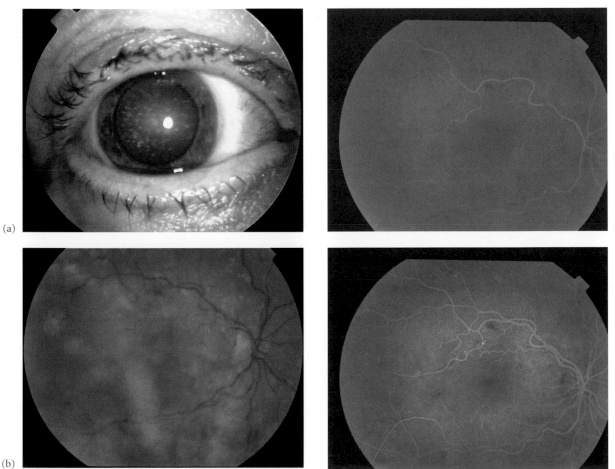

(a) (b) (c) (d)

Fig. 16.9 Case history 4. Asteroid hyalosis. Right macula colour (a,b). Fluorescein angiogram: (c) 24 s after injection of dye; (d) 28 s after injection of dye; (*Continued on p. 190*)

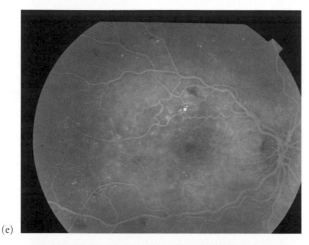

(e)

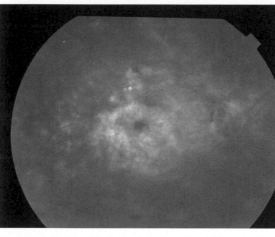

(f)

Fig. 16.9 (*Cont'd*) (e) 47 s after injection of dye; (f) 3 min 30 s after injection of dye showing cystoid macular oedema.

MACROANEURYSM

Retinal macroaneurysms are dilatations of a retinal artery or an arteriole that are larger than the diameter of the vein as it crosses the optic disc margin. They are more common in diabetes, but because they are generally not regarded as microvascular pathology, they do not come under a strict definition of diabetic retinopathy. They are often associated with systemic hypertension as well as diabetes. They are often asymptomatic but can be associated with leakage that threatens the macular area or bleeding producing intraretinal or vitreous haemorrhages. Two examples are given below of macroaneurysms that leaked, threatening the macular area and hence the central vision.

CASE HISTORY 5
Macroaneurysm in type 1 diabetes

This 41-year-old man, with type 1 diabetes since the age of 2, presented at the age of 29 years with exudates threatening the left macular area due to leakage from a macroaneurysm. The left vision was good at 6/6 (20/20). Figure 16.10(a) shows leakage from the macroaneurysm.

He was treated with 45 burns, 100-micron size, power 180–220 mW, 0.1 s, area centralis lens, with approximately 20 burns having been applied directly to the macroaneurysm and 26 burns to the surrounding thickened retina. The photographs taken within a few minutes of treatment show the pale laser burns on the macroaneurysm and some within the surrounding area of exudation (Fig. 16.10b,c).

Four months after treatment, there had been considerable clearing of the exudates and thrombosis of the

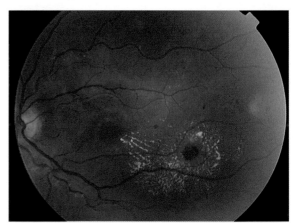

(a)

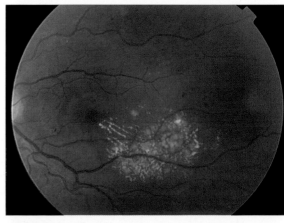

(b)

Fig. 16.10 Case history 5. Macroaneurysm: (a) leaking threatening left macular area; (b) immediately after treatment; (*Continued on facing page*)

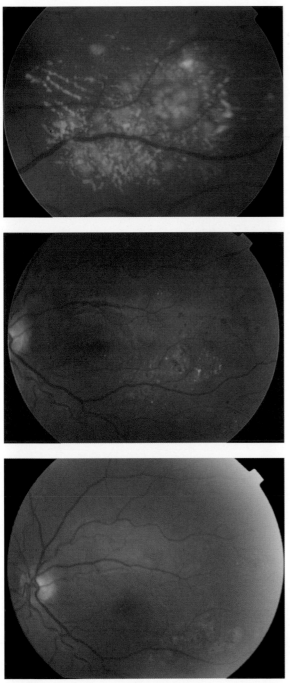

(c)

(d)

(e)

Fig. 16.10 (*Cont'd*) (c) immediately after treatment: magnified view; (d) 4 months after treatment showing clearing of most of the exudate; (e) macroaneurysm 14 years after treatment.

macroaneurysm as shown in Fig. 16.10(d), and 14 years later this improvement had been maintained (Fig. 16.10e).

CASE HISTORY 6
Macroaneurysm in type 2 diabetes

This 87-year-old woman with type 2 diabetes diagnosed 15 years ago, controlled on tablets and with a history of hypertension treated with bendrofluazide 2.5 mg o.d., presented with blurred vision in her right eye, which was reduced to a level of 6/24 (20/120). Colour photographs and a fluorescein angiogram demonstrate a leaking macroaneurysm threatening the right macular area (Fig. 16.11a–e).

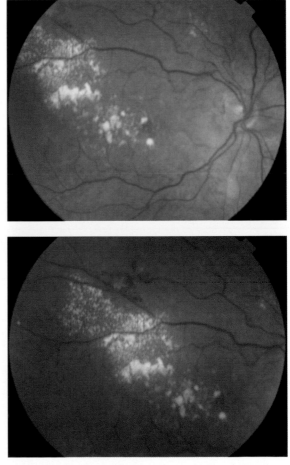

(a)

(b)

Fig. 16.11 Case history 6. Macroaneurysm leaking threatening right macular area: (a) right macula colour photograph; (b) right superior colour photograph; (*Continued on p. 192*)

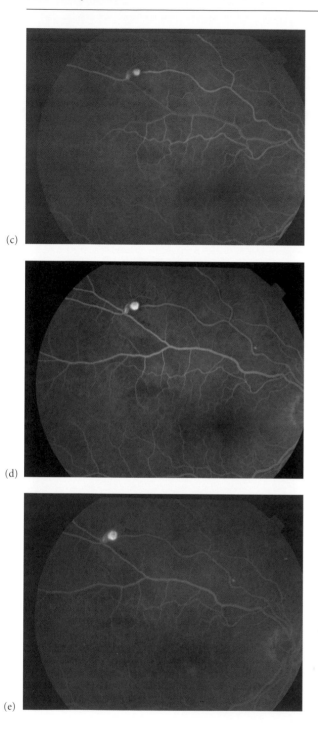

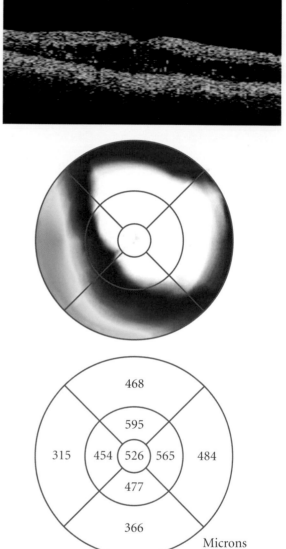

Fig. 16.11 (*Cont'd*) (c) fluorescein angiogram 49 s after injection; (d) fluorescein angiogram 1 min 05 s after injection; (e) fluorescein angiogram 3 min 1 sec after injection. (f) OCT line scan of right macular area before treatment showing thickening. (g) OCT topographic map of right macular area before treatment showing thickening. (*Continued on facing page*)

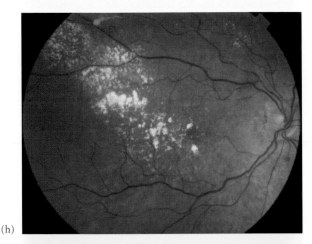

(h)

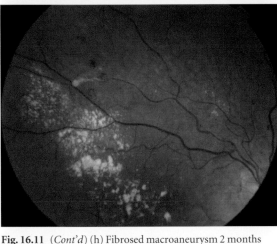

(i)

Fig. 16.11 (*Cont'd*) (h) Fibrosed macroaneurysm 2 months after treatment: right macular colour photograph: exudates starting to clear. (i) Fibrosed macroaneurysm 2 months after treatment: right superior colour photograph: exudates starting to clear.

An OCT scan showed the thickening in the right macular area on both the line scan and the topographic map (Fig. 16.11f,g). Laser treatment was applied directly to the macroaneurysm, resulting in thrombosis of the macroaneurysm; 99 burns were applied, 100-micron size, power 160–450 mW (the higher-powered burns were applied directly to the macroaneurysm and the lower-powered ones to the areas of retinal thickening), 0.1 s, area centralis lens, argon laser.

Figure 16.11(h,i) shows thrombosis of the macroaneurysm and the commencement of clearing of the exudates, which are now in focus because less oedema is present.

PRACTICE POINT

• Diabetic retinopathy is a microvascular disease. However, people with diabetes are also more liable to develop disease of the larger vessels (macrovascular disease) than a person without diabetes. Hence, many of the conditions described in this chapter relate to diseases of the larger vessels.

REFERENCES

1 Winkler J, Lunsdorf H. Ultrastructure and composition of asteroid bodies. *Invest Ophthalmol Vis Sci* 2001; **42**(5): 902–7.
2 Cockburn DM. Are vitreous asteroid bodies associated with diabetes mellitus? *Am J Optom Physiol Opt* 1985; **62**(1): 40–4.
3 Bergren RL, Brown GC, Duker JS. Prevalence and association of asteroid hyalosis with systemic diseases. *Am J Ophthalmol* 1991; **111**(3): 289–93.
4 Moss SE, Klein R, Klein BE. Asteroid hyalosis in a population: the Beaver Dam eye study. *Am J Ophthalmol* 2001; **132**(1): 70–5.

17 Conditions with appearances similar to diabetic retinopathy

Stephen J. Aldington & Peter H. Scanlon

DRUSEN AND AMD

One of the most frequently detected abnormal retinal features are drusen. Principally associated with general ageing, drusen are sufficiently common as to be present and detectable in many people over 50 years of age, particularly in the macular area. They are formed as deposits of lipofuscin, initially within the pigment epithelium and later as deposits between the basement membrane of the pigment epithelium and the inner layer of Bruch's membrane. On examination, they present as yellowish deposits varying in size and appearance from tiny almost crystalline individual hard 'druse' (a common American term for single drusen), to large soft, less defined yellowish white drusen, each often more than twice the diameter of a major vein. Large soft drusen are frequently seen in near-confluent regions around the macula and in the posterior pole generally (Fig. 17.1).

It is important to make a differential diagnosis between drusen (particularly scattered hard drusen) and the presence of any retinal hard exudates which are diabetic in origin. Whilst exudates are caused by leakage of lipid-rich plasma within the middle retinal layers and are frequently associated with other (usually diabetic) retinal features such as microaneurysms, drusen are located much deeper in the eye, are usually less distinct and are unrelated to other (diabetic) retinal lesions. Drusen can of course be present in an eye also affected by intraretinal hard exudates.

A Practical Manual of Diabetic Retinopathy Management.
Peter H Scanlon, Charles P Wilkinson, Stephen J Aldington and David R Matthews. Published 2009 by Blackwell Publishing, ISBN 978-1-4051-7035-2.

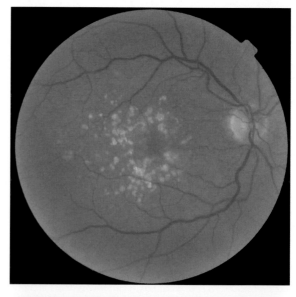

(a)

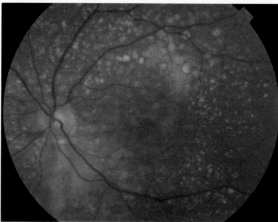

(b)

Fig. 17.1 Drusen: (a) surrounding the central foveal area; (b) scattered throughout the retina. (*Continued on facing page*)

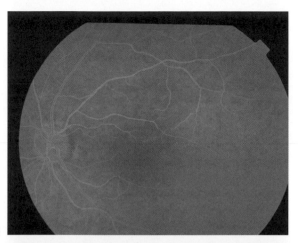

(c)

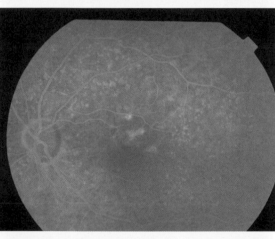

(d)

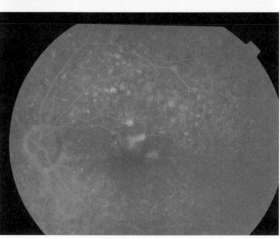

(e)

Fig. 17.1 (*Cont'd*) (c) Minimal uptake of fluorescein by drusen in the early arteriovenous phase. (d) Small uptake of fluorescein by drusen in the midvenous phase. (e) Small uptake of fluorescein by drusen at 3 min 49 s in the late venous phase.

Whilst they are individually asymptomatic and not causative of visual loss, drusen directly affecting the macula are an early feature of age-related macular degeneration (AMD). A full explanation of the development, treatment and outcomes of AMD is beyond the scope of this book. Briefly, however, two main forms of AMD are identified: the 'dry' atrophic type where drusen ultimately cause pigment epithelium atrophy along with associated pigment clumping and possible RPE detachment; and the 'wet' type which leads to significant damage to Bruch's membrane and ultimately to subretinal neovascularization.

AMD presence is most usually bilateral, although the pace of development may be very unequal in the two eyes. Visual loss in one eye has an approximate 12–15% chance of being followed by visual loss in the fellow eye within 1 year.

MYELINATED NERVE FIBRES

The normal adult human eye possesses usually un-observable superficial retinal nerve fibres, connecting the photoreceptors ultimately to the visual cortex. Retinal nerve fibres, unlike those within the optic nerve itself, are usually devoid of a myelin sheath. On occasions however, fetal and very early postnatal development causes the normal myelination to the optic nerve to extend forwards, beyond the normal stopping point of the lamina cribrosa, to involve some of the peripapillary retinal nerve fibres.

On examination, myelinated nerve fibres (MNFs) can be seen as highly reflective whitish-yellow opaque patches surrounding the optic disc with marked striations (caused by the fibres themselves) (Fig. 17.2). Usually these patches are physically connected to the disc margin, although on occasion they can occur as an isolated island development some distance from the margin. It is quite common for the areas of MNF to effectively prevent or obscure an observer's view of retinal vessels in this area.

Large areas of myelinated nerve fibres can cause field defects, although as these are congenital or at least immediately postnatal in terms of longevity, they are effectively asymptomatic and detailed field testing is required to detect their influence.

Correct identification of patches of MNF is important though, to differentiate these from cotton wool spots, hard exudates and in some cases even retinal oedema.

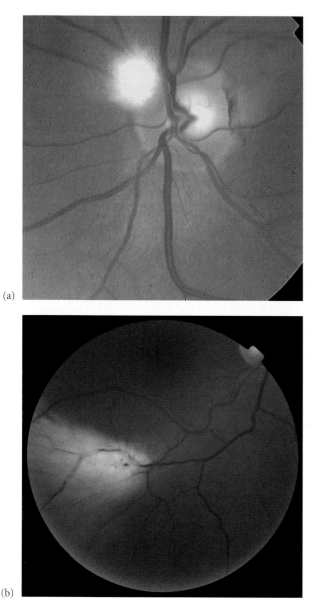

(a)

(b)

Fig. 17.2 (a) Myelinated nerve fibres at left nasal disc margin.
(b) Myelinated nerve fibres: right inferotemporal colour photograph.

SICKLE CELL RETINOPATHY

Sickle cell disease is an inherited blood disorder that affects red blood cells. People with sickle cell disease have red blood cells that contain mostly haemoglobin S, an abnormal type of haemoglobin. Sometimes these red blood cells become sickle-shaped (crescent shaped) and have difficulty passing through small blood vessels.

The different kinds of sickle cell disease and the different traits are found mainly in people whose families come from Africa, the Caribbean, the Eastern Mediterranean, the Middle East and Asia. An example of red blood cells that have become sickle-shaped is shown in Fig. 17.3(a–d).

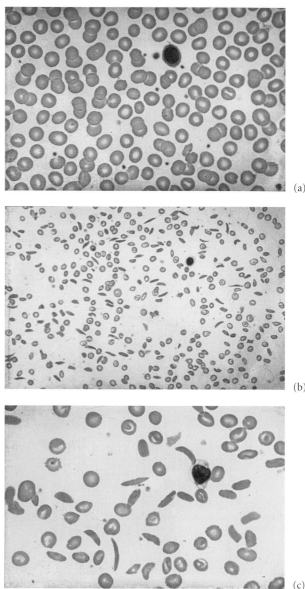

(a)

(b)

(c)

Fig. 17.3 Sickle cell retinopathy. (a) Normal red blood cells with one lymphocyte. (b) Low power film of sickle cells. (c) High power film of sickle cells. (*Continued on facing page*)

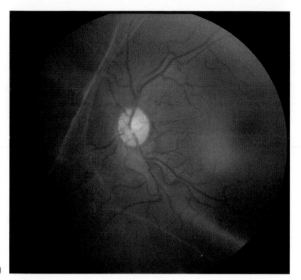

(d)

Fig. 17.3 (*Cont'd*) (d) Fibrotic bands in the peripheral retina of a patient with sickle cell retinopathy.

Ischaemia of the peripheral retina can result in neovascularization and the primary aim of treatment is to prevent visual loss from the complications of the neovascularization.

Although one might expect that peripheral vascular occlusion and ischaemia resulting in neovascularization might be more common in homozygous sickle cell disease (SS genotype), it is in fact commoner in adults with SC disease[1] (SC genotype).

A number of classifications[2–4] have been developed to describe the progression of sickle cell retinopathy. In the recent publication by Sayag[3] they describe an extension of the original classification proposed by Goldberg[4].

Stage 1 – Peripheral arteriolar occlusion is present.

Stage 2 – Peripheral arteriovenous anastamosis.

Stage 3 – Neovascular and fibrous proliferations, subdivided by Sayag into 3A–E, depending on clinical and angiographic characteristics.

Stage 4 – Intravitreal haemorrhage.

Stage 5 – Retinal detachment.

Laser treatment to ischaemic areas of peripheral retina may be required.

A colour photograph of a patient with sickle cell retinopathy, who presented with a vitreous haemorrhage requiring peripheral scatter laser treatment, and who subsequently developed fibrotic bands in the peripheral retina is shown in Fig. 17.3(d).

COATS' DISEASE

Coats' disease is an idiopathic retinal telangiectasia first described by the Scottish ophthalmologist George Coats in 1908, which usually affects only one eye (unilateral) and occurs predominantly in young males, with the onset of symptoms generally appearing in the first decade of life.

A large series of 150 patients referred to the Wills Eye Hospital in Pennsylvania was described by Shields[5] in 2001. In the 150 patients described, Coats' disease was diagnosed at a median age of 5 years (range, 1 month to 63 years), occurred in 114 males (76%), and was unilateral in 142 patients (95%). The first symptom or sign was decreased visual acuity (VA) in 68 cases (34%), strabismus in 37 (23%) and leukocoria in 31 (20%), and 13 patients (8%) were asymptomatic. Visual acuity at presentation was 20/200 to no light perception in 121 eyes (76%).

Shields[6] later described the following stages.

Stage 1 (telangiectasia only).

Stage 2 (telangiectasia and exudate).

Stage 3 (subretinal or retinal detachment).

Stage 4 (total retinal detachment and glaucoma):

Treatment for stages 1 and 2 is usually with laser therapy or cryotherapy.

An example of a fluorescein angiogram of a patient who presented to the eye department at the age of 25 years with blurring of vision in his right eye is shown in Fig. 17.4. This angiogram shows the retinal telangectasia and exudation in the peripheral retina and some central changes of cystoid macular oedema.

RADIATION RETINOPATHY

Radiation retinopathy is occasionally seen in the eye clinic.

Amoaku[7] and Archer described the fluorescein angiographic features, natural course and treatment of radiation retinopathy in a publication in *Eye* in 1990. They described the following grades of severity.

Grade 1 – Small foci of dilated and irregular retinal capillaries with clusters of microaneurysms.

Grade 2 – Multiple foci plus capillary closure plus leakage of dye from defective capillaries.

Grade 3 – Widespread capillary dilatation, telangiectatic-like channels, microvascular incompetence and significant areas of capillary closure. IRMA at borders of non-perfused areas. Significant macular oedema.

Grade 4 – Widespread disorganization of the retinal microvasculature with extensive retinal ischaemia.

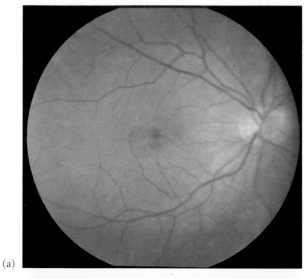

(a)

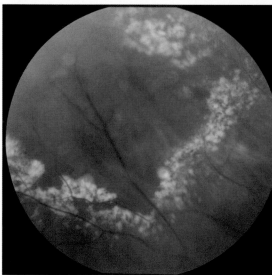

(b)

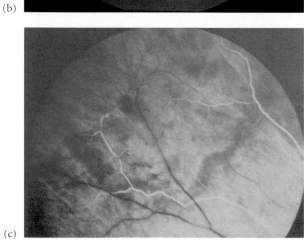

(c)

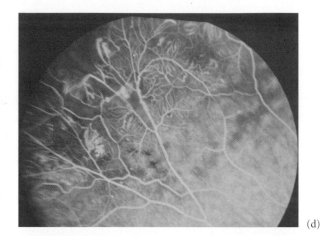

(d)

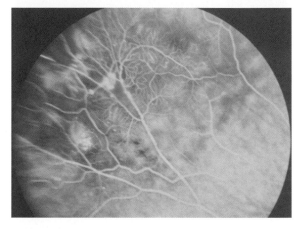

(e)

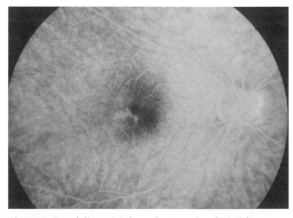

(f)

Fig. 17.4 Coats' disease. Colour photographs of (a) right macula and (b) right peripheral retina. Fluorescein of peripheral retina showing peripheral aneurysms and vascular patterns in: (c) arterial phase; (d) arteriovenous phase. (e) Fluorescein of peripheral retina showing leakage from peripheral aneurysms in early venous phase. (f) Fluorescein of macular area showing some secondary oedema; (*Continued on facing page*)

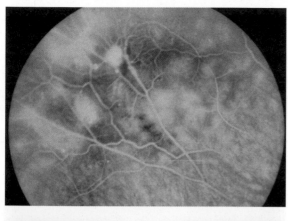

(g)

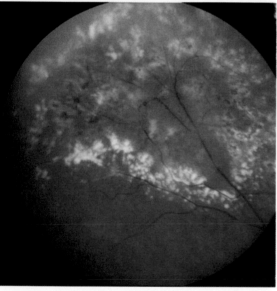

(h)

Fig. 17.4 (*Cont'd*) (g) Fluorescein of peripheral retina showing leakage from peripheral aneurysms in late venous phase. (h) Right peripheral retinal colour photograph showing some clearing of exudate 3 months after first laser treatment.

In a further publication Archer[8] suggested that the following doses and risk factors may give rise to radiation retinopathy.
- The minimum amount administered by teletherapy that will give rise to retinal vasculopathy is unknown; estimates vary from 1500 cGy to 6000 cGy.
- It is unusual under 2500 cGy given in fractions of less than 200 cGy.
- There is a higher risk with diabetes and concomitant chemotherapy.

Parsons[9] studied the effect of high dose radiotherapy on the normal eye in 157 patients followed for a minimum of 3 years treated for primary extracranial tumours.
- Radiation retinopathy developed in 27 eyes of 26 patients.
- The mean time of onset was 2.8 years.
- The risk increased steadily above 45 Gy, especially if fractions were greater than 1.9 Gy.
- There was an increased risk with diabetes and chemotherapy.

Takeda[10] described late retinal complications in a retrospective study of 43 eyes of 25 patients treated with radiation therapy for nasal and paranasal malignancies.
- Radiation retinopathy developed in 7 eyes.
- The mean duration was 32 months (range 16–60).
- There were no retinal complications in patients receiving less than 50 Gy in fractions of 2 Gy.

CASE HISTORY 1
Radiation retinopathy

A 45-year-old man had radiotherapy to his right temple for a recurrence of a basal cell carcinoma and 9 months later presented with a blurring of vision in his right eye. The colour photographs and fluorescein angiogram show the effect of radiation on the right retina and a normal left retina (Fig. 17.5). The right eye shows new vessels forming superotemporally and inferotemporally and areas of vascular occlusion and leakage. These changes are similar to those found in diabetic retinopathy and panretinal photocoagulation was required to treat the right eye.

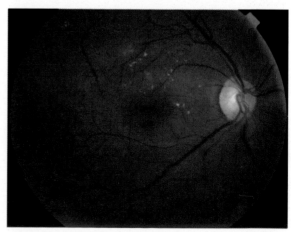

(a)

Fig. 17.5 Case history 1. Radiation retinopathy: (a) right macula colour photograph; (*Continued on p. 200*)

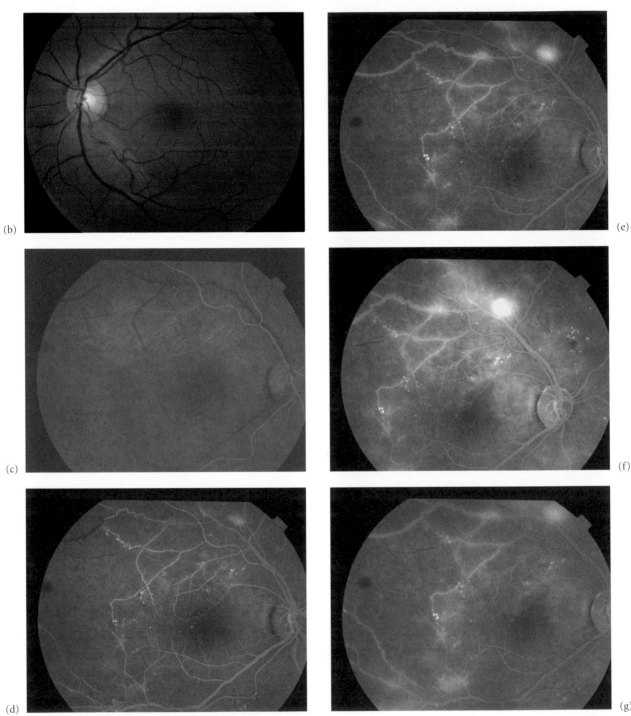

Fig. 17.5 (*Cont'd*) (b) left macula colour photograph. Fluorescein angiogram: (c) 23 s after injection; (d) 33 s after injection; (e) 1 min after injection; (f) 3 min 45 s after injection; (g) 4 min 11 s after injection.

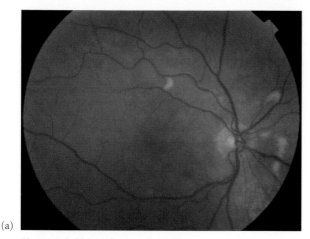

(a)

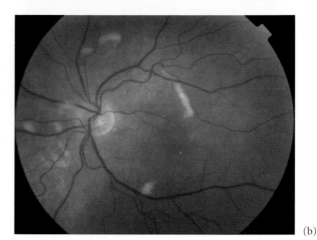

(b)

Fig. 17.6 (a,b) Interferon retinopathy.

INTERFERON RETINOPATHY

Recent literature reports[11–13] have shown retinopathy associated with interferon treatment that is being given for conditions such as chronic hepatitis C, and these patients are beginning to appear in ophthalmology clinics in areas where interferon is being used.

In a prospective study of 81 patients, Saito[12] found that 34.6% (28/81) of patients treated with interferon-alpha therapy for chronic hepatitis C showed cotton wool spots or minor retinal haemorrhage, or both lesions, during therapy, but these lesions were reversed during or after interferon therapy. The occurrence rates of cotton wool spots alone, retinal haemorrhage alone and both lesions were 13.6% (11/81), 6.2% (5/81) and 14.8% (12/81), respectively.

In a prospective study of 107 chronic hepatitis C patients receiving systemic interferon treatment, Kawasaki[13] reported that retinopathy developed in 40 patients (37%) after an average of 77 days of treatment. The incidence of retinopathy was 28% in males and 51% in females, 75% in diabetics and 34% in non-diabetics, and 24% in persons below 55 years. They identified the following risk factors: females (p = 0.04), diabetes (p = 0.002) and advanced age (p = 0.05).

Figure 17.6 shows an example of retinopathy developing in a patient being treated with interferon-alpha therapy for chronic hepatitis C, who did not have diabetes, and developed multiple cotton wool spots that resolved during continuation of the interferon therapy.

PRACTICE POINT

- The conditions described in this chapter can produce lesions very similar to those described in diabetic retinopathy.

REFERENCES

1 Goldberg MF, Charache S, Acacio I. Ophthalmologic manifestations of sickle cell thalassemia. *Arch Intern Med* 1971; **128**(1): 33–9.
2 Penman AD, Talbot JF, Chuang EL, Thomas P, Serjeant GR, Bird AC. New classification of peripheral retinal vascular changes in sickle cell disease. *Br J Ophthalmol* 1994; **78**(9): 681–9.
3 Sayag D, Binaghi M, Souied EH, Querques G, Galacteros F, Coscas G *et al.* Retinal photocoagulation for proliferative sickle cell retinopathy: A prospective clinical trial with new sea fan classification. *Eur J Ophthalmol* 2008; **18**(2): 248–54.
4 Goldberg MF. Classification and pathogenesis of proliferative sickle retinopathy. *Am J Ophthalmol* 1971; **71**(3): 649–65.
5 Shields JA, Shields CL, Honavar SG, Demirci H. Clinical variations and complications of Coats' disease in 150 cases: the 2000 Sanford Gifford Memorial Lecture. *Am J Ophthalmol* 2001; **131**(5): 561–71.
6 Shields JA, Shields CL, Honavar SG, Demirci H, Cater J. Classification and management of Coats' disease: the 2000 Proctor Lecture. *Am J Ophthalmol* 2001; **131**(5): 572–83.
7 Amoaku WM, Archer DB. Fluorescein angiographic features, natural course and treatment of radiation retinopathy. *Eye* 1990; **4**(Pt 5): 657–67.

8 Archer DB. Doyne Lecture. Responses of retinal and choroidal vessels to ionising radiation. *Eye* 1993; **7**(Pt 1): 1–13.

9 Parsons JT, Bova FJ, Mendenhall WM, Million RR, Fitzgerald CR. Response of the normal eye to high dose radiotherapy. *Oncology (Huntingt)* 1996; **10**(6): 837–47; discussion 847–8, 851–2.

10 Takeda A, Shigematsu N, Suzuki S, Fujii M, Kawata T, Kawaguchi O *et al.* Late retinal complications of radiation therapy for nasal and paranasal malignancies: relationship between irradiated-dose area and severity. *Int J Radiat Oncol Biol Phys* 1999; **44**(3): 599–605.

11 Jain K, Lam WC, Waheeb S, Thai Q, Heathcote J. Retinopathy in chronic hepatitis C patients during interferon treatment with ribavirin. *Br J Ophthalmol* 2001; **85**(10): 1171–3.

12 Saito H, Ebinuma H, Nagata H, Inagaki Y, Saito Y, Wakabayashi K *et al.* Interferon-associated retinopathy in a uniform regimen of natural interferon-alpha therapy for chronic hepatitis C. *Liver* 2001; **21**(3): 192–7.

13 Kawasaki A. Risk factors of interferon-associated retinopathy in chronic hepatitis C patients. *Japanese Journal of Clinical Ophthalmology* 2004; **58**(4): 517–20.

Glossary

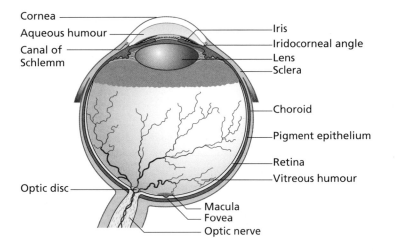

Cornea
Aqueous humour
Canal of Schlemm
Optic disc

Iris
Iridocorneal angle
Lens
Sclera
Choroid
Pigment epithelium
Retina
Vitreous humour
Macula
Fovea
Optic nerve

anterior chamber   the space in the front portion of the eye between the cornea and the iris and lens, which is filled with aqueous humour

aqueous humour   the clear, watery fluid that fills the anterior chamber and the posterior chamber in the front part of the eye and provides nutrients to structures in the anterior chamber

arteriolar sheathing   opacification of the arteriolar wall

arteriovenous nipping   narrowing of the venous diameter where it is crossed by a branch artery. It is often a feature of hypertension

binocular indirect ophthalmoscopy   an examination technique of the retina involving a light source and viewing apparatus placed on the ophthalmologist's head and an indirect lens held between the light source and the eye, with the patient usually lying on a couch

blindness   the WHO definition is visual acuity that does not exceed 20/200 in the better eye with correcting lens

choroid   the middle layer of the eye containing a large and highly vascular bed that provides nourishment to the other parts of the eye, especially the retina

ciliary body   a ring of tissue between the iris and the choroid consisting of muscles and blood vessels that changes the shape of the lens and produces the aqueous humour

conjunctiva   the tissue that lines the inside of the eyelids and covers the front part of the eye except the cornea

contact lens biomicrosopy   an examination technique using a slit lamp biomicroscope to examine retinal detail through a diagnostic fundus contact lens applied to the cornea

cornea   the clear curved structure that comprises the front of the eye, a refractive surface through which light enters

cotton wool spots   the fluffy white opaque areas caused by an accumulation of axoplasm in the nerve fibre layer of the retina

diabetes mellitus   the chronic condition where there is an excess of glucose circulating in the blood stream

diabetic retinopathy   the microvascular complication of diabetes affecting the eye

exudates (or hard exudates)   the small white or yellowish-white deposits with sharp margins, located typically in the outer layers of the retina, but they may be more superficial, particularly when retinal oedema is present

fluorescein angiography an examination technique involving the injection of fluorescein dye in the arm and taking a series of photographs over approximately the next 5 minutes using a blue light source entering the eye and a yellow filter allowing only fluorescent light to be captured, leaving the eye on a monochrome sensor. This enables photographs to be taken of the passage of the fluorescein dye through the retinal vasculature

FPD fibrous proliferations on or within 1DD of the disc margin

FPE fibrous proliferations 'elsewhere'

haemorrhage a red spot, which has irregular margins and/or uneven density, particularly when surrounding a smaller central lesion considered to be a microaneurysm. Flame haemorrhages are superficial haemorrhages just under the nerve fibre layer and blot haemorrhages are deeper haemorrhages

HMa a small haemorrhage or microaneurysm

iris the coloured circular membrane that is in front of the lens and controls the size of the opening at its centre (pupil), thereby regulating the amount of light entering the eye

IRMA intraretinal microvascular abnormality – the tortuous intraretinal vascular segments varying in calibre

laser *l*ight *a*mplification by *s*imulated *e*mission of *r*adiation. Different types of laser are used in the diagnosis and treatment of many eye disorders

LogMar Logarithm of the minimum angle of resolution. This is a modern method used for measurement of visual acuity that has the same number of letters on each line

low-vision aids the optical devices that usually magnify the image to enable people with visual impairment to see print, objects or people at near or far that is not possible with the usual prescription lenses

macula a rod-free area at the centre of the retina that surrounds the fovea and is responsible for best central vision

microaneurysm a red spot less than 125 microns (approx width of vein at disc margin) and sharp margins

MODY maturity-onset diabetes of the young

NVD new vessels at the optic disc or within 1 disc diameter of the optic disc margin

NVE new vessels greater than 1 disc diameter from the optic disc margin

OCT optical coherence tomography – an imaging technique that interprets the 'time of flight' and intensity

of reflected optical waves using interferometry using wavelengths between 600nm and 2000nm

optic disc the head of the optic nerve where it meets the retinal nerve fibres

optic nerve the nerve of sight beginning in the retina at the optic disc, which carries messages from the retina to the brain, resulting in visual images

perimetry the systematic measurement of differential light sensitivity in the visual field by the detection of the presence of test targets on a defined background in order to map and quantify the visual field

PVD posterior vitreous detachment – a common condition of the eye in which the vitreous humour separates from the retina

preretinal haemorrhage boat-shaped haemorrhages and roughly round, confluent or linear patches of haemorrhage just anterior to the retina or under the internal limiting membrane

PRP pan retinal photocoagulation – the type of scatter laser treatment that is given to patients with high risk proliferative diabetic retinopathy and usually involves 1200 to 2000 burns of 500 micron spot size to an oval area of retina defined by a line passing two disc diameters above, temporal to and below the centre of the macula and 500 microns from the nasal one-half of the disc margin

pupil the opening in the centre of the iris that appears as a black dot and through which light enters the eye

retina the innermost layer of the eye containing photoreceptor cells and fibres connecting with the brain through the optic nerve and nourished by a network of blood vessels

sclera the outermost layer of most of the eye, which is the tough protective 'white' of the eye

slit lamp biomicroscopy an examination technique using a slit lamp biomicroscope to examine the anterior segment directly or retinal detail through an indirect lens held between the slit lamp beam and the eye

type 1 diabetes characterized by the absolute deficiency of insulin

type 2 diabetes characterized by the relative deficiency of insulin associated with insulin 'resistance'

ultrasound B-scan examination a means of visualizing the eye and retro-bulbar region involving the placement of a high frequency 10MHz probe onto the eye or eyelid and taking a series of scan sections of the eye

venous loop an abrupt curving deviation of a vein from its normal path

venous reduplication the dilation of a prexisting channel or proliferation of a new channel adjacent to and approximately the same calibre as the original vein

venous sheathing   an opacification of the venous wall

visual acuity   a measurement of the ability of the eye to perceive the shape of objects in the direct line of vision and to distinguish detail; generally determined by finding the smallest symbol on an eye chart that can be recognized at a given distance

20/20 vision   the ability to correctly perceive an object or letter of a designated size from a distance of 20 feet; normal visual acuity

6/6 vision   the ability to correctly perceive an object or letter of a designated size from a distance of 6 metres; normal visual acuity

vitreous body   the transparent colourless mass of soft, gelatinous material filling the globe of the eye between the lens and the retina

vitreous haemorrhage   a haemorrhage that is in the vitreous gel, having penetrated through the internal limiting membrane

Index